Eating Disorders in Special Populations

Eating Disorders in Special Populations

Medical, Nutritional, and Psychological Treatments

Edited By

Jonna Fries, PsyD
Veronica Sullivan, PhD

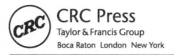

CRC Press
Taylor & Francis Group
Boca Raton London New York

CRC Press is an imprint of the
Taylor & Francis Group, an **informa** business

CRC Press
Taylor & Francis Group
6000 Broken Sound Parkway NW, Suite 300
Boca Raton, FL 33487-2742

First issued in paperback 2021

ISBN-13: 978-1-03-209664-3 (pbk)
ISBN-13: 978-1-4987-5936-6 (hbk)

This book contains information obtained from authentic and highly regarded sources. Reasonable efforts have been made to publish reliable data and information, but the author and publisher cannot assume responsibility for the validity of all materials or the consequences of their use. The authors and publishers have attempted to trace the copyright holders of all material reproduced in this publication and apologize to copyright holders if permission to publish in this form has not been obtained. If any copyright material has not been acknowledged, please write and let us know so we may rectify in any future reprint.

Publisher's Note
The publisher has gone to great lengths to ensure the quality of this reprint but points out that some imperfections in the original copies may be apparent.

Library of Congress Cataloging-in-Publication Data

Names: Fries, Jonna, editor. | Sullivan, Veronica, 1980-editor.
Title: Eating disorders in special populations : medical, nutritional, and
psychological treatments / [edited by] Jonna Fries and Veronica Sullivan.
Description: Boca Raton : Taylor & Francis, 2017. | Includes bibliographical
references and index.
Identifiers: LCCN 2016052455 | ISBN 9781498759366 (hardback : alk. paper)
Subjects: | MESH: Feeding and Eating Disorders--therapy | Feeding and Eating
Disorders--psychology | Diet Therapy--methods | Population Groups
Classification: LCC RC552.EI8 | NLM WM 175 | DDC 362.196/8526--dc23
LC record available at https://lccn.loc.gov/2016052455

Visit the Taylor & Francis Web site at
http://www.taylorandfrancis.com

and the CRC Press Web site at
http://www.crcpress.com

Dedication

To our husbands, children, grandchildren, parents, friends, mentors, students, and colleagues, we thank you for your love and support and the delight you bring to our lives.

We dedicate this book to those who battle eating disorders every day and to the providers who support them in the fight. We stand beside you.

Jonna and Veronica

Contents

SECTION I A Multidisciplinary Approach to Treatment

SECTION II Special Populations

Editors

Dr. Jonna Fries is a psychologist and director of Counseling and Psychological Services at California State University, Los Angeles. She is an adjunct faculty at the Chicago School of Professional Psychology, a certified integrative body psychotherapist, a certified IBP instructor, an EMDR-approved consultant, and chair of the International Association of Eating Disorder Professionals (IAEDP) consultation group. She maintains a private practice in Los Angeles where she focuses on trauma and eating disorders. Dr. Fries is a recipient of the Cal State Los Angeles Distinguished Women Award and the IAEDP Member of the Year Award. Her doctoral project was the development of a multicultural group therapy treatment for those at the intersection of binge-eating disorder, obesity, and body image distress. Her doctoral concentration was on diversity, which she continues to teach at the graduate level.

Dr. Veronica Sullivan is a licensed psychologist and group therapist at Kaiser Permanente in Portland, Oregon. Prior to this, she was a tenure-track professor and staff psychologist at California State University, Northridge, where she served as a faculty advisor and group therapy coordinator for the Joint Advocates on Disordered Eating (JADE) peer education program. Dr. Sullivan has presented at national conferences on multiple topics and was a participant at the 2014 National Eating Disorders Association (NEDA) conference. She earned her PhD from the State University of New York at Albany, where her dissertation research examined the intersections of emotional eating, coping, and obesity. Her clinical specialties in private practice include body image and eating disorders, with a focus on the treatment of binge-eating disorder.

Contributors

Anna M. Bardone-Cone, PhD, is an associate professor in the Department of Psychology and Neuroscience at the University of North Carolina at Chapel Hill (UNC), Chapel Hill, North Carolina. She attended Williams College for her BA in mathematics and French and the University of Wisconsin-Madison for her doctoral degree in clinical psychology. Her research in the realm of eating disorders and body image focuses on race and ethnicity, with a particular interest in African American and Latina experiences; sociocultural factors, such as peers, family, and social media; perfectionism in relation to bulimic symptoms and its interactions with constructs such as self-efficacy and social comparison; and defining recovery and remission from eating disorders. At UNC, she teaches undergraduate courses on eating disorders and psychopathology as well as a graduate course on multiculturalism and clinical psychology.

Maggie Baumann, LMFT, CEDS, is a certified eating disorders specialist and trauma therapist who dedicates part of her Newport Beach, California, private practice to treating pregnant women and moms with eating disorders. Maggie has been a featured guest on nationwide talk shows, HuffPost Live, CNN.com, and TV segments profiling eating disorders in pregnant women and moms. Maggie is also a guest eating disorder video expert for KidsinTheHouse.com, a resource promoting over 9000 parenting videos. In 2014, Maggie cofounded, with Timberline Knolls Treatment Center, the first online support group for pregnant women and moms with eating disorders called "Lift the Shame."

Kate Bennett, PsyD, is a clinical sport psychologist and the director of Athlete Insight, PC. She combines her experiences as an athlete, coach, and athletic trainer with her psychological expertise to meet the clinical and performance needs of athletes. As a coach, Dr. Bennett coached several national champions as well as earned two national championships herself. During her graduate and postdoctoral training, Dr. Bennett specialized in the treatment of eating disorders. She presented at both the American Psychological Association and Association for Applied Sport Psychology Annual Conferences on the treatment of athletes struggling with eating disorders.

Vicki Berkus, MD, PhD, CEDS, is currently the medical director for the first Joint Commission on the Accreditation of Healthcare Organizations (JCAHO) certified telemedicine intensive outpatient program (IOP) for eating disorders called Bright Heart Health. She is also a fellow for Remuda Ranch at the Meadows. She has been in the eating disorders field for over 20 years and has authored numerous articles as well as a book, titled *10 Commitments to Mental Fitness.* Dr. Berkus is the past president of the International Association of Eating Disorder Professionals (IAEDP) and currently a member of the IAEDP senior advisory board. She had been a featured presenter for multiple eating disorder organizations including the

IAEDP, Academy of Eating Disorders (AED), and NEDA. Dr. Berkus has been the medical director of the eating disorders programs at several treatment centers and has had a private outpatient practice. She is now a speaker for the US Journal Training seminars and continues to see patients with eating disorders.

Carolyn Costin, MA, MEd, LMFT, CEDS, is a renowned clinician, author, and speaker acclaimed for her expertise, passion, and accomplishments in eating disorders. Recovered herself, Carolyn recognized her calling while treating her first eating disorder client in 1979. She founded several inpatient programs until opening Monte Nido, the first home-like residential facility. Carolyn pioneered the notion that sufferers could be fully "recovered" and openly hired recovered staff. Monte Nido's outcome study (Brewerton and Costin) and Carolyn's five books helped Monte Nido grow into 14 facilities prior to her departure. Carolyn maintains a private practice and shares her insight and wisdom with the public and professionals, lecturing, teaching, and supervising.

Mandy Golman, PhD, MS, MCHES, is an assistant professor in the Health Studies Department at Texas Woman's University (TWU), Denton, Texas, and is a multi-faceted educator, researcher, trainer, and consultant whose work spans the health spectrum to include women's wellness, eating disorder prevention, teen pregnancy, parenting, adolescent sexuality, nutrition, and the importance of positive body image. In addition, her expertise includes needs assessment, program planning, and evaluation. She routinely consults and conducts workshops for major school districts, private schools, and health-care providers. Dr. Golman is the principal investigator (PI) and evaluator on several grants, including a $4.9 million grant from the Office of Adolescent Health.

M. K. Higgins Neyland, PhD, graduated with honors from the University of Virginia with a BA in psychology. She received her PhD in clinical psychology with a quantitative psychology minor from the University of North Carolina at Chapel Hill (UNC). Katy's dissertation centered on Latina women and their experience of treatment and recovery from an eating disorder; she was supported in this work by a National Institute of Mental Health Diversity Supplement. She is currently completing a clinical postdoctoral fellowship in Arlington, Virginia, where she uses evidence-based practices to treat teenagers and adults with eating disorders. She is also working as a research postdoctoral fellow at UNC where she has published articles on racial/ethnic minorities' eating disorder treatment, and recovery experiences, as well as mechanisms of binge eating.

Susan Karpiel, MS, RDN, LD, is a registered dietitian nutritionist (RDN). She earned her master's degree in nutrition from Texas Woman's University (TWU) and is currently pursuing her doctorate in health studies, with a minor in nutrition. Susan has a diverse background. She has worked as director of food and nutrition in both hospital and long-term care settings. She also has experience in worksite wellness, weight loss, and community health. Susan is very passionate about health and wellness and loves helping others reach their personal health goals. She currently teaches at TWU, has a consulting business, and is opening a private practice as an RDN/wellness coach. Susan lives in Denton with her husband, two dogs, and a cat. They have three adult children who live in Austin, Texas and Toronto, Canada. When not studying, she loves to travel, exercise, and work in her organic garden.

Sondra Kronberg, MS, RD, CDN, CEDRD, is a nutrition therapist with 30 years of experience and a recognized leader in the field of eating disorders. She is the founder and the executive director of the Eating Disorder Treatment Collaborative, FEED, IOP, CONNECT, and CONCIERGE programs. Sondra specializes in treatment and training of the collaborative approach to eating disorders. She is the founding member and past Board Trustee of the National Eating Disorders Association (NEDA). She is the author of *Comprehensive Learning/Teaching Handout Series Manual for Eating Disorders* and is a contributing author to *Eating Disorders: Clinical Guide to Counseling and Treatment.* Sondra received the IAEDP's 2010 Certified Eating Disorder Specialists Award, the NEDA 2004 Excellence in Treatment Award, and the 2002 SCAN Excellence in Practice Award. She is currently a national speaker, treatment consultant, and media spokesperson. Sondra's greatest passion is helping people learn to nourish their minds and bodies in order to reclaim their lives and thrive.

Stacy L. Lin, MA, is a doctoral candidate in clinical psychology in the Department of Psychology and Neuroscience at the University of North Carolina (UNC) at Chapel Hill. She attended the University of Southern California where she earned her BA in health and humanity. Her research focuses on individual- and cultural-level psychosocial factors that affect eating disorder risk and body image, with emphases on perfectionism and culturally related risk and protective factors in racial/ethnic minorities. She has a strong interest in issues of diversity in clinical psychology training, practice, and research, and is active in the UNC clinical psychology department Diversity Training Committee.

Dr. Margo Maine is a founder and adviser of the NEDA and Founding Fellow of the Academy for Eating Disorders. She has authored the following books: *Pursuing Perfection: Eating Disorders, Body Myths, and Women at Midlife and Beyond; Treatment of Eating Disorders: Bridging the Research-Practice Gap; Effective Clinical Practice in the Treatment of Eating Disorders*; *The Body Myth*; *Father Hunger;* and *Body Wars.* In addition, she is senior editor of *Eating Disorders: The Journal of Treatment and Prevention.* She is the 2007 recipient of the Lori Irving Award for Excellence in Eating Disorders Awareness and Prevention and the 2015 recipient of the NEDA Lifetime Achievement Award. A member of the Renfrew Foundation Conference Committee, its Clinical Advisory Board, and the Walden Clinical Advisory Board, Dr. Maine lectures nationally and internationally on eating disorders and maintains a private practice, Maine & Weinstein Specialty Group, West Hartford, Connecticut.

Dr. Marilyn Massey-Stokes is an associate professor in the Department of Health Studies at Texas Woman's University, Denton, Texas. She is also a certified health education specialist and a certified health and wellness coach. Dr. Massey-Stokes has over 27 years of experience as a health educator at the university level and has published several book chapters concerning body image and eating disorder prevention. She has also published journal articles and book chapters on other health topics, and she has numerous years of experience presenting at state and national health education conferences. In addition to her role as a teacher-scholar at the university level, Dr. Massey-Stokes is focused on helping others achieve personal goals through her role as a health and wellness coach.

Jacque Mular, MS, RD, MFTI, has devoted the last two decades to specializing in the treatment of disordered eating using an intuitive eating, nondiet approach. She earned her MS in nutrition at California State University at Northridge and her MA in psychology at Antioch University. She has extensive experience working with people suffering from anorexia, bulimia, binge-eating disorder, compulsive exercise, and polycystic ovary syndrome (PCOS). She has worked as both director of nutrition as well as assistant clinical director in facilities that encompass residential, inpatient, partial hospitalization, and intensive outpatient eating disorder treatment. Jacque's passion for helping others heal is infectious, and she continues to find inspiration in her daily interactions with her clients. Jacque truly believes that relationships bridge the gap between "disordered" and "recovered" and transcend the isolating effects of disordered eating and compulsive exercise. Jacque originally hails from a small town in Northwestern Montana but she now lives in Portland, Oregon with her husband, twin boys, and two cats.

Helen B. Murray is a doctoral student in clinical psychology at Drexel University, Philadelphia, Pennsylvania. She received her BA in psychology from Georgetown University. Prior to entering graduate school, Helen worked with the Eating Disorders Clinical and Research Program at Massachusetts General Hospital and the Psychiatry Department at Children's National Medical Center. Her clinical work involves the treatment of eating disorders in a variety of populations including comorbid disordered feeding behavior such as symptoms of rumination disorder. Helen focuses her research on the identification of neurocognitive and neurobiological maintenance factors and examination of mechanisms of change in psychological treatment for eating disorders.

Gail Prosser, RD, CDE, is a registered dietitian and certified diabetes educator with nearly 30 years of experience working in the field of pediatric nutrition and dietetics. She lives in Northern California and works full time at Kaiser Permanente, Oakland, California specializing in pediatric eating disorders and diabetes. Following an internship at Touro Infirmary, New Orleans, Louisiana, Gail was employed at Texas Children's Hospital, becoming highly experienced in pediatric medical nutrition therapy. Later, she worked in private practice and also as a certified product trainer for Medtronic, training clients on the use of insulin pump therapy and continuous glucose monitoring systems for diabetes. In 2004, Gail became part of the Healthy

Bodies Healthy Minds outpatient eating disorder treatment team at Santa Rosa, Kaiser Permanente.

Dr. Adelaide S. Robb is a professor of child and adolescent psychiatry at George Washington University and Children's National Health System. She is board certified in adult and child and adolescent psychiatry. She did her medical training and general psychiatry residency at Johns Hopkins, fellowship training at the National Institute of Mental Health (NIMH) in psychiatric genetics, and child and adolescent psychiatry fellowship at the Children's National Medical Center. She sees children and adolescents with a variety of psychiatric disorders in inpatient and outpatient settings. Her focus is on psychopharmacology including the study of new medications in children and adolescents with a variety of psychiatric disorders. She has served as PI on both National Institutes of Health (NIH) and industry registration trials. She ran an inpatient eating disorders unit for adolescents for over 15 years where they manualized treatment that incorporated the use of nocturnal nasogastric refeeding and served young men and women on a mixed disorder unit.

Karen Samuels, PhD, is a psychologist in Ormond Beach, Florida and Founder/Director of COPE: Community Outreach to Prevent Eating Disorders. She serves as a consultant for the Family Residency Program, Halifax Medical Center, and is affiliated with the Jean Baker Miller Training Institute as well as the Wellesley Centers for Women. A lifelong yogi, she is a guide and psychologist providing education and outreach for the continuum of disordered eating, body image disturbance, and utilizing yoga as an adjunct for treatment. She has developed middle school outreach media literacy programs, trains physicians in interprofessional eating disorder teams, and conducts eating disorder group therapy with midlife/aging women. She has published articles and been interviewed on HuffPost Live, lectures nationwide, and blogs and tweets about eating disorders and body image disturbance. Dr. Samuels received the 2014 NEDA Westin Family Award for Activism and Advocacy.

Jessica Setnick, MS, RD, CEDRD, envisions a world where no one is ashamed to talk about their eating issues. Her work includes *The Eating Disorders Clinical Pocket Guide*, *The American Dietetic Association Pocket Guide to Eating Disorders*, and *Eating Disorders Boot Camp: Training Workshop for Professionals*, each of which is known to professionals around the globe. In 2011, Jessica cofounded IFEDD, the International Federation of Eating Disorder Dietitians, with the mission of improving access to nutrition counseling and achieving insurance coverage for individuals with eating disorders. In 2013, Jessica created the first ever Certified Eating Disorder Registered Dietitian (CEDRD) prep class to prepare dietitians for certification as an Eating Disorder Specialist through the IAEDP. Based in Dallas, Texas, Jessica currently works as a Senior Fellow with Remuda Ranch Eating Disorder Treatment Center.

Cathey Soutter, PhD, LPC, is the director of counseling services in the Dr. Bob Smith Health Center at Southern Methodist University (SMU) in Dallas, Texas. She has a 27-year affiliation with SMU having served as associate director of the

Women's Center and then moving to counseling services in 1995 serving in various roles until assuming the position as director in 2010. She teaches Psychology of Women to undergraduates and administers the Elisa Ruth McCall Foundation at SMU that promotes healthy body image as well as awareness and prevention of eating disorders.

Therese Waterhous, PhD/RDN, CEDRD, an IAEDP-Approved Supervisor, is the owner of Willamette Nutrition Source, LLC, Corvallis, Oregon, a private outpatient practice devoted to eating disorders care. Therese has formal training in basic research, clinical nutrition, and multidisciplinary team treatment of pediatric disorders. Therese coauthored the American Dietetic Association (ADA) practice paper on nutrition intervention in treatment of eating disorders; she is immediate past director of the sports, cardiovascular, and wellness nutrition practice group's eating disorder subunit and she is a professional advisor for FEAST-ED.org. She is the credentialing chair for the Oregon IAEDP chapter, has served as cochair of the Family Based Treatment Special Interest Group within the AED, and currently serves on the Medical Care Standards committee for the AED. Therese enjoys conducting trainings for health-care professionals on eating disorder research and treatment and educating the general public about eating disorders.

Introduction

Medical providers, psychotherapists, dieticians and nutritionists, body workers, practitioners of eastern medicines, coaches and trainers, advisors, eating disorder sufferers, family members, and more will benefit from the depth and breadth of information within these pages.

Internationally respected leaders in the field of eating disorders have collaborated to present the latest information on eating disorders in special populations. Imagine a multifaceted diamond representing a person with an eating disorder, with each facet representing a different way to view the person, the problem, and a sophisticated method to restore the sufferer to mental, physical, and spiritual well-being. Now imagine treating a sufferer by shining light through only one facet; then, re-imagine treating someone with brilliant light entering through all the facets. Collectively, our trailblazing authors represent a highly valuable spectrum of cutting-edge perspectives.

The goal of this text is to demonstrate that there is no "typical" person who suffers from an eating disorder, to emphasize that this disease affects a broad diversity of subgroups, each with unique needs and challenges, and to lend guidance in the treatment of special populations. You may notice a consistent theme in that often there is a call for more research, which is needed to fully understand and provide informed treatment to these special populations. However, it is our hope that this text will bring a deeper understanding of a multidisciplinary approach to treatment planning in a culturally sensitive way.

Eating disorders are notoriously complex in terms of etiology, mind–body complications, and requirements in the healing process. We know that we cannot treat eating disorders from our professional silos. While it is impossible to be an expert in every discipline, when we understand various approaches to healing and open our minds to learn from one another, we can better develop effective interventions, develop relevant research protocols, and, most importantly, maintain our compassion for the suffering on the often long and arduous journey to healing.

Our hope is that readers will have a better capacity to shine the light through all facets in order to provide the most effective and best tailored treatment possible.

Jonna Fries and Veronica Sullivan

Section I

A Multidisciplinary Approach to Treatment

1 What Are Eating Disorders?

Therese Waterhous, PhD/RDN, CEDRD

CONTENTS

LEARNING OBJECTIVES

After reading this chapter, the reader should be able to do the following:

- Discuss eating disorders as viewed and identified throughout history and through various cultural lenses
- Identify and discuss historical challenges to reaching consensus among professionals about (1) the definition of eating disorders, (2) etiology, and (3) appropriate treatment
- Synthesize a working definition of eating disorders based on current biochemical, neurodevelopmental, and psychological research

- Describe genetic, epigenetic, and biochemical advances in the understanding of eating disorders and summarize how genetic and epigenetic
  contributions to eating disorder etiology are related to environmental and
  psychological theories of eating disorders

INTRODUCTION

As a lead-in to this text on treatment of eating disorders, it is important to discuss
what eating disorders are from a historical perspective and as explained through
recent research. This is necessary because, as the reader will see, how one conceptualizes and views eating disorders greatly affects the type of treatment that follows.
Treatment of eating disorders has mirrored the evolution of thought about etiology;
many practitioners realize that there has been considerable debate among treatment
professionals about types of effective treatment. That debate continues today yet
slowly there seems to be the formation of some consensus about what eating disorders are and therefore the best way to treat them.

HISTORY

THE RESTRICTING DISORDERS: AN EVOLUTION OF THOUGHT

The Early Accounts

In the late nineteenth century, anorexia nervosa (AN) was first described in separate
texts by Lasègue (1873) in France and Gull (1874) in England. However, fasting and
self-starvation have been recorded since the sixth century BC when Vardhamana, the
founder of Jainism, died of self-starvation or fasting behavior. Jainism embraced the
idea that the soul is separate from the body, with the ultimate goal to release the soul
by willful and extreme self-control (Bemporad 1996). Fasting has been described
throughout history and used for a variety of purposes. Ritual fasting was used to
achieve trance-like states, to show devotion to one's gods, and as a means of purifica-
tion. Both Hinduism and Buddhism have accounts of gods and goddesses giving up
food to engage in the ascetic control of one's body (Bemporad 1996). The Gnostic
thesis, which means that the body is a material evil force and separate from the godly
world, led to beliefs that separating the body from the soul required giving up all
things worldly, including food. Early Christianity incorporated some of the Gnostic
beliefs, as shown by the hermits who gave up much of the comforts of daily living in
order to purify themselves, and during the Dark Ages self-starvation was considered
a form of satanic possession. Throughout this early history, self-starvation was not
considered a disease but rather was linked to religion or philosophy and frequently
seen as a positive attribute (Halse et al. 2008). From the thirteenth to the seventeenth centuries, a form of self-starvation resembling AN emerged in Europe and
was called "holy fasting" (Bell 2014).

Holy fasting became popular following the example of Saint Catherine who
seemed to become what now would be described as depressed, following the death
of one of her sisters. She became withdrawn, started to eat less, and devoted herself

to prayer. Eventually, she became a nun and devoted her life to serving others. She died of malnutrition at age 32. During this time, other women followed Catherine's example and theories emerged about this behavior, including that women were trying to escape the traditional female role of that time, which included marriage and childbirth (especially given that many women of that era died in childbirth); that women felt they could communicate directly with God by fasting or self-torture; and that they felt superior in being close to God. Self-denial in the name of piety continued until the church itself began to change. That an individual could become close to God by self-starvation gave way to the thinking that an intermediary, such as a priest, was necessary to help one to attain a relationship with God. Over time, self-denying individuals were no longer seen as desirable or holy. Yet, in spite of the prevailing views that evolved since the late Middle Ages, there have been recent reported cases of AN in people who seemed to feel that their self-starvation and denial of personal needs brought them closer to God; thus, religion seems to serve as a platform from which AN can evolve or be maintained (Banks 1996; Morgan et al. 2000).

From Self-Denial to a Medical Model

During the seventeenth and eighteenth centuries, a metamorphosis of thought regarding self-starvation ensued. Instead of considering fasting holy, thought transformed to consider fasting as self-serving and in need of attention, and then to the possibility of fasting as a somatic illness. The "miraculous maids" came into being during this time. These were young girls and women who claimed to be able to exist without nourishment. One case was described in 1669 by Thomas Hobbes, who wrote that a girl claimed to exist by "wetting her lips from a feather dipped in water" and "she became so emaciated her belly touched her backbone" (Bemporad 1996). She drew the attention of many curious townspeople who paid her family for the privilege of viewing her. Indeed, many of the starving young women attracted a circus-like atmosphere and could earn income for their families by being displayed for a fare. During this era, John Reynolds wrote the *Discourse on Prodigious Abstinence* which argued for a medical model of the disease in contrast to prevailing theories rooted in supernatural or religious causation. Reynolds offered several theories about how or why people would or could self-starve. He thought perhaps that fermentation took place within the bowels of the starving and therefore could create an internal source of nourishment, and he also had theories about an abnormal condition of the blood (Brumberg 2000).

Other theories that emerged between 1600 and 1800 were that AN was due to "insufficient bathing of the gastric nerves by the bodily fluids or the brain's insensitivity to messages from the stomach" (Bemporad 1996). Some of the theses written during the late 1600s describe starvation as one of the disorders of consumption, and at least one thesis described a woman who began to starve after learning that her beloved brother died (Bemporad 1996; Brumberg 2000).

Moving toward a Differential Diagnosis

The nineteenth century is noteworthy for medical literature beginning to develop a differential diagnosis for a number of ailments, including eating disorders. There were efforts to collect statistics on the numbers of people displaying "insanity," laying the groundwork that would lead to the development of the *Diagnostic and Statistical Manual (DSM)*. Within the body of literature coming out of this time are accounts of people beginning to self-starve after romantic breakups or other anxiety-producing life events, as well as people beginning to eat less and less, stating that they just felt discomfort with eating. In *The Body Project*, Joan Brumberg (2000) cites the findings of W.S. Chipley reported in the *Journal of Insanity* in 1859. Chipley described a disorder called sitophobia or dread of food among patients in psychiatric asylums and considered this condition to be part of overall psychosis. Another disease associated with lack of adequate food intake was chlorosis or chloroanemia, often called "green sickness" for the greenish skin tone exhibited by those afflicted. Symptoms included lack of appetite, lack of energy, headache, and shortness of breath; in approximately 1870, anemia was described in this population. The green sickness had been described since the 1600s and at one time was given the name the "virgin's disease" because it was thought that with the absence of menses, a variety of toxins were being retained that typically would be discharged with menstruation (Loudon 1984).

The mid- to late-nineteenth century ushered in many theories and beliefs about women, their body functions, and their appetites, including notions that women had frailer digestive systems, that meat eating would encourage "heat production and arousal of the passions" and that appetite was a "barometer of sexuality" (Brumberg 2000). The "professional hunger artists" who self-starved reportedly for money and who were predominantly male came into being in the nineteenth century as did several well-written accounts of female "fasting girls." This group of individuals appears to have various motives for their behavior with a general theme being that of attraction-seeking or money-making. Reports detail that some of these individuals did die of malnutrition while others were found to be secretly eating, yet they maintained a public persona of being able to exist without eating.

From Medical Model to the Beginnings of Psychological Illness

In 1859, Louis-Victor Marce described a condition observed in young women who "arrive at a delirious conviction that they cannot or ought not to eat" and who present with "oppositionalism and an obsession with food." Marce recommended force-feeding if necessary and interestingly he advised extended follow-up as relapse often occurred. Gull and Lasègue did not give credit to Marce, but they did add to his original description of AN: amenorrhea, anosognosia, restlessness, and onset during adolescence or early adulthood. Gull and Lasègue also made a number of treatment recommendations, including gradual refeeding along with removal from the family, as family members were seen as interfering with treatment. These early descriptions and recommendations for treatment did not speculate much on why predominantly young women developed the disorder. Later in the nineteenth century, Freud offered that "the well-known AN of girls seems to me on careful observation to be a melancholia occurring where sexuality is underdeveloped" (Brumberg 2000). Ideas like this persisted. In the early twentieth century, the disease was thought to be mainly of psychiatric origin because if a therapist could persuade the patient to eat, then the disease process halted; also, no physical findings were thought to exist to explain the disease. This changed when in 1919 Simmonds described the similarities between the lack of appetite in women with AN and those with pituitary atrophy, discovered at autopsy. For over 20 years, AN was considered a disease of the pituitary and so treated with endocrinological preparations (Brumberg 2000).

In 1948, Sheenan and Summers made more careful observations and distinguished between AN and pituitary atrophy, removing the disease once again from that of a physical disorder and returning the disease again to the realm of psychiatry (Sheenan and Summers 1948). Adding to this speculation was the fact that when individuals died of AN, at autopsy no obvious physical pathology would be seen, and so at this time in history the disorder was again thought to be purely psychiatric in origin.

The mid-twentieth century was a time of great psychoanalytic speculation, thus AN was viewed from this perspective. Unconscious motives were thought to be the underlying force behind the disease. These motives included oral fixations, maybe in response to difficulty adapting to puberty, and repression of sexual desire. Theoretically, a vulnerable girl who experienced a "narcissistic blow" during puberty would regress to oral modes of fulfillment and wish for oral impregnation and the self-starvation was interpreted as a defense against gratifying this wish. Over time, psychoanalysis did not support this theory, so it was dropped and psychiatry moved toward theories involving relationships.

In the early 1960s, theories once again began to emerge about the etiological role of the family. One theory postulated that the anorexic adolescent was unable to differentiate from his or her mother because the mother had sabotaged the child's identity and prevented individuation. The "maternal object" was identified with the anorexic's own body and the body needed to be controlled as it contained a plethora of "malevolent powers" that threatened the fragile and helpless ego of the patient (Bemporad 1996). At this time, many theories stressed the sense of helplessness and weakness experienced by people with AN. Hilde Bruch in 1973 discussed not only these personality features but also described the distorted body image common for people with AN (Bruch 1962). From the 1970s to the 1980s, theories about the need for control in a family that neither allowed self-control nor the autonomy needed for separation tasks of adolescence became popular and psychodynamics focused on the premorbid relationships of the family (Bruch 1985).

Hilde Bruch also differentiated "primary anorexia" from what she described as "me too" anorexics with the primary anorexic person representing the true psychological entity and the "me too" anorexic person simply representing copycat-type illnesses (Bruch 1986). Bruch and Russell described how the central psychological features of AN changed over time. Russell noted that the focus of individuals with AN seemed to be fear of becoming fat rather than rebelling against the demands of adult life, and Bruch noted that the more recent patients with AN "seemed to lack the passion of her earlier patients." Bruch speculated that her early career patients with AN had "invented" their illness because they had no knowledge of the illness prior to getting it, while her more recent patients picked up the illness after becoming aware of AN. Bruch went on to say the disease could lose much of its psychodynamic meaning, which was so clearly present in her earlier patients, as the disorder became more commonplace and was now seen in patients with many different personality issues.

Importantly, only recently has the fear of becoming fat been introduced into diagnostics. The early holy fasters and diseases of consumption or diseases of hysteria

were believed as not being associated with fear of weight gain, yet once this preoccupation was discovered and clinicians then thought to inquire about it, it became
increasingly noted as a central feature of the disease (Habermas 1989, 1996). It is
also noteworthy that the diseases of restriction had a culture-bound feature in that
people who engaged in self-starvation seemed to take on what the current culture
deemed important to prove one's worth, or what the culture recognized as a deter-
minant of religious or social standing. Thus, a central element of disorders involving
restriction of food intake, when physical reasons for lack of appetite are ruled out,
seems to be that of focusing on things within the current society that are considered
important either for social standing, or enhancement of spiritual or physical qualities. This over-focus would then take on an obsessive quality. Gordon discusses the
culture-bound aspects of restricting and purging disorders and also how these disorders might be considered developmental in nature (Gordon 2000). One can appreciate that there would have to be, within individuals who are capable of severe food
restriction, something contributing to the ability to ignore hunger and other physical
and mental discomforts that come with self-starvation.

Binging and Purging Disorders

Bulimia nervosa (BN) was first described and named as a clinical disease in 1979
by Gerald Russell and was initially thought of as a complicated form of AN (Russell
1979). Russell did a lot of work describing the features of BN and the "Russell signs"
are named after him. BN has been described since in numerous texts and publications as an eating disorder with considerable consequences and morbidity.

Historically, self-induced vomiting and other forms of purging to accomplish either
bodily cleansing or to atone for overeating were once considered positive behaviors
(Russell 1979). From the Egyptian Eber Papyrus to the Syriac Book of Medicine
and on to Hippocrates, one can find numerous prescriptions for self-induced vomiting for the betterment of one's health. There existed ideas that too much food could
cause illness, or that purging was necessary to relieve oneself of the desire to "binge,"
although excessive food intake at that time was considered more self-indulgence
rather than a psychiatric condition. Avicenna, the Arabic doctor, wrote about how
to induce vomiting if one ate to excess stating "the use of a finger or a feather will
incite the movement" and he went on to prescribe emesis one to two times per month
as it was beneficial "for the flabbiness of the body" (Nasser 1993). Purging by use of
cathartic drugs, including mercury, was common from the Middle Ages through the
seventeenth century, as it was widely believed that purging rid the body of toxins.

Nasser asked the intriguing question that if purging in various forms has been
common and prescribed throughout history, then how does this fact inform what we
now call eating disorders (Nasser 1993). Some accounts in ancient times reported
a ravenous hunger associated with exhaustion and fainting. Reports of a "powerful
appetite" have existed since the fourth century BC (Ziolko 1996) when a disorder
termed kynorexia was described as an utterly uncontrollable appetite and ravenous
eating to the point of uncomfortable fullness with vomiting following to relieve the
discomfort. The appetite of kynorexia was sometimes referred to as *appetites cani-
nus* or appetite of dogs, resembling the manner in which hungry dogs will eat and

then vomit due to the rapidity of food ingestion. In 1736, BN was described as the eating of a large amount of food that was retained, and kynorexia was described as the eating of a large amount of food that was purged. Later, both disorders were considered one and the same, but by 1772, seven differentiated subtypes of BN were described ranging from mere gluttony, to eating a large amount of food to avoid fainting, to eating a large amount of food secondary to parasitic infection, to eating a large amount of food and then vomiting. In the nineteenth century, BN was thought to co-occur with several organic maladies such as double pancreatic duct, enlarged liver or stomach, or infarcted mesentery. It was considered to be associated with other diseases such as tuberculosis, epilepsy, diabetes, scurvy, and cerebral lesions; at this point in history, BN was considered part of somatic diseases.

Gradually, from the early to mid-twentieth century, the concept of BN as a psychiatric disorder developed with purging recognized as a compulsive act to avoid weight gain (Ziolko 1996). Purging behaviors seem to have retained the motivations of improving the general health and avoiding weight gain as a central feature throughout history.

GUIDELINES, CLASSIFICATIONS, AND DIAGNOSTIC MANUALS

Attempts to classify mental disorders, including eating disorders, date back to the 1840 census in the United States where, for the first time, data were gathered on the number of people with "idiocy or insanity." In the early 1920s, the American Medico-Psychological Association, which later became the American Psychiatric Association (APA), developed a set of psychiatric classifications that would be incorporated in the first edition of the American Medical Association's *Standard Classified Nomenclature of Disease*.

Following World War II, there was a need to describe the various psychological conditions observed in military personnel. The World Health Organization's *International Classification of Diseases* (ICD) was developed to meet this need, and for the first time it incorporated descriptions of mental illness, using many of the US Army's descriptions of mental disorders.

The *ICD* comprises the global health information standards and continues to be used for epidemiological and health information purposes as well as for diagnostic and clinical purposes. The APA created a variant of the sixth version of the *ICD* manual, *ICD-6*, and this was in fact the first *DSM* (APA 2016). This first *DSM* described AN as a neurotic illness. *DSM-II* described AN as a special feeding disturbance and it was placed in the same category as pica and rumination. Several revisions to the first two *DSMs* occurred post–World War II and *DSM-III* was published in 1975. *DSM-III* described more explicit diagnostic criteria for mental conditions, including eating disorders, it incorporated the multiaxial diagnostic assessment system, and it moved away from the strictly psychodynamic view of etiology. *DSM-III* contained newly constructed and validated diagnostic criteria and psychiatric interviews for research and clinical uses. *DSM-IV* was published in 1994 with the intention of aligning it with the 1992 *ICD-10*, in terms of descriptions of illnesses and disorders. A text revision, *DSM-IV-TR*, was published in 2000. More recently, *DSM-5* was released in 2013 following significant revisions and is currently being used as of this publication date. The *DSMs* have closely followed the *ICD* systems and *ICD-11* is expected by 2018 (World Health Organization 2016).

COMPARING EATING DISORDERS CHANGES BETWEEN *DSM-IV* AND *DSM-5*

Work on the fifth major revision of *DSM* (*DSM-5*) started in 2000, with the formation of work groups to create an agenda guiding revisions. The work groups provided the field with a summary of the state of the science relevant to all psychiatric diagnoses and identified where gaps existed in the current research. In 2007, APA formed the *DSM-5* Task Force, composed of 13 work groups focusing on various disorder areas, and began revising the manual with the hope of it deriving more from research. *DSM-5* was published in 2013. There are important differences between *DSM-IV* and *DSM-5* in how the eating disorders are defined.

DSM-5 does not specify a weight criterion in the diagnosis of AN but rather describes behaviors leading to a low body weight according to age and gender specific norms. Using weight as a diagnostic criterion has been criticized as arbitrary and insensitive to issues of gender, ethnicity, frame size, and age (Wilfley et al. 2007). Weight may be irrelevant to medical compromise in individuals who start out at a high weight but lose weight rapidly and thus might be normal or clinically overweight yet still very ill with AN. The *DSM-IV* diagnostic criteria for AN stated "refusal to maintain body weight" at a certain level, and the term "refusal" was removed from the updated *DSM-5* as it is potentially misleading (Becker et al. 2009). The term refusal implies an act of will or stubbornness, while current research suggests an inability to maintain weight, rather than frank refusal (Hebebrand and Bulik 2011). *DSM-5* also does not include the cessation of menses criteria (also called amenorrhea) because it is irrelevant in cases of young children and males and is inconsistently a marker of physical wellness in adult females.

For BN, the frequency of bingeing and purging behaviors, whether self-induced vomiting, use of diet pills, laxatives, or compulsive exercise has been reduced from twice per week to once per week in *DSM-5*, allowing inclusion of more people with this disorder. Perhaps the biggest change is that binge-eating disorder (BED) is recognized as a distinct eating disorder in *DSM-5*, whereas it previously fell under the broad category of eating disorders not otherwise specified (EDNOS). Avoidant, restrictive food intake disorder has also been added, which describes food-refusing behaviors and food avoidance without the accompanying weight and shape concerns. The EDNOS category has been replaced with the category of other specified feeding and eating disorders.

CONTROVERSIES CONCERNING *DSM* CRITERIA

It is argued that the current diagnostic systems, including *DSM-5*, do not fully describe the gray areas in the eating disorder spectrum and may define eating disorders too rigidly to be clinically useful (Fairburn and Cooper 2011). Some researchers have stated that future eating disorder diagnoses will rely on the genetic and neuroimaging studies to parcel out the variants of the disorders (Brooks et al. 2012). It could be that eating disorder subgroups can be developed based on neurobiological mechanisms (Frank 2015).

Recently, Nicholls and Arcelus compiled an excellent review of comments from child, adolescent, and eating disorder psychiatrists about *DSM-5* and the upcoming *ICD-11*, both of which classify eating disorders (Nicholls and Arcelus 2010). Some important issues that have been raised about classification systems include developmental sensitivity, specific markers of underweight or starvation and their limitations, and significant eating problems that do not have within them the concerns about body image, weight, or shape. Comments from experts revealed that there is still a great deal of discrepancy in how eating disorders are defined and seen by professionals. Some psychiatrists believe they should not be categorized under "behavioral syndromes associated with physiological disturbances and physical factors" but rather with emotional/anxiety disorders similar to obsessive-compulsive disorders (OCDs; Nicholls and Arcelus 2010).

Eating disorders are thought by some to be driven by anxiety, and the disordered eating and behaviors function to control the anxiety. Other proposed classifications would place eating disorders under mood disorders or under neurodevelopmental disorders Nicholls and Arcelus 2010). Some respondents suggested that eating disorders be classed according to weight, placing eating disorders in an underweight, normal weight, or overweight classification scheme. Removing body image concerns and fear of weight gain was suggested although many professionals seemed to prefer to retain those concerns as part of the diagnosis for typical AN and BN and develop some new diagnoses for what were called atypical AN and BN (Nicholls and Arcelus 2010).

New diagnoses suggested include purging disorder, atypical eating disorder, and other disorders seen in pediatrics such as selective feeding disorder, food avoidance, and functional dysphasia, which are associated with anxiety, mood disturbance, or obsessive thinking but do not have weight and shape concerns (Nicholls and Arcelus 2010). Research has been conducted to look at various subgroupings within the current diagnostic schemes (Turner et al. 2010). The identification of subgroups might aid in explaining the lack of fit between the *DSM-IV* diagnosis and treatment outcome. A simple diagnostic scheme that does not identify subgroups might list all persons meeting a general set of criteria as having AN, but within that diagnosis there might be several subcategories. For example, in subcategories related to disease severity, each might respond differently to different treatment plans. Subcategorizing might also provide a means of describing the frequent crossover states seen between AN and BN (Hebebrand and Bulik 2011). Subcategories and clusters have been identified based on measurements of coping styles, general medical health, functional impairment, depression, eating pathology, and attachment (Turner et al. 2010).

By creating more specific criteria in *DSM-5*, such as BED, the hope is that this will reduce the number of EDNOS cases, which are often seen as being less serious and therefore might receive less attention from clinicians (Machado et al. 2013). Another proposed scheme for diagnosing eating disorders, the broad categories for the diagnosis of eating disorders (BCD-ED) almost eliminates the EDNOS category (Sysko and Walsh 2011). The BCD-ED has three major categories of eating disorder, similar to *DSM-5*, and then has categories for behaviorally similar disorders to the major three with various subgroups to define atypical clinical presentations. The evolution of methods to diagnose and treat eating disorders has come from ongoing research in the field. Undoubtedly there will be further revisions to the *DSM* and other classification systems, with resulting improvements in treatment modalities, incorporating new findings such as biomarkers of disease.

CURRENT RESEARCH

PSYCHOLOGICAL CHARACTERISTICS OF ANOREXIA AND BULIMIA

Eating disorders collectively can be described as distorted thoughts and behaviors involving food selection, food preparation, food consumption, exercise execution, weight control, and perception of body shape and/or size. There is a growing body of research attempting to link the behaviors seen in eating disorders with genetics, stress, the interaction of environmental stressors on neurodevelopment, and how collectively these factors can give rise to certain temperaments or personality traits.

Eating disorders often co-occur with certain personality traits and behaviors. In both AN and BN, there are high rates of comorbidity with anxiety, depression, and OCD (Klump et al. 2009). Other traits and diagnoses frequently seen in individuals with AN and/or BN include neuroticism, negative emotionality, harm avoidance, low self-directedness, low cooperativeness, and traits associated with avoidant personality disorder (Lock et al. 2015). Individuals with BN are more likely to have high impulsivity, are more sensation- and novelty-seeking, and are more likely to engage in substance abuse and display traits associated with borderline personality disorder (Kaye 2008). Global childhood rigidity and expression of perfectionist traits often appear in children in advance of weight-related concerns and pathological eating behaviors (Halmi et al. 2012).

People with restricting AN show more traits such as low novelty-seeking, constriction of affect and emotional expressiveness, anhedonia, and reduced social spontaneity. An interesting difference between AN and BN is that Theory of Mind ability, or the ability to "read" or perceive other people's emotions and mental states, supposedly remains intact in individuals with BN but not in individuals with AN (Kenyon et al. 2012).

Anorexia and BN are characterized by what appear to be obsessions about food, eating, and body size, leading some researchers to ask whether eating disorders are a type of OCD. Since the late 1930s, the similarities between OCD and eating disorders have been noted. Kaye reported that 64% of people diagnosed with an eating disorder have some form of anxiety disorder and of those individuals, 41% have OCD (Kaye 2008). Clinicians familiar with AN notice the common and recurring symptoms that are obsessive in nature, such as various rules about food and eating, and excessive concern about weight and appearance.

Hildebrandt and others present very intriguing information about AN and its overlap with other anxiety disorders, in particular OCD (Hildebrandt et al. 2012). Personality traits elevated in AN include perfectionism, compulsivity, harm avoidance, and trait anxiety, and these traits are seen in family members as well. There is strong evidence that these anxiety traits are carried genetically and further evidence from twin studies of genetic overlap between AN and other anxiety disorders (Keel et al. 2005). The anxious perfectionist temperament may give rise to unattainable demands for thinness, perfectionism regarding diet and food choice, and catastrophic thinking about weight gain, fatness, and eating behaviors. Predictors of compulsive exercise include a drive for thinness, perfectionism, and obsessive-compulsiveness (Goodwin et al. 2011). Strober posed the hypothesis that AN, anxiety disorders, and anxious temperaments are related genetic phenotypes and Pallister and Waller suggest a common anxiety-based etiology for AN with core behavioral features similar to obsessions and compulsions (Pallister and Waller 2008; Strober 2004). OCD and anxiety are frequently seen in family members of individuals diagnosed with AN (Strober 2004).

Hildebrandt et al. discuss the anxiety, fear, and worry of AN in terms of triggers for anxiety (Hildebrandt et al. 2012). The authors explain the anxiety of AN as a central psychological feature, aroused by triggers in five domains. These domains include food, eating, interoceptive cues, shape and weight, and finally, social evaluation. As explained by Hildebrandt et al., these domains have within them many potential triggers that could elicit an anxious response. Food, for example, can be triggering due to its caloric or fat content, or the fact that it is composed mainly of carbohydrate or is labeled a dessert. The interoceptive or physiological perceptions might include hunger or sense of fullness, while the social evaluation cues can include any social setting in which the person with an eating disorder either actually experiences something judgmental, which could include a remark about weight, or perceives themself to be judged during mealtime. Shape and weight concerns include actual or perceived weight gains, changes in appearance, or perceived changes in appearance. Shape and weight concerns as well as social evaluation concerns can be worries placed in the future or distal concerns, meaning they are not occurring presently but concerns over what could happen in the future, for example, after one gains weight.

Other comorbid disorders seen with AN include social phobia and other specific phobias. Fear is a common emotion experienced by individuals with AN and many have theorized about how fear is learned and retained in AN. Several researchers have postulated that there is reduced pleasure associated with eating, in patients with AN. The response to foods in underweight versus weight-restored patients with AN differed in terms of their peripheral ghrelin levels. A derangement in the ghrelin response is thought to reduce motivation to eat (Maria Monteleone et al. 2016). The fact that food is not rewarding could make it easier to develop fear or concerns about food, more rigidity, and habits to avoid negative consequences of eating. Again, this is similar to what is seen in OCD where one repeats behaviors to avoid that which is fearful or anxiety producing.

Worry is another feature seen in AN and can manifest as hypervigilance over things such as weight, body shape, or clothing size (Hildebrandt et al. 2012). Hildebrandt and others describe avoidance behaviors as a response to the anxiety and worry of AN. Avoidance can be a safety behavior, a prevention strategy, or a compulsion and is similar to the avoidance behaviors seen in OCD that are ritualized and repetitive (Núñez-Navarro et al. 2011). In summary, people with AN may experience and then evaluate a concern or threat from one of the five domains, including food, eating, interoceptive cues, shape and weight, and finally, social evaluation. In their evaluation of the threat, a fear response is learned, and then behaviors to avoid the fear and discomfort associated with the threat are developed.

As research has uncovered more information about genetics, neurobiology, and environmental interactions, it has become clear that individuals do not choose to have eating disorders (Bulik 2016), nor is overcoming them a matter of simple will-power. Extinguishing the real fear involved in changing how one eats is similar to overcoming the fear of being in a small space for those with claustrophobia. The fear is very real and needs to be respected. This does not mean a person with an eating disorder is helpless.

Personal motivation to change eating disorder behaviors is frequently thought necessary and many therapies attempt to bolster motivation to change. If the personal motivation is not enhanced, the client is deemed "not ready to change," even though ambivalence toward treatment is a common characteristic of eating disorders. Research has only recently begun examining the role that personal motivation plays in the recovery process for eating disorders (Waller 2012).

Waller discusses some of the potential myths that currently underlie the use of motivational strategies in therapy for eating disorders. He proposes that it is indeed a myth that motivation fits into "neat stages" or that current motivational strategies are based on solid evidence. Waller proposes some alternatives involving active behavioral change strategies, and perceiving motivation in terms of behavioral outcomes. Instead of perceiving that clients are "not ready to change," clinicians need to be aware of the characteristics of eating disorders that may present as being unwilling to change and see these instead as being unable to change, without appropriate intervention. This is crucial to understanding the nature of eating disorders and it will affect how clinicians choose to treat their patients.

Recently, another review examined the evidence in support of motivational interviewing in eating disorder treatment and found little evidence to support its use. It was argued that people do not choose to have eating disorders; therefore, enhancing motivation to change was based on an ill-conceived conceptualization of the problem (Knowles et al. 2013). One study looked at how patients feel about being pressured to admit to a hospital for treatment. Researchers found that when first hospitalized, patients did not see the need for treatment and displayed the characteristic ambivalence toward treatment. After being in treatment for 2 weeks, patients believed that their admission was necessary (Guarda et al. 2007). Another study demonstrated lack of insight into one's illness and lack of motivation to recover in adolescents with AN when compared to healthy adolescents in terms of reasoning skills and capacity to make informed decisions regarding their illness versus a hypothetical illness. Adolescents with AN were less able to think about consequences of their illness, and experienced more difficulty with comparative and overall reasoning (Turrell et al. 2011).

Perhaps the ability to "choose" to change is compromised by the fact that a starved brain cannot create the chemical signals necessary to "motivate" them. The Minnesota starvation study showed that many of the symptoms of AN were symptoms of starvation and once starvation was corrected by refeeding, the person's overall affect changed. Symptoms such as depression and anxiety also generally improved with feeding (Kalm and Semba 2005). With this in mind, it may be that clinicians need to catalyze the initial changes in behavior by using interventions aimed at refeeding first.

Alexithymia, or the diminished ability to identify or differentiate emotions, frequently co-occurs with eating disorders, with a representative prevalence of 63% in AN and 56% in BN (Cochrane et al. 1993). Alexithymia is correlated with certain physical illnesses, such as inflammatory bowel disease, cardiac disorders, gastrointestinal problems, immune suppression, and pain frequency (Verissimo et al. 1998). It is theorized that failure to regulate emotions cognitively might result in prolonged stimulation of the autonomic nervous system and neuroendocrine systems, which can lead to somatic diseases. Recent research has demonstrated that people with AN show blunted positive response to film clips, and therefore may not show a full range of emotions (Davies et al. 2011).

AN is characterized by lack of insight into the illness, or anosognosia, in spite of increasing wasting and medical consequences (Vandereycken 2006). Dysphoria, or the overall feeling of discontent, is another feature seen in eating disorders and there is evidence that restrictive eating behavior, seen in both AN and BN, may provide respite from the dysphoria, thus creating positive reinforcement for restriction (Kaye 2008). Recent research using neuroimaging has shown that women who are recovered from AN continue to have decreased sensitivity to hunger and blunted reward signaling processes when hungry (Wierenga et al. 2015).

THE PSYCHOLOGY OF BINGE EATING

Binge eating is a behavior common to both BN and BED. It has been suggested that restrictive eating coupled with the resultant excessive hunger may precede binge-eating behaviors. People with BN and BED have reported higher levels of hunger compared to controls, which may suggest that they have an altered physiological perception of hunger or a greater drive to eat (Stice et al. 2000). Haedt-Matt and Keel (2011) examined hunger as a precursor to binge-eating episodes and found that excessive hunger did not seem to precipitate binge eating. Further, they found that actual hunger or rating of degree of hunger was higher before consumption of a normal meal or regular amount of food as compared to what is described as a binge. This is supported by other research indicating that bingeing may not be directly related to physical hunger (Haedt-Matt and Keel 2011). Impulsiveness and impulsivity-related traits are also associated with bingeing and with BN. One of these traits—negative urgency—or the predisposition to act in a rash manner when under distress has been strongly linked to binge eating (Combs et al. 2011).

There are important distinctions between BN and BED related to type of dietary restraint. Cognitive restraint applied to food intake can be divided into rigid cognitive restraint, or "black and white" and "all or nothing" type of thinking, and flexible restraint, which would translate into a moderate approach to dietary restraint. BN is associated with many levels of dietary restraint, including very restrictive eating behaviors, while BED features less restrictive eating and less overall restraint (Blomquist and Grilo 2011).

Recently, a group of researchers studied the clinical presentation and personality traits of individuals diagnosed with BED, BN-nonpurging type, or BN-purging type to determine different characteristics of these diagnostic categories and found that disease severity differed with BN-purging being most severe, followed by BN-nonpurging and then BED. Clinical presentation differed; however, personality traits did not differ between these disorders.

A description of BED has been proposed as "overeating associated with other psychological disturbances" (Wolfe et al. 2009) and loss of a sense of control over eating. Ideas that overeating might fall into the realm of "normal" or a normal response to a large available food supply have yet to be explored. Humans learn that eating is associated with pleasure, and that one eats or distresses in response to the discomfort of hunger. This is illustrated by the infant response to hunger, which is to show distress by fidgeting, sucking on a fist, and crying. Without these signs of distress, which parents respond to by feeding, a species would die out due to starvation. Typically in the brain's response to food, hunger mechanisms become aroused. In primitive cultures, it was normal to "binge" when food became abundant after days or weeks of suboptimal food availability. Clinicians should question how hunger responses differ in an environment replete with vast amounts of food, and perhaps explore answers to this question prior to assigning pathology to overeating. Studies have demonstrated that women under stress vary in terms of their food preferences, with those under more stress choosing higher fat and sweet foods in comparison to those who are under less stress (Habhab et al. 2009). Recently, researchers have shown in a sample of over 65,000 adults that self-reported or perceived stress was associated with greater intake of fast foods and high-fat foods but not with a higher intake from carbohydrate (Barrington et al. 2014). Why this occurs is not clear although several theories have been proposed. When the body is in anticipation of a probable flight or fight response or possible increased fuel need, which can occur in stressful situations, maybe there is intrinsic modification of food preference toward those foods that would provide increased fuel, such as high-fat foods. Again, clinicians might need to differentiate between psychopathology and physical response in assessing food preferences in a given situation. That said, there is usually psychological distress when a person binges, whether a subjective or objective binge.

Moreno and Tendon (2011) provide a comparison of addiction and substance use disorders to overeating, as there is discussion that overeating might fit the definition of an addiction. Their conclusion is that "food addiction" would not fit as an addictive disorder but that night eating syndrome and binge eating deserve further consideration as being included as addictive behaviors (Moreno and Tandon 2011). The reader is referred to an excellent chapter on the relationship between feeding and drug-seeking behaviors, which discusses the interwoven nature of reward-seeking behaviors (Carrol and Nathan 2014). Some clinicians state food components themselves may not have addictive qualities like drugs can have, such as development of tolerance and withdrawal symptoms upon removal. However, "food addiction" or other food-related behaviors may fit into the category of a process addiction. There is implied tolerance to binge-eating and bulimic behaviors, such as the observed increasing amounts of food eaten during binges or the impaired satiety, thought to be related to low-functioning brain reward circuitry.

Evidence from animal studies, neuroimaging, and genetics has further shown the addictive qualities of many behaviors seen in the eating disorders (Brewerton 2014).

GENETICS, NEUROBIOLOGY, AND THE INTERACTION OF STRESS

As detailed later in this chapter, some researchers have stated that eating disturbances are a manifestation of sociocultural influences and/or psychological disturbances, and often the psychological disturbances have been attributed to past trauma, abuse, or abandonment (Delvecchio et al. 2014).

Given what we know about the biology of eating as well as the genetic component of eating disorders, this brings up the age-old question of nature versus nurture. This line of thought and inquiry may explain why some providers see eating disorders through a lens of past experiences and learned behaviors, while some clinicians see the disorders through the lens of biology. Certainly, there are some patients who seem to fall ill without any notable past history of trauma/abuse, which has further complicated theories on causality and then treatment that follows.

Genetic variations certainly give rise to differences in eating behaviors, hunger, hunger perception, and anxiety traits. Polymorphisms in the leptin and/or leptin receptor gene are associated with increased snacking behaviors (de Krom et al. 2007). Alterations in cholecystokinin (*CCK*) and serotonin receptor 2C genes are associated with eating patterns and satiety (de Krom et al. 2007). The expression of key regulatory hormones, active in satiety signaling, and synthesis of neurotransmitters in the enteric nervous system are affected by nutrient composition of the diet (Neunlist and Schemann 2014). Evidence shows that varying levels of methylation of the oxytocin receptor gene are associated with disease severity in AN (Kim et al. 2014).

The "circadian clock" or period 2 gene is positively associated with greater stress experienced when restricting calories, higher dropout rate from behavioral weight loss programs, increased snacking behaviors, increased boredom eating, and skipping breakfast (Garaulet et al. 2010). It has been shown that sleep deprivation, shift work, and exposure to bright lights in the evening are associated with insulin resistance, abdominal adiposity, and metabolic syndrome. The period 2 gene is a major component of the molecular mechanism that generates circadian rhythms in mammals and a missense mutation in this gene in humans is linked to diurnal preference, advanced sleep phase syndrome, and psychological disturbances related to seasonal variation, such as seasonal affective disorder (Garaulet et al. 2010).

It is known that light and food are the two main regulators of central and peripheral oscillators, which serve to regulate circadian rhythms, and extreme snacking is said to disrupt the oscillators' capacity to provide accurate feedback (Garaulet et al. 2010). A single-nucleotide polymorphism in the Circadian Locomotor Output Cycles Kaput (*CLOCK*) gene is linked to mood disorders, shorter sleep duration, increased weight, higher energy intake, and difficulties in losing weight (López-Guimerà et al. 2014). These important findings may offer a novel way to view variations in eating behaviors as not simply a means to reduce inner stress but that stress is affected by the eating itself, and that these behaviors are heavily influenced by genetics.

Higher order neural circuitry associated with appetite may be involved in restrictive eating seen in AN and also the overeating observed in BN. Using functional magnetic resonance imaging to measure brain response to sweeteners, research showed that people recovered from AN had decreased sensitization to sucrose while those recovered from BN had a heightened sensitization to sucrose (Wagner et al. 2015). This emerging neurophysiological perspective might help demystify what has been called emotional eating, and alleviates the need to blame the individual for variations in eating behavior, as is often done in weight loss programs as well as in the media.

There are important questions regarding the role of genetics, especially with epigenetic research providing new information about environment–gene interactions. Do genes determine entirely the physical and emotional outcome or is it ever the other way around? Can stress affect the outcome of genetics?

Some events would cause stress in almost every human, such as being chased by a mountain lion or witnessing a horrific act of violence. There are also events that would most likely not cause stress in most people, such as being in a relaxing vacation atmosphere. The very attempt to try to describe a situation where almost no people would feel stress is somewhat difficult and leads one immediately to the conclusion that stress is subjective in many ways or that people have varying levels of susceptibility to anxiety and stress. In looking at eating disorder risk factors identified by researchers over the past 15 years, one appreciates the wide array of risk factors related to environment (Mazzeo and Bulik 2009). This list includes those environmental factors that can be measured or documented in some way, but may not evaluate the perception of or susceptibility to stress by individuals.

Epigenetic changes can be environmentally induced, modulate gene expression independent of the deoxyribonucleic acid (DNA) sequence, and can be passed on from either parent through the germ cell line. DNA methylation and histone modification are both epigenetic mechanisms that alter gene expression and epigenetic processes can give rise to variable phenotypes from identical cells. Epigenetic alterations are dynamic, can be reversible, coordinate gene expression throughout development, and may confer susceptibility to or reaction to stress. Epigenetically sensitive developmental periods such as the prenatal and perinatal period have been identified, and many of the epialleles (identical genes that vary between individuals in degree of methylation) are altered due to environmental signals such as maternal stress and nutrition (Campbell et al. 2011). It is interesting that "obstetrical complications" are listed as a risk factor associated with eating disorder development in offspring and that obstetric complications might also cause the mother stress. Transgenerational stress experiences are thought to be passed on through epigenetic changes in parents.

Epidemiological studies show a strong association between gestational stress (including infection, starvation, and hypoxia) and neurodevelopmental disorders such as schizophrenia and autism spectrum disorders. Animal models have shown that maternal stress changes the offspring's hypothalamic–pituitary–adrenal (HPA) stress axis and stress reactivity, and results in cognitive impairment (Banks 1996). Animal models have also shown that epigenetic alteration occurs in males and can persist through several generations. Using a murine model of stress response, researchers found that sperm could be reprogrammed and produce offspring of either gender with hypofunctioning HPA stress axis (Bale 2014). These researchers postulated that stressing a father prior to breeding altered offspring reactivity to future stressors and that this might be an evolutionary advantage in that it allowed offspring to react less to a stressful environment. Research suggests that alterations in one generation's germ cell line may be passed on to several future generations and may underlie risk for posttraumatic stress disorder. Polymorphisms in the methylenetetrahydrofolate reductase gene have been shown to result in developmental disorders in humans and they may be implicated as increasing susceptibility to neonatal stress (Kezurer et al. 2013).

Epigenetics might offer a bridge to some of the gaps in knowledge about how specific risk factors translate into increased risk for eating disorder development, and they may also offer a way to explain the common theory that parental behaviors are a causative agent in eating disorder development. For example, stress during pregnancy may increase fetal glucocorticoid exposure, which could have adverse health consequences including alterations in function of the HPA axis. Candidate genes for study in terms of epigenetics and risk for eating disorders include the fat mass and obesity-related (*FTO*) gene, implicated in increased risk of obesity, the leptin and leptin receptor genes, the proopiomelanocortin gene, and the brain-derived neurotrophic factor gene (Campbell et al. 2011). Heightened activity of the *FTO* gene, for example, may increase DNA methylation of genes involving resting energy expenditure. Individuals with two copies of a common polymorphism of the *FTO* gene are at increased risk of clinical obesity (Campbell et al. 2011). Researchers have looked at polymorphisms in the *FTO* gene to see if these correlated with eating disordered behaviors and thus far have not found this to be the case, rather the *FTO* gene is thought to influence energy metabolism or modulate the effects of energy expenditure (Jonassaint et al. 2011).

Twin studies have shown that there is an inherited component to restrained eating attempts and there are genetic as well as hormonal contributions involved in overeating and choice of energy dense foods (Schur et al. 2009; Cecil et al. 2008). Deficits in satiation have been associated with hormones involved in pre- and posteating, such as CCK and glucagon-like peptide-1 (GLP-1), which is released from intestinal cells in response to a meal and increases satiation, with corresponding reduction in food intake in humans (Dossat et al. 2015). Individuals with BN report feeling less satisfied and full after a standardized meal and they show reduced levels of both CCK and GLP-1 postprandially.

Polymorphisms in the serotonin transporter gene promoter region (5-HTTLPR) affecting serotonin transporter transcription have been linked to development of eating disorders. A lower expressing 5-HTTLPR genotype (S allele) is found in individuals who may be more sensitive to early stressors in life and is considered a risk factor for eating disorders. In women who reported binge eating, the S allele was associated with more binge eating and higher levels of anxiety. Exposure to early life stressors seems to modulate the effects of 5-HHTLPR leading some researchers to say that there is an interaction between childhood trauma and the S allele that confers risk for eating disorder development (Stoltenberg et al. 2012).

Serotonin transporter binding abnormalities are found in people during the acute stage of BN as well as in individuals recovered from bulimic symptoms (Pichika et al. 2012). These and other findings support earlier research describing certain personality characteristics as being present prior to illness onset and remaining after eating disorder behaviors have been extinguished (Kaye 2008).

Additional work on serotonin dysfunction, genetic polymorphisms, and the effects of estrogens on bulimic symptoms has shown that polymorphisms of serotonin genes are seen in OCD and low serotonin is seen in several behaviors associated with impulsivity such as substance abuse disorders, BN, and binge eating. Estrogens and serotonin are thought to modulate and contribute to maintenance of bulimic symptoms and it has been suggested that estrogen is a regulator of the serotonin system (Hildebrandt et al. 2012). Exposure to reproductive hormones in utero may alter risk of development of eating disorders. Increased levels of prenatal exposure to testosterone, measured by digit ratios, may be protective for men and women as far as future development of eating disorders (Smith et al. 2010).

The biological response to stressors is the activation of the HPA axis. Glucocorticoids, in part, mediate many of the effects of HPA activation and individual's response to stress. These hormones also regulate the basal control of HPA axis activity, integrate much of the response to stress, and have a key role in the termination of the stress response. Lo Sauro et al. (2008) examined literature regarding the relation between HPA axis functioning and eating disorders. In summarizing their finding, the authors note that HPA axis hyperactivity is well documented for both AN and BN, although it is less so for BN. They cannot state whether the HPA axis hyperactivity modified eating behaviors or if eating behaviors modified HPA axis activity or both. They further note that many studies have examined stress and stressful life events as preceding eating disorder development and have come to the conclusion that chronic stress is associated with eating disorder development. Additionally, there is evidence that some people diagnosed with eating disorders might perceive life events as more stressful than control subjects (Lo Sauro et al. 2008).

Using a questionnaire developed to measure sensitivity to reward and punishment, Jappe et al. (2011) were able to show that women diagnosed with AN were more sensitive to both reward and punishment as compared to control subjects and this may be supported now by genetic research. AN may have a feature of impaired interoception. Functional brain imaging studies have shown a heightened response in terms of anticipating a painful stimulus yet a blunted response in terms of rating a pain stimuli, in people recovered from AN (Strigo et al. 2013). Finally, there is intriguing research showing an association between the intestinal microbiome and levels of depression, anxiety, and eating disorder psychopathology in patients with AN. The microbe–gut–brain axis is a fruitful area of exploration in the field of eating disorders (Kleiman et al. 2015).

Genetics, epigenetics, and neurobiological research have given us tools to explain the links between experiences, stress, perception of stress, and environmental factors. Recently, acquired knowledge of brain function, neurobiological development, and epigenetic alterations, as well as insight into stress and environmental influences and how these can change with various therapies due to neuroplasticity, provide hope for advancing effectiveness of treatments.

SOCIAL AND CULTURAL CONSIDERATIONS

The eating disorders collectively are very puzzling disorders and as such, have lent themselves to many theories about causation. As detailed above, there are biological tendencies that contribute to the vulnerability to developing an eating disorder.

Research shows that there are a number of social and cultural factors that may enhance the biological predisposition and promote development of an eating disorder. It is useful for clinicians to examine what social/cultural domains might contribute to promoting an eating disorder. If it is accepted that stress promotes eating disorders, then clinicians need to examine the environment of an affected individual for factors contributing to stress. Parenting styles and family dynamics have frequently been blamed for eating disorders, and they might contribute to stress, but family environment and dynamics are not considered causative in eating disorders.

Conceptualization of the etiology of eating disorders has evolved from believing outside forces, trauma, or poor parenting were causative, to thinking genetics and biology were solely responsible, to a new synthesis of thought. Currently, there is a holistic appreciation of genetic susceptibility, neurobiology, and the inherent resilience of an individual within an environment supplying a great deal of stress. Stress is also appreciated to be subjective in nature (Mazzeo and Bulik 2009). Cultures bring varying ideas about food, feeding behaviors, or evaluation of body types, and these values can influence children, some of whom might hardly notice and some of whom may be genetically susceptible to eating disorders (Mazzeo and Bulik 2009). Many have postulated that cultural factors, including the relatively recent thin idealization, might play a role in the development of eating disorders, and programs targeting reduction in thin ideal internalization have been developed to prevent eating disorders (Shaw et al. 2009). If pressure to conform to an ideal body type creates anxiety or stress in a given individual, and if we accept that stress lays the foundation for genetic activation leading to eating disorder pathology, one might state that cultural pressures play a role in eating disorder development. There is evidence that over the past 50 years the thin ideal has been adopted by cultures and that this fact could account for increased anxiety in people (Mazzeo and Bulik 2009). One study examined women in Miss America contests and Playboy centerfold photos across several decades and noted that in the United States, women have been depicted with increased emphasis on thinness over time (Wiseman et al. 1992). Interestingly, this same study counted the number of weight-loss diet, weight-loss exercise, and weight-loss diet/exercise articles in several popular magazines, replicating an earlier study, and found a dramatic increase in the number of articles for weight reduction between the years 1959 and 1988 (Garner et al. 1980).

What a culture deems important to pay attention to, as discussed above, is relevant to the emergence of eating disorders. Throughout history, some have argued that weight phobia was not a central defining feature of AN or binge-purge disorders until recently, when there has been more focus on body shape and promotion of the thin ideal (Thompson and Stice 2001). However, weight phobia as a central defining motive at least in AN has been defended (Habermas 1996). It might be that weight phobia has been cleverly hidden behind other motives. During history and in other cultures, religious beliefs and the desire to become close to God might have served as justifications for restricting food but may have been masking a fat phobia. Today, the justification that a person "just wants to eat healthfully" is often used for the beginning of food restriction.

CONCLUSION

What has history, research, and experience told us about eating disorders? How have we been informed recently about what eating disorders are? Throughout history, eating disorders have been present and theories about their nature have run the gamut. However, in looking at historical accounts one cannot help but notice the common thread concerning the temperament of those with AN or the underlying rationale for self-induced vomiting. The importance of cultural contributions is notable, particularly as they define what is important or valued for a given culture. Witztum and coworkers have posed the idea of eating disorders as idioms of distress. This intriguing idea postulates that people in different cultures express their anxiety in ways that reflect the meaning a culture gives to distress, and also that culture might dictate how people display their distress (Witztum et al. 2008). Emerging epigenetic research is illuminating the process by which cultural realities may contribute to the environmental and emotional stressors, which in turn cause alterations in genetic expression.

Ultimately, as research offers new information supplanting some of the theories that have tried to explain eating disorders, clinicians will gain a greater understanding of just what these disorders really are. As clinicians' clarity evolves, people diagnosed with eating disorders will experience less discrimination and enjoy unbiased, fully informed, and effective treatment.

REFERENCES

American Psychiatric Association. *History of the DSM*. 2016. Available at http://www.psychiatry. org/psychiatrists/practice/dsm/history

Bale, TL. Lifetime stress experience: Transgenerational epigenetics and germ cell programming. *Dialogues in Clinical Neuroscience* 16, no. 3 (2014): 297.

Banks, CG. There is no fat in heaven: Religious asceticism and the meaning of anorexia nervosa. *Ethos* 24, no. 1 (1996): 107–135.

Barrington, WE, Beresford SAA, McGregor BA, and White E. Perceived stress and eating behaviors by sex, obesity status, and stress vulnerability: Findings from the vitamins and lifestyle (Vital) study. *Journal of the Academy of Nutrition and Dietetics* 114, no. 11 (2014): 1791–1799.

Becker, AE, Eddy KT, and Perloe A. Clarifying criteria for cognitive signs and symptoms for eating disorders in DSM. *International Journal of Eating Disorders* 42, no. 7 (2009): 611–619.

Bell, RM. *Holy Anorexia*. Chicago, IL: University of Chicago Press, 2014.

Bemporad, JR. Self-starvation through the ages: Reflections on the pre-history of anorexia nervos. *International Journal of Eating Disorders* 19, no. 3 (1996): 217–237.

Blomquist, KK, and Grilo CM. Predictive significance of changes in dietary restraint in obese patients with binge eating disorder during treatment. *International Journal of Eating Disorders* 44, no. 6 (2011): 515–523.

Brewerton, TD. Are eating disorders addictions? In *Eating Disorders, Addictions, and Substance Use Disorders*, edited by TD Brewerton and AB Dennis, pp. 267–299. Heidelberg, Berlin: Springer-Verlag, 2014.

Brooks, SJ, Rask-Andersen M, Benedict C, and Schiöth HB. A debate on current eating disorder diagnoses in light of neurobiological findings: Is it time for a spectrum model? *BMC Psychiatry* 12, no. 1 (2012): 76.

Bruch, HC. Anorexia nervosa: The therapeutic task. In *Handbook of Eating Disorders: Physiology, Psychology and Treatment of Obesity, Anorexia and Bulimia*, edited by KD Brownell and JP Foreyt, pp. 328–350. New York, NY: Basic Books, 1986.

Bruch, HC Four decades of eating disorders. In *Handbook of Psychotherapy for Anorexia Nervosa and Bulimia*, edited by DM Garner and PE Garfinkel, pp. 7–18. New York, NY: Guilford Press, 1985.

Bruch, HC. Perceptual and conceptual disturbances in anorexia nervosa. *Psychosomatic Medicine* 24, no. 2 (1962): 187–194.

Brumberg, JJ. *Fasting Girls: The History of Anorexia*. New York, NY: Random House, 2000.

Bulik, CM. Towards a science of eating disorders: Replacing myths with realities: The fourth Birgit Olsson lecture. *Nordic Journal of Psychiatry* 70, no. 3 (2016): 224–230.

Campbell, IC, Mill J, Uher R, and Schmidt U. Eating disorders, gene-environment interactions and epigenetics. *Neuroscience and Behavioral Reviews* 35, no. 3 (2011): 784–793.

Carrol, ME, and Nathan AH. The relationship between feeding and drug-seeking behaviors. In *Eating Disorders, Addictions, and Substance Use Disorders*, edited by TD Brewerton and AB Dennis, pp. 23–45. Heidelberg, Berlin: Springer-Verlag, 2014.

Cecil, JE, Tavendale R, Watt P, Hetherington MM, and Palmer CN. An obesity associated FTO gene variant and increased energy intake in children. *New England Journal of Medicine* 359, no. 24 (2008): 2558–2566.

Cochrane, CE, Brewerton TD, Wilson DB, and Hodges EL. Alexithymia in the eating disorders. *International Journal of Eating Disorders* 14, no. 2 (1993): 219–222.

Combs, JL, Pearson CM, and Smith GT. A risk model for preadolescent disordered eating. *International Journal of Eating Disorders* 44, no. 7 (2011): 596–604.

Davies, H, Schmidt U, Stahl D, and Tchanturia K. Evoked facial emotional expression and emotional experience in people with anorexia nervosa. *International Journal of Eating Disorders* 44, no. 6 (2011): 531–539.

de Krom, M, van der Schouw YT, Hendriks J, Ophoff RA, van Gils CH, Stolk RP, Grobbee DE, and Adan R. Common genetic variations in CCK, leptin, and leptin receptor genes are associated with specific human eating patterns. *Diabetes* 56, no. 1 (2007): 276–280.

Delvecchio, E, Di Riso D, Salcuni S, Lis A, and George C. Anorexia and attachment: Dysregulated defense and pathological mourning. *Frontiers in Psychology* 5 (2014): 1218.

Dossat, AM, Bodell LP, Williams DL, Eckel LA, and Keel PK. Preliminary examination of glucagon-like peptide-1 levels in women with purging disorder and bulimia nervosa. *International Journal of Eating Disorders* 48, no. 2 (2015): 199–205.

Fairburn, CG, and Cooper Z. Eating disorders, DSM-5, and clinical reality. *British Journal of Psychiatry* 198, no. 1 (2011): 8–10.

Frank, GK. Recent advances in neuroimaging to model eating disorder neurobiology. *Current Psychiatry Reports* 17, no. 4 (2015): 1–9.

Garaulet, M, Corbalán-Tutau MD, Madrid JA, Baraza JC, Parnell LD, Lee YC, and Ordovas JM. PERIOD2 variants are associated with abdominal obesity, psycho-behavioral factors, and attrition in the dietary treatment of obesity. *Journal of the American Dietetic Association* 110, no. 6 (2010): 917–921.

Garner, DM, Garfinkel PE, Schwartz D, and Thompson M. Cultural expectations of thinness in women. *Psychological Reports* 47, no. 2 (1980): 483–491.

Goodwin, H, Haycraft E, Willis AM, and Meyer C. Compulsive exercise: The role of personality, psychological morbidity, and disordered eating. *International Journal of Eating Disorders* 44, no. 7 (2011): 655–660.

Gordon, RA. *Eating Disorders: Anatomy of a Social Epidemic*. Malden, MA: Blackwell Publishers, 2000.

Guarda, AS, Pinto AM, Coughlin JW, Hussain S, Haug NA, and Heinberg LJ. Perceived coercion and change in perceived need for admission in patients hospitalized for eating disorders. *American Journal of Psychiatry* 164, no. 1 (2007): 108–114.

Gull, WW. Anorexia nervosa. *Transaction of the Clinical Society* 7 (1874): 22–28.

Habermas, T. In defense of weight phobia as the central organizing motive in anorexia nervosa: Historical and cultural arguments for a culture-sensitive psychological conception. *International Journal of Eating Disorders* 19, no. 4 (1996): 317–334.

Habermas, T. The psychiatric history of anorexia nervosa and bulimia nervosa: Weight concerns and bulimic symptoms in early case reports. *International Journal of Eating Disorders* 8, no. 3 (1989): 259–273.

Habhab, S, Sheldon JP, and Loeb RC. The relationship between stress, dietary restraint, and food preferences in women. *Appetite* 52, no. 2 (2009): 437–444.

Haedt-Matt, AA, and Keel PK. Hunger and binge eating: A meta-analysis of studies using ecological momentary assessment. *International Journal of Eating Disorders* 44, no. 7 (2011): 573–578.

Halmi, KA, Bellace D, Berthod S, Ghosh S, Berrettini W, Brandt HA, Bulik CM, Crawford S, Fichter MM, Johnson CL, Kaplan A, Kaye WH, Thornton L, Treasure J, Blake Woodside D, and Strober M. An examination of early childhood perfectionism across anorexia nervosa subtype. *International Journal of Eating Disorders* 45, no. 6 (2012): 800–807.

Halse, C, Honey A, and Boughtwood D. *Inside Anorexia: The Experiences of Girls and Their Families*. Philadelphia, PA: Jessica Kingsley Publishers, 2008.

Hebebrand, J, and Bulik CM. Critical appraisal of the provisional DSM-5 criteria for anorexia nervosa and an alternative proposal. *International Journal of Eating Disorders* 44, no. 8 (2011): 665–678.

Jappe, LM, Frank GK, Shott ME, Rollin MD, Pryor T, Hagman JO, Yang TT, and Davis E. Heightened sensitivity to reward and punishment in anorexia nervosa. *International Journal of Eating Disorders* 44, no. 4 (2011): 317–324.

Jonassaint, CR, Szatkiewicz JP, Bulik CM, Thornton LM, Bloss C, Berrettini W, Kaye WH, Bergen AW, Magistretti P, Strober M, Keel P, Brandt H, Crawford S, Crow S, Fichter MM, Goldman D, Halmi KA, Johnson C, Kaplan A, Klump K, La Via M, Mitchell J, Rotondo A, Treasure J, and Woodside DB. Specific common variants of the obesity-associated FTO gene are not associated with psychological and behavioral eating disorder phenotypes. *American Journal of Medical Genetics Part B: Neuropsychiatric Genetics* 154B, no. 4 (2011): 454–461.

Kalm, LM, and Semba RD. They starved so that others be better fed: Remembering Ancel Keys and the Minnesota experiment. *Journal of Nutrition* 135, no. 6 (2005): 1347–1352.

Kaye, W. Neurobiology of anorexia and bulimia nervosa. *Physiology and Behavior* 94, no. 1 (2008): 121–135.

Keel, PK, Klump KL, Miller KB, McGue M, and Iacono WG. Shared transmission of eating disorders and anxiety disorders. *International Journal of Eating Disorders* 38, no. 2 (2005): 99–105.

Kenyon, M, Samarawickrema N, Dejong H, Van den Eynde F, Startup H, Lavender A, Goodman-Smith E, and Schmidt U. Theory of mind in bulimia nervosa. *International Journal of Eating Disorders* 45, no. 3 (2012): 377–384.

Kezurer, N, Galron D, and Golan HM. Increased susceptibility to mild neonatal stress in MTHFR deficient mice. *Behavioural Brain Research* 253 (2013): 240–252.

Kim, YR, Kim JH, Kim MJ, and Treasure J. Differential methylation of the oxytocin receptor gene in patients with anorexia nervosa: A pilot study. *PLoS One* 9, no. 2 (2014): e88673.

Kleiman, SC, Watson HJ, Bulik-Sullivan EC, Huh EY, Tarantino LM, Bulik CM, and Carroll IM. The intestinal microbiota in acute anorexia nervosa and during renourishment: Relationship to depression, anxiety, and eating disorder psychopathology. *Psychosomatic Medicine* 77, no. 9 (2015): 969–981.

Klump, KL, Bulik CM, Kaye WH, Treasure J, and Tyson E. Academy for eating disorders position paper: Eating disorders are serious mental illnesses. *International Journal of Eating Disorders* 42, no. 2 (2009): 97–103.

Knowles, L, Anokhina A, and Serpell L. Motivational interventions in the eating disorders: What is the evidence? *International Journal of Eating Disorders* 46, no. 2 (2013): 97–107.

Lasègue, C. De L'anorexie histerique. *Archives Générales de Médicine* (1873): 385–403.

Lo Sauro, C, Ravaldi C, Cabras PL, Faravelli C, and Ricca V. Stress, hypothalamic-pituitary-adrenal axis and eating disorders. *Neuropsychobiology* 57, no. 3 (2008): 95–115.

Lock, J, La Via MC, and American Academy of Child and Adolescent Psychiatry (AACAP) Committee on Quality Issues (CQI). Practice parameter for the assessment and treatment of children and adolescents with eating disorders. *Journal of American Academy of Child and Adolescent Psychiatry* 54, no. 5 (2015): 412–425.

López-Guimerà, G, Dashti HS, Smith CE, Sánchez-Carracedo D, Ordovas JM, and Garaulet M. CLOCK 3111 T/C SNP interacts with emotional eating behavior for weight-loss in a Mediterranean population. *PLoS One* 9, no. 6 (2014): e99152.

Loudon, I. The diseases called chlorosis. *Psychological Medicine* 14, no. 1 (1984): 27–36.

Machado, PP, Gonçalves S, and Hoek HW. DSM-5 reduces the proportion of EDNOS cases: Evidence from community samples. *International Journal of Eating Disorders* 46, no. 1 (2013): 60–65.

Maria Monteleone, A, Monteleone P, Dalle Grave R, Nigro M, El Ghoch M, Calugi S, Cimino M, and Maj M. Ghrelin response to hedonic eating in underweight and short-term weight restored patients with anorexia nervosa. *Psychiatry Research* 235 (2016): 55–60.

Mazzeo, SE, and Bulik CM. Environmental and genetic risk factors for eating disorders: What the clinician needs to know. *Child and Adolescent Psychiatric Clinics of North America* 18, no. 1 (2009): 67–82.

Moreno, C, and Tandon R. Should overeating and obesity be classified as an addictive disorder in DSM-5? *Current Pharmaceutical Design* 17, no. 12 (2011): 1128–1131.

Morgan, JF, Marsden P, and Lacey JH. " Spiritual starvation?": A case series concerning Christianity and eating disorder. *International Journal of Eating Disorders* 28, no. 4 (2000): 476–480.

Nasser, M. A prescription of vomiting: Historical footnotes. *International Journal of Eating Disorders* 13, no. 1 (1993): 129–131.

Neunlist, M, and Schemann M. Nutrient-induced changes in the phenotype and function of the enteric nervous system. *Journal of Physiology* 592, no. 14 (2014): 2959–2965.

Nicholls, D, and Arcelus J. Making eating disorders classification work in ICD-11. *European Eating Disorders Review* 18, no. 4 (2010): 247–250.

Núñez-Navarro, A, Jiménez-Murcia S, Alvarez-Moya E, Villarejo C, Díaz IS, Augmantell CM, Granero R, Penelo E, Krug I, Tinahones FJ, Bulik CM, and Fernández-Aranda F. Differentiating purging and nonpurging bulimia nervosa and binge eating disorder. *International Journal of Eating Disorders* 44, no. 6 (2011): 488–496.

Pallister, E, and Waller G. Anxiety in the eating disorders: Understanding the overlap. *Clinical Psychology Review* 28, no. 3 (2008): 366–386.

Pichika, R, Buchsbaum MS, Bailer U, Hoh C, Decastro A, Buchsbaum BR, and Kaye W. Serotonin transporter binding after recovery from bulimia nervosa. *International Journal of Eating Disorders* 45, no. 3 (2012): 345–352.

Russell, G. Bulimia nervosa: An ominous variant of anorexia nervosa. *Psychological Medicine* 9, no. 3 (1979): 429–448.

Schur, E, Noonan C, Polivy J, Goldberg J, and Buchwald D. Genetic and environmental influences on restrained eating behavior. *International Journal of Eating Disorders* 42, no. 8 (2009): 765–772.

Shaw, H, Stice E, and Becker CB. Preventing eating disorders. *Child and Adolescent Psychiatric Clinics of North America* 18, no. 1 (2009): 199–207.

Sheenan, ML, and Summers VK. The syndrome of hypopituitarism. *Quarterly Journal of Medicine* 18, no. 72 (1948): 319–378.

Smith, AR, Hawkeswood SE, and Joiner TE. The measure of a man: Associations between digit ratio and disordered eating in males. *International Journal of Eating Disorders* 43, no. 6 (2010): 543–548.

Stice, E, Telch CF, and Rizvi SL. Development and validation of the eating disorder diagnostic scale: A brief self-report measure of anorexia, bulimia, and binge-eating disorder. *Psychological Assessment* 12, no. 2 (2000): 123.

Stoltenberg, SF, Anderson C, Nag P, and Anagnopoulos C. Association between the serotonin transporter triallelic genotype and eating problems is moderated by the experience of childhood trauma in women. *International Journal of Eating Disorders* 45, no. 4 (2012): 492–500.

Strigo, IA, Matthews SC, Simmons AN, Oberndorfer T, Klabunde M, Reinhardt LE, and Kaye WH. Altered insula activation during pain anticipation in individuals recovered from anorexia nervosa: Evidence of interoceptive dysregulation. *International Journal of Eating Disorders* 46, no. 1 (2013): 23–33.

Strober, M. Pathologic fear conditioning and anorexia nervosa: On the search for novel paradigm. *International Journal of Eating Disorders* 35, no. 4 (2004): 504–508.

Sysko, R, and Walsh BT. Does the broad categories for the diagnosis of eating disorders (BCD-ED) scheme reduce the frequency of eating disorder not otherwise specified? *International Journal of Eating Disorders* 44, no. 7 (2011): 625–629.

Thompson, KJ, and Stice E. Thin-deal internalization: Mounting evidence for a new risk factor for body image disturbance and eating pathology. *Current Directions in Psychological Science* 10, no. 5 (2001): 181–183.

Turner, H, Bryant-Waugh R, and Peveler R. A new approach to clustering eating disorder patients: Assessing external validity and comparisons with DSM-IV diagnoses. *Eating Behaviors* 11, no. 2 (2010): 99–106.

Turrell, SL, Peterson-Badali M, and Katzman DK. Consent to treatment in adolescents with anorexia nervosa. *International Journal of Eating Disorders* 44, no. 8 (2011): 703–707.

Vandereycken, W. Denial of illness in anorexia nervosa-a conceptual review: Part 2 different forms and meanings. *European Eating Disorders Review* 14, no. 5 (2006): 352–368.

Verissimo, R, Mota-Cardoso R, and Taylor G. Relationships between alexithymia, emotional control, and quality of life in patients with inflammatory bowel disease. *Psychotherapy and Psychosomatics* 67, no. 2 (1998): 75–80.

Wagner, A, Simmons AN, Oberndorfer TA, Frank GK, McCurdy-McKinnon D, Fudge JL, Yang TT, Paulus MP, and Kaye WH. Altered sensitization patterns to sweet food stimuli in patients recovered from anorexia and bulimia nervosa. *Psychiatry Research: Neuroimaging* 234, no. 3 (2015): 305–313.

Waller, G. The myths of motivation: Time for a fresh look at some received wisdom in the eating disorder? *International Journal of Eating Disorders* 45, no. 1 (2012): 1–16.

Wierenga, CE, Bischoff-Grethe A, Melrose AJ, Irvine Z, Torres L, Bailer UF, Simmons A, Fudge JL, McClure SM, Ely A, and Kaye WH. Hunger does not motivate reward in women remitted from anorexia nervosa. *Biological Psychiatry* 77, no. 7 (2015): 642–652.

Wilfley, DE, Bishop ME, Wilson GT, and Agras WS. Classification of eating disorders: Toward DSM-V. *International Journal of Eating Disorders* 40, no. S3 (2007): S123–S129.

Wiseman, CV, Gray JJ, Mosimann JE, and Ahrens AH. Cultural expectations of thinness in women: An update. *International Journal of Eating Disorders* 11, no. 1 (1992): 85–89.

Witztum, E, Latzer Y, and Stein D. Anorexia nervosa and bulimia nervosa as idioms of distress: From the historical background to current formulations. *International Journal of Child and Adolescent Health* 1, no. 4 (2008): 283–294.

Wolfe, BE, Baker CW, Smith AT, and Kelly-Weeder S. Validity and utility of the current definition of binge eating. *International Journal of Eating Disorders* 42, no. 8 (2009): 674–686.

World Health Organization. International Classification of Diseases. 2016. Available at www.who.int/classifications/icd/en/.

Ziolko, HU. Bulimia: A historical outline. *International Journal of Eating Disorders* 20, no. 4 (1996): 345–358.

2 The Psychology of an Eating Disorder
Etiology and Risk Factors

Cathey Soutter, PhD, LPC

CONTENTS

LEARNING OBJECTIVES

After reading this chapter, the reader should be able to do the following:

- Identify and understand the role of general risk factors for eating pathology
- Determine the role of specific risk factors or vulnerabilities implicated in the onset and maintenance of eating disorders
- Understand the comorbidity of psychiatric disorders in onset and maintenance of eating pathology

INTRODUCTION

It was a brilliant spring morning and a little girl and her grandmother were walking down an ivy-covered walkway. Her dress was pink, her hair was shiny and curly; she was wearing white tights and black patent Mary Janes and everyone who saw her said: "Oh my gosh, how beautiful you look—twirl around and let me look at you." As enchanting as this may sound, this is often how it begins—a "let me see how you look" moment where we move from being the subject of our lives to seeing ourselves as objects—how we "look" to others. Recently, a commercial aired in which a mother was looking in a floor-length mirror holding a pair of jeans in front of her and imagining herself wearing them. . . . Would they fit. . .? Her teenage daughter walks in and says "Are those my jeans?" Mom looks startled and the scene cuts to her in the kitchen wearing her daughter's jeans and eating a bowl of cereal with the voice over saying that "anything is possible" if you eat brand X cereals. Other phrases come to mind—watching your weight, watching your figure. Even our fairy tales teach us that we are constantly being watched and evaluated—"Mirror, Mirror on the wall, who's the fairest of them all?"

Are we set up to believe from an early age that our success and happiness in life depends on how we "look" more than who we are? Examples like those above point out the early and ongoing influence of the culture in which we live, where we are systematically taught to question how we look to others and to feel that our worth depends on the answers we receive. Our cultures consist of many layers beginning with family environment, immediate and extended, and then broaden as schools and the wider community begin to play a larger role in the life of the individual.

These two experiences described involve girls and women, and indeed many more females than males are likely to be challenged by issues within themselves and their cultures that may lead to disordered eating behaviors and eating disorders. Girls in particular experience significant challenges in our changing world and are dealing with far more complex issues than in previous generations (Deak 2002). It has been suggested more strongly that repressive cultural forces are developmentally disabling to young females and interact with individual and familial environments, which may make engaging in eating-disordered behaviors an attractive and adaptive strategy (Steiner-Adair 1991). Similar challenges face men and boys but in far fewer numbers (Mitchison and Mond 2015; Muise et al. 2003). What are these repressive and cultural forces, that is, risk factors that subtly and not-so-subtly may serve as a threat to healthy development in adolescent males and females as they navigate this challenging period of their lives?

GENERAL RISK FACTORS

Risk factors are variables that increase the probability of an adverse outcome. The following will address the elements that may serve to influence the development of disordered eating and eating disorders. These include gender, puberty, self-esteem, body dissatisfaction, drive for thinness and/or muscularity, and dietary restraints.

GENDER

Gender is a social symbolic structure that is not necessarily innate or stable, rather it is acquired through interaction in a social world that changes as it evolves, a complex set of interrelated cultural ideas that stipulate the social meanings of many things including what constitutes masculinity and femininity. Moreover, gender is a relational concept because masculinity and femininity makes sense as we compare and contrast various aspects of it (Wood 2001). The cultures we live in have much to say in defining these concepts, structures, and practices that communicate norms and expectations, and construct or shape day-to-day interactions and personal experiences. Those who participate in these various cultures bring with them their own "expectations, resources, scripts, and vested interests . . . fostering and supporting ways of understanding the world about them replete with their own assumptions that are made about themselves and others with whom they interact" (Travis 2006). Often these assumptions foster an "us-versus-them" stance, which casts the other in a state of strangeness— different from us. It has been argued that gender is the major risk factor in the development of eating disorders and other types of mental health concerns for women and girls particularly, with gender described as "everywhere but nowhere . . . so embedded in everyday details as to be invisible" (Travis 2006). The social context of gender is viewed as fundamental to the analysis of threats to healthy development (Travis 2006).

In past years, when thinking of those suffering with eating disorders, the picture that came to mind for most people was a perfectionistic, affluent, young, white woman. Today, eating disorders are known to occur across age, gender, race and ethnicity, class, culture, and place, found in over 40 countries including developing nations (Gordon 2001; Samuels and Maine 2012) leading many clinicians and researchers to conclude that gender alone is the best predictor of risk for developing an eating disorder (Travis 2006). Gender has been identified as the major risk factor in the development of anorexia nervosa (AN)—with the female-to-male diagnosis ratio estimated as being 10:1 (Garfinkel et al. 1995; National Association of Anorexia Nervosa and Associated Disorders 2016). The American Psychological Association Guidelines for Psychological Practice with Girls and Women asserts that despite many complex changes in access to education, career opportunities, and in personal areas of reproductive health and relational life, girls and women are still at risk for higher rates of depression than boys and men, more subject to discrimination than men, at higher risk for anxiety disorders than men, and nine times more likely than boys and men to develop an eating disorder (American Psychological Association 2007; Stice et al. 2004). It is estimated that only 5%–15% of those diagnosed with anorexia, bulimia, or binge-eating disorder are male (National Association of Anorexia Nervosa and Associated Disorders 2016). In adolescent and young adult males, similar incidence of cases of anorexia and bulimia nervosa (BN) were found, and 40% of those diagnosed with binge-eating disorders were male (Muise et al. 2003). A recent review of the literature further confirms that AN and BN rates tend to be lower and more variable in males in contrast to females (Mitchison and Mond 2015).

Emergent Themes in Gender Issues

Gender socialization. There are, of course, the obvious physical differences between boys and girls but some psychosocial differences have emerged as interest and research grows in the study of gender (Shaffer 1996). A pattern of gender social-ization is reinforced by an overall devaluation of women in comparison to men, and women are often socialized into roles involving compliance, care giving, help-lessness, as well as a preoccupation with body image and appearance (American Psychological Association 2007). Differential devaluing of girls and women can contribute to higher risks for the development of depression (Jack 1993), anxiety, and eating disorders, as well as poorer outcomes for treatment and recovery (Johnson 2009; Travis 2006). Gender socialization may contribute to lower numbers of eat-ing disorder diagnoses for boys and men because eating disorders are considered by many to be a "woman's issue," not something that boys or men develop. As a result, males are less likely to report disordered eating concerns and many doctors are likely to underdiagnose eating disorders in males which then results in fewer males being referred for treatment. This delay in diagnoses in males may lead to more serious medical complications. This "female-centric nature of current classi-fication schemes and the consequent lack of appropriate assessment instruments" is a challenge to more effective diagnosis in males of eating disorders as well as body image disorders (Mitchison and Mond 2015).

Emotional sensitivity and internalization. In comparison with boys, girls are more likely to report a bias toward empathy and emotional expressiveness, particu-larly in late childhood and early adolescence (Gilligan 1982; Shaffer 1996), so much so that young women have been described as "empathy sick" (Pipher 1994), that is, invested in others to the neglect of their own needs, wishes, and desires, a shift from internal standards to emphasis on external ones (Surry 1991). In contrast to boys, prepubescent girls report internalized feelings of distress such as anxiety (Epkins 2002), and as they move through adolescence become less willing to articulate those feelings despite reporting higher levels of sadness and hopelessness.

Weight and appearance. From elementary school years onward, girls become more aware of their appearance and express more concern about how they appear to others. Girls as young as second and third grade are reporting being on diets, are dissatisfied with their bodies (Field et al. 1999; La Greca et al. 2006), and are more likely to engage in behavior that is risky for their health (Stice and Shaw 2003). Adolescent boys at later ages may be equally dissatisfied with their bodies but more often than not, the dissatisfaction is not about numbers on a scale indicating weight but about the desire to obtain an ideal masculine physique, that is, wider shoulders, slimmer waist, and thighs with more muscularity (Núñez-Navarro et al. 2012).

PUBERTY

Puberty is a time of rapid physical changes as the body reaches maturation (Piran and Ross 2006) occurring with gradual onset from approximately age 9 through 13. Awaiting adolescence is a series of developmental tasks or crises involving one's rela-tionship with oneself and body, and relationships to others and to the cultures in which they are living. An older medical meaning of the word "crisis" suggests a turning point for better or worse—similar to the Chinese symbol for crisis that incorporates opportunity with danger (Erickson 1968). There is a long-standing body of literature that identifies puberty as a time of just such a crisis (or task) for adolescent girls in particular. By the late 1800s, early mental health professionals such as Josef Breur, a colleague of Freud's, described girls who would later be diagnosed with hysteria stating that "for the most part, these girls were lively, gifted, and full of intellectual interests before they fell ill" (Showalter 1985). A number of similar comments from clinicians of the same era indicated that girls are more likely than boys to experience a narrowing or psychic constraint during puberty, that is, a disavowal of self or repression (Deutsch 1944; Freud 1905/1962; Horney 1926; Petersen 1998; Thompson 1964). Throughout time, girls were more likely to suffer from depression in contrast to boys, be diagnosed with eating disorders and poor body image, reported higher levels of suicidal ideation, and experienced a significant decrease in sense of self-worth. It was found that boys and girls enter elementary schools with similar self-esteem scores but by graduation from high school, girls' self-esteem scores are significantly lower than boys (American Association of University Women 1994).

Freud has described girls undergoing a fresh wave of repression beginning in adolescence (Stern 1991). Others researchers at that time concurred by noting the disturbing increase in passivity in adolescent girls in contrast to boys, as well as the increased tendency of girls, previously seen as strong preadolescents, to renounce their own judgment (Deutsch 1944; Horney 1926; Thompson 1964). A corresponding sudden drop in resiliency has been noted in girls just as they enter puberty (Block 1990). Prepubescent girls were found more likely to be optimistic than boys but this changes by the time they reach their adult years, with women being two times more likely be depressed than men (Seligman 1991). It has been surmised that whatever is going on, it does not begin in childhood: "Something must happen at or shortly after puberty that causes a flip-flop—and this hits girls very hard indeed" (Seligman 1991). Researchers found striking similarities in conversations with fourth- through eighth-grade girls, describing the crisis as a disavowal of self, going underground, or into hiding. This has been termed a relational crisis, a time when girls seem to be in danger of drowning or disappearing, a time of individuation to be sure but one in which the importance of strong, supportive relationships does not change (Brown and Gilligan 1992; Gilligan et al. 1990). The question for these girls becomes—can a sense of self develop without relinquishing connections or can they maintain connections while establishing a sense of a separate self?

What is going on with girls during this crucial developmental period and, more importantly, what does it have to do with eating disorders? Some researchers postulate that the crisis girls are experiencing is due to a failure to separate and individuate. It is speculated that as girls enter into this period of growth and challenge, their experience of the inner self may be at variance or discordant with the cultural scripts they see for girls and women in families, school, and the wider community (Rieger et al. 2010). Girls are observed to be leaving a childhood rich with relational images and entering a more repressive state of development (Brown 1989; Brown and Gilligan 1992; Debold and Brown 1991; Gilligan et al. 1990; Rogers and Gilligan 1988; Rogers 1994). As she ages, a young woman's self-perception may conflict with what she sees as she looks into the cultural mirrors available to her. Are the images reflected back to young women accurate or do they function as fun-house mirrors? In puberty as girls look for ways to be themselves and to be successful in the culture in which they live, move, and have their being, "they are pressed to take on images of perfection as the model of the pure or perfectly good woman: the woman whom everyone will promote and value and want to be with" (Brown and Gilligan 1992; Gilligan et al. 1990; Jack 1993). This pressure can cause some girls to begin an internal desertion, that is, a disavowal of self, in order to take on the images of the culture of the successful woman (Steiner-Adair 1991; Stern 1991).

Some women choose a way to fit the outer mold or script and/or to numb, silence, or quiet the authentic self through strategies such as adjusting the self to an internalization of the thin idea through the mechanisms of eating-disordered behavior or eating pathology.

Initially what begins as an attempted solution to a problem quickly takes on a life of its own, often reinforced by praise, even adulation of a sort—"Oh you look great, have you lost weight?" The problem with this strategy of striving for outward perfection means girls and women are not able to relate authentically to others in ways that lead to growth. Instead, they keep important parts of themselves out of connection while the eating disorder becomes the only way of communicating with themselves and with others. This has been described as a silencing of the self, a time during which young women may begin to speak with their bodies (Jack 1993). Girls and women who suffer with eating disorders talk about the sense of control and peace that comes through the numbing of the self in order to fit in rather than to communicate directly, reinforcing what our culture suggests—you are only as good as you look. One young woman is quoted as saying

> It's pretty hard being a girl nowadays. You can't be too smart, too dumb, too pretty, too ugly, too friendly, too coy, too aggressive, too defenseless, too individual, or too programmed. If you're too much of anything, then others envy you or despise you because you intimidate them or make them jealous. It's like you have to be everything and nothing all at once, without knowing which you need more of....

Nora, twelfth grade (Deak 2002)

This is a tall order for anyone at any time. As girls' lives continue to expand with more opportunities for freedom of choice about their lives, they are freer than ever to dream big dreams that are actually within reach for them. However, clearly there is a darker side to growing up female. As stated previously, there are many girls who do not develop depression, anxiety, and eating disorders; however, they do understand the reality of these issues in their daily lives and in the lives of girls they know (Deak 2002). Adolescence has been described as a time when the brightest and the best of girls react with strategies of withdrawing, conforming, and becoming angry and/or depressed (Pipher 1994).

Interpersonal psychotherapy for eating disorders postulates that disturbances of the self, consistent with those described above, are "linked to the individual's experiences and perceptions of his/her social world . . . and that functions pertaining to the self (i.e. self-esteem maintenance and associated positive affect) come to be performed by the eating disorder . . . which acts as a de facto social agent" (Rieger et al. 2010). It is further proposed that eventually the eating disorder becomes a more dependable source of both self-esteem and affect regulation (Rieger et al. 2010).

For boys and adolescent males, similar cultural pressures to have the ideal body type can lead to unhealthy diet and exercise habits. Given that boys are particularly concerned about appearing muscular, this can lead to the use of over-the-counter supplements and/or steroids. Parents and physicians may ignore the use of such strategies by young men, seeing them as harmless rather than a possible source of dangerous side effects. Moreover, the lack of concern can lead to inattentiveness of medical and mental health professionals in recognizing behaviors in males as possible precursors to disordered eating and eating disorders (Wagner 2012).

Self-Esteem, Body Dissatisfaction, and Drive for Thinness

Many clinicians and researchers identify self-esteem, body dissatisfaction, and drive for thinness as three significant factors implicated in the development of eating-disordered behaviors and/or eating disorders in both females and males (Polivy and Herman 2002; Rieger et al. 2010). It might be useful to first define these concepts and provide information as to how they relate to the psychology of an eating disorder.

Self-esteem is particularly difficult to untangle since most individuals have a specific idea of what this means. Carl Rogers (1965) defined self-esteem as the extent to which an individual likes, values, and accepts himself or herself and involves cognitive and affective components (i.e., self-knowledge and self/other evaluation) (Rogers 1965). This differs from self-confidence and/or self-efficacy both of which are related to beliefs in one's abilities to obtain desired outcomes (Bandura 1997). Others define self-esteem as an experience of competence that is related to social feedback, particularly from significant others in one's life (Harter 1993a, 1993b). Proponents of interpersonal psychotherapy for eating disorders (IPT-ED) see self-esteem as "essentially an internal psychological gauge that monitors how well one is faring in interpersonal situations" (Rieger et al. 2010).

Body dissatisfaction (sometimes called body esteem) relates to body image—how boys, men, girls, and women feel about their body shape and weight. As detailed earlier in this chapter, the pressure to meet the cultural ideal for both males and females begins early; even very young children understand the stigma of being labeled "fat" (Smolak 2006). However, girls and women are more likely to describe their image as "inferior to that of the cultural ideal" (Smolak 2006). It is startling to note that preadolescent girls as early as 5 years of age report dissatisfaction with their bodies and weight (Bruch 1973; Davison et al. 2000; Smolak 2006). Girls' body esteem decreases steadily in the middle school; over 60% report dissatisfaction with shape and weight (Field et al. 1999). Moreover, approximately 50% of adult women report body dissatisfaction (Muise et al. 2003). More recent studies would add that males who endorse body dissatisfaction may have an early diagnosis of obesity or be more concerned about gaining a more muscular body (Muise et al. 2003).

Drive for thinness involves the internalization of "the thin ideal." Boosted by images of ever-thinner models in the media and denigration of being labeled over-weight or obese, individuals can become obsessed with being slim. One only has to watch a few minutes of a popular television show such as *The Biggest Loser* to have a clear picture of the power of the thin ideal for men and women in contrast to those who are labeled as fat or obese.

Though drive for thinness can affect both men and women, men are less likely to focus on thinness or low weight and more likely to focus on the ideal masculine body shape, that is, broader shoulders, trimmer waist, and thighs (Mitchison and Mond 2015; Muise et al. 2003). Some studies postulate that boys are generally less concerned about their weight in adolescence and suggest that body mass is viewed differently for boys than girls (Gila et al. 2005; Ohzeki et al. 1993).

However, for women the pervasive cultural message is clear:

1. Women must be attractive in order to be successful in work and in relationships.
2. Women must be thin to be attractive.
3. Any woman can become thin and hence attractive if she works hard enough.

Perhaps not surprisingly, internalization of the thin ideal has been found to be a risk factor for both poor body image and eating disturbances; fortunately, women who reject these messages are less likely to become dissatisfied with their weight (Thompson and Stice 2001).

Interactions of Self-Esteem, Body Dissatisfaction, and Drive for Thinness

As detailed above, self-esteem is a delicate balance between the relationship with oneself and relational life with others. Liking, accepting, and valuing oneself is part and parcel of self-esteem (Erickson 1968) and has both cognitive and affective elements—that of self-knowledge and evaluative aspects. These aspects operate in both relational arenas. As girls and boys moves from early childhood to puberty, they transition from experiencing themselves as the subject of one's life to perceiving oneself as an object during a period of intensive physical and social changes. These changes occur within the relationship with oneself and in the interpersonal realm in an increasingly complex social context. If one has a fairly stable and resilient sense of self, she or he can explore, assimilate, and experience mastery within one's surroundings (Deci and Ryan 1995). However, the push/pull of knowing oneself as the subject of one's life in contrast to seeing oneself as an object in Western culture is strong. A resultant sense of dissatisfaction with the body is considered normative in Westernized culture for women and girls. For many, the idealized images in media convey the messages to young women that they will not do as they are; every part of the body requires some type of modification—the right hair style, makeup to hide and enhance, and the need to be thinner (Kilbourne 1999). For men and boys, the message is often to be muscular and fit with an idealized masculine body.

For some, competition and comparison to "perfect" images can trigger a drive toward thinness or muscularity creating a deprivation or dieting mentality. It may be through this mechanism of being a "good or bad" dieter that self-esteem becomes related to how successful one is in restriction of calories, controlling food intake, weight loss/gain, and needs (Surry 1991).

Most theories of the development of the self—male and female—occur in a relational context, that is, in the context of and through healthy connections beginning from earliest childhood experiences (Banks 2010). These early relational images within each individual become the template or concept we use to order our relational experience—"to determine our expectations about what will occur in relationship then guide our actions. They are the inner pictures we devise of what's happened to us, they become the framework by which we determine who we are, what we do and how we can do and how worthwhile we are" (Miller and Stiver 1997).

SPECIFIC RISK FACTORS

As we move to addressing more specific and individual risk factors, it must be stated that clinicians and researchers have many different ideas about what constitutes general versus specific factors that lead to increased vulnerability for developing an eating disorder. For example, some consider dietary restriction and body dissatisfaction as prodromal, symptoms that can indicate the future onset of a disorder that are also features of the disorder (Stice et al. 2010), and would include them in a more general factor list, while others view these factors as more individual in nature. However, since risk factors such as body dissatisfaction, internalization of the thin or body ideal, and dieting are reported to affect 30%–70% of adolescent girls, whereas eating disorders are reported in only 10%, it has been suggested that these figures represent vulnerability factors rather than prodromes (Stice et al. 2010). For adolescent males, enhanced muscularity and the pressure to be physically strong may function similarly as vulnerability factors (Dominé et al. 2009).

DIETARY RESTRICTION

A number of studies report on the triggering effects of dieting and calorie restriction, suggesting that those who report higher dietary restriction are subsequently at greater risk for onset of threshold AN or BN (Patton et al. 1990, 1999; Stice et al. 2010). However, dieting is widespread in Western culture, yet not everyone who engages in this behavior develops disordered eating, suggesting it is likely far more complex than a simple correlation. In fact, studies looking at the correlation between dietary restriction and eating pathology are divided in their findings (Evans et al. 2005). One theory is that body dissatisfaction may influence dietary restriction in pursuit of the desired thin ideal (Stice 1994).

PERSONALITY CHARACTERISTICS

The immediate personality characteristics in those exhibiting eating pathology are perfectionism in those diagnosed with AN, low negative affect, compliance, obsessive thoughts, impulsivity in those with BN, and to some degree dissociation, particularly in those with a trauma history (Evans et al. 2005; Polivy and Herman 2002). In fact, impulsive behavior (such as suicidal attempts, sexual acting out, drug abuse, and shoplifting) is one correlation that has been found to differentiate BN from AN (Polivy and Herman 2002). Harm avoidance and fear of change may play significant roles as well (Johnson 2009). Many of these personality characteristics and traits are viewed from a recovery model that looks at those characteristics that are present after recovery and assumes that these were present before the onset of eating pathology, suggesting they may create a vulnerability to development of eating disorders.

FAMILY ENVIRONMENT

Family environment may also play a role in the development of eating disorders. It is hypothesized that families may maintain eating pathology by praising slenderness and making self-control/discipline a positive trait (Polivy and Herman 2002). Furthermore, problematic attachment may be implicated as well; those engaging in eating pathology often describe insecure attachment. Other eating-disordered patients describe a family environment that is often critical and controlling with parental caring and expectations low; as detailed below, those who report physical and/or sexual abuse are also at higher risk for developing an eating disorder (Ackard et al. 2008; Polivy and Herman 2002). Poor family connections are reported in males with disordered eating and weight control issues (Ackard et al. 2008). Negative evaluation of daughters by parents—more often mothers than fathers—may encourage weight loss (Hill and Franklin 1998) and mothers who have eating disorders tend to feed their children irregularly and focus negatively on their children's weight and body shape (Polivy and Herman 2002).

CHILDHOOD SEXUAL AND/OR PHYSICAL ABUSE HISTORY

It appears that there is a connection between childhood sexual and/or physical abuse and eating disorders. Posttraumatic stress disorder (PTSD) and mood disorder are implicated as well with evidence that childhood sexual abuse is more prevalent in women with anorexia, bulimia, and binge eating disorder when compared to the general population of women (Herzog et al. 1993; Micali et al. 2017; Mitchell 2015). Researchers argued that childhood abuse of any sort induces "intolerable emotions and undermines self-identity . . . through refocusing one's attention onto weight, shape and eating thus gaining a domain that offers some emotional control" (Polivy and Herman 2002). Researchers report an association between disordered eating in males with depression, body dissatisfaction, lower self-esteem, and alcoholism (Keel et al. 1998; Soundy et al. 1995), as well as past physical abuse in their families (Kinzl et al. 1997). Other studies suggest that males who report serious childhood physical abuse are at greater risk to develop eating disorders than those who endorse stronger family connections and no physical abuse (Ackard et al. 2008; Kinzl et al. 1997).

SEXUAL ORIENTATION

Several studies looking specifically at sexual orientation and eating disorders postulate that individuals who identify as gay, lesbian, or bisexual may be at higher risk for eating disorders than individuals who identify as heterosexual (Ackard et al. 2008; Carlat et al. 1997; Keel et al. 1998; Muise et al. 2003; Soundy et al. 1995).

SPORT ACTIVITIES AND PROFESSIONAL PURSUITS INVOLVING WEIGHT AND BODY IMAGE FOCUS

There are any number of professional and sports activities that focus on weight and body shape—in sports such as swimming, track, wrestling, and gymnastics, as well as professions such as acting or performance art.

Ballet in particular has been the focus of much research attention due to the extreme emphasis on appearance and athleticism (Garner and Garfinkel 1980; Vaisman et al. 1996). In fact, the prevalence rates for diagnosable eating disorders among ballet dancers are 4–25 times higher than in the general population (Garner and Garfinkel 1980; Vaisman et al. 1996), and it has been found that disturbed eating attitudes persist after ballet dancers retire from active professional life (Khan et al. 1996).

Elite athletes as well as those pursuing a career path in the entertainment field are striving for the "sure thing or the perfect look" in order to attain success. Obtaining the perfect look or body size and shape often begins in sports that are seen as "lean sports" particularly in women (NCAA 2014) and in those involved in performance activities such as acting, dance, modeling, and other entertainment industry pursuits. It can involve internalizing the thin ideal and becoming dissatisfied with one's body at the same time and can render an athlete or performance artist vulnerable to engaging in restricting calories or engaging in disordered eating, which can lead to developing an eating disorder.

Given that the most prevalent ages for onset of eating disorders corresponds with peak times of training in either sports or performance art, it is not surprising that we are beginning to see a growing emphasis on early detection and prevention in these adolescents and young adults. The New York State Commissioner of Labor in 2009 requested that the Child Performer Advisory Board to Prevent Eating Disorders recommend guidelines for employers of child performers and models for preventing, early diagnosing, and treatment of eating disorders (The Child Performer Advisory Board 2009). The advisory board suggested that in addition to oversight by parents, child performers (those under 18) seeking to gain a permit to work in New York State must be evaluated "by a pediatrician, adolescent medicine specialist, family practice physician, or internist which would include an eating disorder screening" among other stipulations (The Child Performer Advisory Board 2009).

Vulnerability is not limited to professional or elite (Ravaldi et al. 2003) athletes. One study compared eating disorders and body image disturbances among ballet dancers, gymnasium users, and body builders and found that nonprofessionals performers of sport that have an emphasis on thinness, strength, and body building show a "high degree of body uneasiness and inappropriate eating attitudes and behaviors" (Ravaldi et al. 2003).

MEDIA

What if any role does mass media play in the psychology of eating disorders? Most would agree that the mass media does play a significant role in the relentless pursuit of the beauty ideal, but does that imply causality as some would assert? Is the industry of image-making part of the social and cultural forces that aid in the development of eating pathology? These questions have been raised in the search for a model of the relationship between media and anorexia (Williams et al. 2003).

Media images play an important role in gender role learning and identity formation, as well as in presenting a standard of values and beliefs about the ideal body type in women (Harrison and Cantor 1997; Levine and Murnen 2009; Stice 1994) and in men (Ackard et al. 2008). In a meta-analysis of the literature on the effect of media images displaying the thin ideal or body image, it was concluded that they activate rather than cultivate a "thinness schema in females who are highly motivated and cognitively prepared to think about themselves in relation to weight, shape, and beauty" (Groesz et al. 2002). Other studies assert that it is specifically individuals who are already highly concerned about their body image who are more likely to be affected by media images (Ackard et al. 2008; Levine and Smolek 1996; Stice et al. 2001).

The relationship between "media and anorexia has been suggested to be circular in nature; that as young women grow more dependent on the control of eating as a solution to life's challenges, they turn more frequently to the media in an effort to find solutions or to strengthen their resolve to control their eating" (Williams et al. 2003). It is further proposed that many young people lack other role models to provide healthier coping strategies and instead use mass media for comfort and instruction (Polivy and Herman 2002). Although our culture may value thinness, additional factors contribute to the degree that a particular individual would take this valuation to a pathological extreme (Polivy and Herman 2002). In a review of the literature, Levine and Murnen (2009) conclude that "engagement with mass media is probably best considered a variable risk factor that might well be later shown to be a causal risk factor."

COMORBIDITY

A number of psychiatric disorders commonly are seen in individuals with eating disorders. Mood disorders, anxiety disorders (specifically social phobia [now known as social anxiety disorder] and obsessive compulsive disorder), substance abuse, personality disorders (Johnson et al. 2002), and traumatic stress disorder are the ones most commonly identified. In early adolescence and young adulthood, depressive disorders are associated with an increased onset of eating disorders (Johnson et al. 2002). Depressive symptoms combined with low self-esteem co-occur with eating and weight problems as well as dietary restriction, purging behavior, and fluctuations in body weight (Fairburn 1997). Depression during these vulnerable times may play a contributory role to the development of eating pathology.

CONCLUSION

Eating disorders are serious psychiatric disorders that are currently described as complex biopsychosocial disorders indicating a group of illnesses, adjustments, or adaptations that have biological and genetic components as well as psychological and sociocultural aspects (Ice 2006). This chapter has focused on general risk factors in addition to looking at some of the more specific vulnerabilities that may create an environment in which eating pathology can thrive. As the literature suggests, the research has yielded some new and important findings that suggest the growing importance of biological and genetic factors. Despite these gains as well as the introduction of new and innovative treatment methods, eating disorders continue to be a disease with the highest mortality rate of any psychiatric disorder. Moreover, the prevalence rate continues to rise in all groups—younger and older, men and women—indicating that there is still much that is unknown and much left to do in order to develop more prevention and modes of treatment.

REFERENCES

Ackard, DM, Fedio G, Neumark-Sztainer D, and Britt HR. Factors associated with disordered eating among sexually active adolescent males: Gender and number of sexual partners. *Psychosomatic Medicine* 70, no. 2 (2008): 232–238.

American Association of University Women. *Shortchanging Girls, Shortchanging America: Executive Summary*. Washington, DC: American Association of University Women, 1994.

American Psychological Association. Guidelines for psychological practice with girls and women and women. *American Psychologist* 62, no. 9 (2007): 949–979.

Bandura, A. *Determinants of Self-Esteem in African-American and White Adolescent Girls*, Compiled by O Malanchuk and JS Eccles. Albuquerque, NM, 1997.

Banks, AM. *Developing the Capacity to Connect. Works in Progress, No 107*. Wellesley, MA: Center for Research on Women Working Paper Series, 2010.

Block, J. Ego resilience through time: Antecedents and ramifications. In *Resilience and Psychological Health*. Boston, MA: Symposium of the Boston Psychoanalytic Society, 1990.

Brown, L. *Narratives of Relationship: The Development of a Care Orientation in Girls 7 to 16*. Cambridge, MA: Harvard University, 1989.

Brown, LM, and Gilligan C. *Meeting at the Crossroads: Women's Psychology and Girls' Development*. New York, NY: Ballantine Books, 1992.

Bruch, H. *Eating Disorders*. New York, NY: Basic Books, 1973.

Carlat, DJ, Camargo CA, and Herzog DB. Eating disorders in males: A report on 135 patients. *American Journal of Psychiatry* 154, no. 8 (1997): 1127–1132.

Davison, KK, Markey CN, and Birch LL. A longitudinal examination of patterns in girls' weight concerns: Body dissatisfaction from ages 5–9 years. *International Journal of Eating Disorders* 33, no. 3 (2000): 320–332.

Deak, JM. *Girls Will Be Girls: Raising Confident and Courageous Daughters*. New York, NY: Hyperion, 2002.

Debold, E, and Brown LM. Losing the body of knowledge: Conflicts between passion and reason in the intellectual development of adolescent girls. In paper presented at the Annual Meeting of the Association for Women in Psychology, March 1991, Hartford, CT.

Deci, EL, and Ryan, RM. Human agency: The basis for true self-esteem. In *Efficacy, Agency, and Self-Esteem*, edited by HM Kernis, 31–50. New York, NY: Plenum Press, 1995.

Deutsch, H. *The Psychology of Women, Volume One: A Psychoanalytic Interpretation*. New York, NY: Grune & Stratton, 1944.

Dominé, F, Berchtold A, Akré C, Michaud PA, and Suris JC. Disordered eating behaviors: What about boys? *Journal of Adolescent Health* 44, no. 2 (2009): 111–117.

Epkins, CC. A comparison of two self-report measures of children's social anxiety in clinical and community samples. *Journal of Clinical Child and Adolescent Psychology* 31, no. 1 (2002): 69–79.

Erickson, E. *Identity, Youth and Crisis*. New York, NY: W.W. Norton and Company, 1968.

Evans, DL, Foa EB, Gur RE, Hendin H, O'Brien CP, Seligman MEP, and Walsh BT. Eating disorders: Commission on adolescent eating disorders. In *Treating and Preventing Adolescent Mental Health Disorders: What We Know and What We Don't Know. A Research Agenda for Improving the Mental Health of Our Youth*, edited by CM Bulik, CG Fairburn, NH Golden, KA Halmi, DB Herzog, AS Kaplan, RE Kreipe, JE Mitchell, KM Pike, E Stice, RH Striegel-Moore, C. Barr Taylor, TA Wadden, GT Wilson, and BT Walsh. New York, NY: Oxford University Press, 2005.

Fairburn, CG. Interpersonal psychotherapy for bulimia nervosa. In *Handbook of Treatment for Eating Disorders*, edited by DM Garner and PE Garfinkel, pp. 278–294. New York, NY: Guilford Press, 1997.

Field, AE, Camargo CA, Taylor CB, Berkey CS, Frazier AL, Gillman MW, and Colditz GA. Overweight, weight-conscious and bulimic behavior among girls and boys. *Journal of the American Academy of Child and Adolescent Psychiatry* 38, no. 6 (1999): 754–760.

Freud, S. The transformation of puberty. In *Three Essays on the Theory of Sexuality*, edited by S Freud. New York, NY: Basic Books, 1905/1962.

Garfinkel, PE, Lin E, Goering P, Spegg C, Goldbloom DS, Kennedy S, Kaplan AS, and Woodside DB. Bulimia nervosa in a canadian community sample: Prevalence and comparison of sub-groups. *American Journal of Psychiatry* 152, no. 7 (1995): 1052–1058.

Garner, DM, and Garfinkel PE. Socio-cultural factors in the development of anorexia nervosa. *Psychological Medicine* 10, no. 4 (1980): 647–656.

Gila, A, Castro J, Cesena J, and Toro J. Anorexia nervosa in male adolescents: Body image, eating attitudes, psychological traits. *Journal of Adolescent Health* 36, no. 3 (2005): 221–226.

Gilligan, C. *In a Different Voice, Psychological Theory and Women's Development*. Cambridge, MA: Harvard University Press, 1982.

Gilligan, C, Brown LM, and Rogers A. Psyche embedded: A place for body, relationships, and culture in personality theory. In *Studying Persons and Lives*, edited by R Zucker, R Emmons, and S Frank AI Rabin. New York, NY: Springer, 1990.

Gilligan, CA, Lyons NP, and Hanmer TJ. *Making Connections: The Relational World of Adolescent Girls at Emma Williard School*. Cambridge, MA: Harvard University Press, 1990.

Gordon, RA. Eating disorders east and west: A culture bound syndrome unbound. In *Eating Disorders and Cultures in Transition*, edited by MA Katzman, RA Gordon, and M Nasser, pp. 1–23. New York, NY: Brunner-Routledge, 2001.

Groesz, LM, Levine MP, and Murnen SK. The effects of experimental presentation of thin media images on body satisfaction: A meta-analytic review. *International Journal of Eating Disorder* 31, no. 1 (2002): 1–16.

Harrison, K, and Cantor J. The relationship between media consumption and eating disorders. *Journal of Communications* 47, no. 1 (1997): 40–67.

Harter, S. Causes and consequences of low self-esteem in children and adolescents. In *Self-Esteem: The Puzzle of Low Self-Regard*, edited by RF Baumeister, pp. 87–116. New York, NY: Plenum Press, 1993a.

Harter, S. Causes, correlates, and the functional role of global self-worth: A life span perspective. In *Competence Considered*, edited by J Killigan, and RJ Sternberg, pp. 67–97. New Haven, CT: Yale University Press, 1993b.

Herzog, B, Staley JE, Carmody S, Robbins WN, and van der Kolk BA. Childhood sexual abuse in anorexia nervosa and bulimia nervosa. *Journal of the American Academy of Child and Adolescent Psychiatry* 32, no. 5 (1993): 962–966.

Hill, AJ, and Franklin JA. Mothers, daughters, and dieting: Investigating the transmission of weight control. *British Journal of Clinical Psychology* 37 (1998): 3–13.

Horney, K. The flight from womanhood. *International Journal of Psychoanalysis* 7 (1926): 324–339.

Ice, S. A medical director's perspective on eating disorders: Enduring wisdom, new frontiers. *Perspective, A Professional Journal of the Renfrew Center Foundation* Winter (2006): 13–15.

Jack, DC. *Silencing the Self: Women and Depression*. New York, NY: Harper Perennial Press, 1993.

Johnson, C. Something new…something old: Six of the most useful concepts for patients, families, and clinicians. In Annual Professional Symposium for the Prevention and Treatment of Eating Disorders, 2009.

Johnson, JG, Cohen P, Kotler L, Kasen S, and Brook JS. Psychiatric disorders associated with risk for development of eating disorders during adolescence and early adulthood. *Journal of Consulting and Clinical Psychology* 70, no. 5 (2002): 1119–1128.

Keel, PK, Klump KL, Leon GR, and Fulkerson JA. Disordered eating in adolescent males from a school-based sample. *International Journal of Eating Disorders* 23, no. 2 (1998): 125–132.

Khan, KM, Green RM, Saul A, Bennell KL, Crichton KJ, Hopper JL, and Wark JD. Retired elite female ballet dancers and nonathletic controls have similar bone mineral density at weight bearing sites. *Journal of Bone and Mineral Research* 11, no. 10 (1996): 1566–1574.

Kilbourne, J. *Deadly Persuasion: Why Women and Girls Must Fight the Addictive Power of Advertising*. New York, NY: Free Press, 1999.

Kinzl, JF, Mangweth B, Traweger CM, and Biebl W. Eating disordered behavior in males: The impact of adverse childhood experiences. *International Journal of Eating Disorders* 22, no. 2 (1997): 131–138.

La Greca, AM, Mackey ER, and Miller KB. The interplay of physical and psychosocial development. In *Handbook of Girls' and Women's Psychological Health: Gender and Well-Being across the Lifespan*, edited by J Worrell, and CD Goodheart, pp. 251–262. New York, NY: Oxford University Press, 2006.

Levine, MP, and Murnen SK. Everybody knows that mass media are/are not [pick one] a cause of eating disorders: A critical review of evidence for a causal link between media, negative body image, and disordered eating in females. *Journal of Social and Clinical Psychology* 28, no. 1 (2009): 9–42.

Levine, MP, and Smolek L. Media as a context for the development of disordered eating. In *The Developmental Psychopathology of Eating Disorders: Implications for Research, Prevention, and Treatment*, edited by MP Levine, R Striegel-Moore, and L Smolek, pp. 235–257. Mahwah, NJ: Laurence Ehrlbaum and Associates, 1996.

Micali, N, Martini MG, Thomas JJ, Eddy KT, Kothari R, Russell E, Bulik CM, and Treasure J. Lifetime and 12-month prevalence of eating disorders amongst women in midlife: A population-based study of diagnoses and risk factors. *BMC Medicine* 15, no. 12 (2017): 1–10.

Miller, JB and Stiver, I. *The Healing Connection: How Women Form Relationships in Therapy and in Life*. Boston, MA: Beacon Press, 1997.

Mitchell, K. Comorbid eating disorders and posttraumatic stress disorder: Implications for etiology and treatment. *Eating Disorders Review*, 26, no. 4 (2015): 3.

Mitchison, D, and Mond J. Epidemiology of eating disorders, eating disordered behavior, and body image disturbance in males: A narrative review. *Journal of Eating Disorders* 3, (2015): 20.

Muise, AM, Stein DG, and Arbess G. Eating disorders in adolescent boys: A review of the adolescent and young adult literature. *Journal of Adolescent Health* 33, no. 6 (2003): 427–435.

National Association of Anorexia Nervosa and Associated Disorders. 2016. Available at http://www.eatingdisorderhope.com/information/statistics-studies (accessed November 30, 2012).

NCAA. *Mind, Body and Sport Understanding and Supporting Student-Athlete Mental Wellness*, edited by GT Brown. Indianapolis, IN: National Collegiate Athletic Association, 2014.

Núñez-Navarro, A, Agüera Z, Krug I, Jiménez-Murcia S, Sánchez I, Araguz N, Gorwood P, Granero R, Penelo E, Karwautz A, Moragas L, Saldaña S, Treasure J, Menchón JM, and Fernández-Aranda F. Do men with eating disorders differ from women in clinics, psychopathology and personality? *European Eating Disorders Review* 20, no. 1 (2012): 23–31.

Ohzeki, T, Otahara H, Hanaki K, Motozumi H, and Shiraki K. Eating attitudes test in boys and girls 6–18 years: Decrease in concerns with eating in boys and the increase in girls with their ages. *Psychopathology* 26, no. 3–4 (1993): 117–121.

Patton, GC, Johnson-Sabine E, Wood K, Mann AH, and Wakeling A. Abnormal eating attitudes in London schoolgirls—A prospective epidemiological study: Outcome at twelve month follow-up. *Psychological Medicine* 20, no. 2 (1990): 383–394.

Patton, GC, Selzer R, Coffey C, Carlin JB, and Wolfe R. Onset of adolescent eating disorders: Population based cohort study over 3 years. *British Medical Journal* 318, no. 7186 (1999): 765–768.

Petersen, A. Adolescent development. *Annual Review of Psychology* 39 (1998): 583–607.

Pipher, M. *Reviving Ophelia: Saving the Selves of Adolescent Girls.* New York, NY: Berkeley Publishing Group, 1994.

Piran, N, and Ross E. From girlhood to womanhood: Multiple transitions in context. In *Handbook of Girls' and Women's Psychological Health*, edited by CD Goodheart and J Worrell, pp. 301–310. New York, NY: Oxford University Press, 2006.

Polivy, J, and Herman CP. Causes of eating disorders. *Annual Review of Psychology* 53, no. 1 (2002): 187–213.

Ravaldi, C, Vannacci A, Zucchi T, Mannucci E, Cabras PL, Boldrini M, Murciano L, Rotella CM, and Ricca V. Eating disorders and body image disturbances among ballet dancers, gymnasium users and body builders. *Psychopathology* 36, no. 5 (2003): 247–254.

Rieger, E, Van Buren DJ, Bishop M, Tanofsky-Kraff M, Welch R, and Wilfley DE. An eating disorder-specific model of interpersonal psychotherapy (IPT-ED): Causal pathways and treatment implications. *Clinical Psychology Review* 30, no. 4 (2010): 400–410.

Rogers, A. *Exiled Voices: Dissociation and the "Return of the Repressed" in Women's Narratives, Paper No. 67.* Work in Progress, 1994.

Rogers, A, and Gilligan C. *Translating the Language of Adolescent Girls: Themes of Moral Voice and Stages of Ego Development. Monograph No. 6.* Cambridge, MA: Harvard Graduate School of Education, Center for the Study of Gender, Education, and Human Development, 1988.

Rogers, C. *Client Centered Therapy.* Boston, MA: Houghton Mifflin, 1965.

Samuels, KL, and Maine MD. *Treating Eating Disorders at Midlife and Beyond: Help, Hope, and Relational-Cultural Theory, Works in Progress: 110.* Wellesley, MA: Jean Baker Miller Training Institute at the Wellesley Centers for Women, 2012.

Seligman, MEP. *Learned Optimism.* New York, NY: Random House, 1991.

Shaffer, DR. *Developmental Psychology: Childhood and Adolescence* (4th ed.), Pacific Grove, CA: Brooks/Cole, 1996.

Showalter, E. *The Female Malady.* New York, NY: Penguin, 1985.

Smolak, L. Body image. In *Handbook of Girls and Women's Psychological Health: Gender and Well-Being across the Life Span*, edited by J Worell and CD Goodheart. New York, NY: Oxford University Press, 2006.

Soundy, TJ, Lucas AR, Suman VJ, and Melton LJ. *Psychological Medicine* 25, no. 5 (1995): 1065–1072.

Steiner-Adair, C. When the body speaks: Girls, eating disorders and psychotherapy. In *Women, Girls, and Psychotherapy: Reframing Resistance*, edited by AG Rogers, DL Tolman, and CA Gilligan. New York, NY: Harrington Park Press, 1991.

Stern, L. Disavowing the self in female adolescence. In *Women, Girls and Psychotherapy: Reframing Resistance*, edited by AG Rogers, DL Tolman, and C Gilligan. New York, NY: Routledge, 1991.

Stice, E. Review for the evidence for a sociocultural model of bulimia nervosa and exploration of mechanisms of action. *Clinical Psychology Review* 14, no. 7 (1994): 633–661.

Stice, E, Burton M, and Shaw H. Prospective relations between bulimic pathology, depression, and substance abuse: Unpacking comorbidity in adolescent girls. *Journal of Consulting and Clinical Psychology* 72, no. 1 (2004): 62–71.

Stice, E, Ng J, and Shaw H. Risk factors and prodromal eating pathology. *Journal of Child Psychology and Psychiatry* 51, no. 4 (2010): 518–525.

Stice, E, Schupak-Neuberg E, Shaw HE, and Stein RI. Relation of media exposure to eating disorder symptomology: A examination of mediating mechanisms. *Journal of Abnormal Psychology* 103, no. 4 (1994): 836–840.

Stice, E, and Shaw H. Prospective relations of body image, eating and affective disturbance to smoking onset in adolescent girls: How Virginia slims. *Journal of Consulting and Clinical Psychology* 71, no. 1 (2003): 129–135.

Stice, E, Spangler D, and Agras WS. Exposure to media-portrayed thin-ideal images adversely affects vulnerable girls: A longitudinal experiment. *Journal of Social and Clinical Psychology* 20, no. 3 (2001): 270–288.

Surry, J. Eating patterns as a reflection of women's development. In Women's Growth in Connection: *Writings from the Stone Center*, edited by JV Jordan, AG Kaplan, J Baker Miller, I Stiver, and J Surrey. New York, NY: Guilford Press, 1991.

The Child Performer Advisory Board. The Child Performer Advisory Board to Prevent Eating Disorders: Recommendations to the New York State Commissioner of Labor. 2009. Available at http://www.labor.ny.gov/workerprotection/laborstandards/secure/child_performer_advisory_board_recommendations.pdf (accessed April 15, 2009).

The Little Mermaid. Directed by R. Clements and Musker J. Clements. Produced by H, and Musker J Ashman. 1989.

Thompson, C. *Interpersonal Psychoanalysis*. New York, NY: Basic Books, 1964.

Thompson, JK, and Stice, E. Thin-ideal internalization: Mounting evidence for a new risk factor for body-image disturbance and eating pathology. *Current Directions in Psychological Science* 10, no. 5 (2001): 181–183.

Travis, CB. Risks to healthy development: The somber planes of life. In *Handbook of Girls and Women's Psychological Health. Gender and Well-Being across the Life-Span*, edited by J Worell and P Goodheart. New York, NY: Oxford University Press, 2006.

Vaisman, N, Voet H, Akivis A, and Sive-Ner I. Weight perception of adolescent dancing school students. *Archives of Pediatrics and Adolescent Medicine* 150, no. 2 (1996): 187–190.

Wagner, R. The silent victims: More men have eating disorders than ever before. *The Atlantic*, April 2012.

Williams, MS, Thomsen SR, and McCoy JK. Looking for an accurate mirror: A model for the relationship between media use and anorexia. *Eating Disorders* 4, no. 2 (2003): 127–134.

Wood, JT. *Gendered Lives: Communication, Gender, and Culture*. Belmont, CA: Wadsworth Thomson Learning, 2001.

3 Physiology of an Eating Disorder

Vicki Berkus, MD, PhD, CEDS

CONTENTS

LEARNING OBJECTIVES

After reading this chapter, the reader should be able to do the following:

- Understand the medical and physiological consequences of anorexia nervosa (AN), bulimia nervosa (BN), and binge-eating disorder (BED)
- Describe the physiological presentation of patients suffering from each of these eating disorders
- Assess appropriate levels of care based on eating-disorder patients' clinical needs

PHYSIOLOGICAL PRESENTATION OF PATIENTS WITH EATING DISORDERS

ANOREXIA NERVOSA

The mortality rates of eating disorders are two times higher than for any other mental health disorder, and the fatality rate for AN is six times higher (Schmidt et al. 2016). It is critical for providers to understand the importance of physiological consequences of eating disorders, and AN in particular.

Patients with AN are identifiable based on low weight. They may be wearing layers of clothing and have just loaded up on fluids prior to their visit to increase the "number" on the scale. One of the laboratory tests ordered is a urine specific gravity. If the patient is water loading, the specific gravity will show urine that is concentrated or diluted. This is important to know because the patients can change the levels of electrolytes in their blood. Patients will have a symptom list that they may or may not be willing to share initially. Patients usually present for help because their way is not working and they are experiencing the negative consequences of their behaviors. Several patients may have had emergency room (ER) visits for low potassium or sodium levels that can cause fainting or a feeling of weakness and dizziness. This gets the attention of the family, physician, and ER staff. The reality of their behaviors starts to attract medical attention. Medical providers are learning to identify several physical features associated with all of the major eating disorders in addition to low body weight, restricted food intake, compulsive exercising, or purging (see Table 3.1).

Often patients present with a history of restricting food, yet their laboratory values do not reflect the level of disease that is present. The body has an ability to maintain homeostasis. The body will adjust to a decreased number of calories but, at some point, this ability starts to decline. This "hypometabolic" state is consistent with a series of changes in laboratory values (see Table 3.2) (Forbes et al. 1984; Ornstein et al. 2003; Vaisman et al. 1988).

The body focuses on keeping the major organs (heart, lungs, and kidneys) functioning and uses whatever nutrients are taken in to allow it to function. When a patient

TABLE 3.1
Transdiagnostic Physical Complications

Delayed puberty	Oligo- or amenorrhea	Lanugo	Hair loss
Brittle hair and nails	Acrocyanosis	Tooth decay	Gingivitis
Russell's sign[a]	Swelling of the face and cheeks[b]	Enlargement of the salivary glands	Dental erosions, tooth decay, and gingivitis
Chest pain and heartburn	Headaches	Nausea	Abdominal bloating
Muscle cramps	Diarrhea, sometimes bloody from laxative abuse	Bruising	

[a] Calluses on the back of the hand secondary to abrasions from the teeth when the fingers are used to induce vomiting.

[b] Including the lower eyelids due to increased pressure of blood in the face during vomiting.

TABLE 3.2
Hypometabolic Laboratory Findings

Low sodium	Low potassium	Low phosphate
Low hormone levels (estradiol, FSH, LH, testosterone)	Low red blood cells (anemia)	Low white blood cells (leukopenia)
Low blood glucose	Low magnesium	High cholesterol
High amylase		

LH, luteinizing hormone; FSH, follicle-stimulating hormone.

arrives in an ER with a low heart rate or blood pressure, the first impulse is to replace fluids to raise these values. However, someone who has a history of AN needs to have these fluids replaced slowly so their body metabolism (Forbes et al. 1984; Ornstein et al. 2003; Vaisman et al. 1988) does not cause a fluid overload taxing the heart and lungs further. Many patients are secretive about their eating, purging, laxative use, or compulsive exercising. They are already feeling out of control based on the attention of concerned treatment providers and they know they may be losing even more of that control.

The initial studies on starvation came from the Minnesota study involving conscientious objectors who were given the option of losing 25% of their body weight (Keys et al. 1950). Symptoms experienced by the participants are shared with the symptoms of AN. The psychological change included obsessive thinking about food with a heightened focus on what they and others were eating. Several participants turned to bingeing after they were allowed to normalize their weight. Emotional changes included depression, isolating behaviors, and antisocial behaviors. Physiological changes included decreases in heart rate, gastrointestinal discomfort, weakness, decreased need for sleep, hair loss, cold hands and feet, inability to focus, and prickling sensations in their hands and feet (Boag et al. 1985; Birmingham et al. 2005). The physiological changes are accounted for by the body's struggle to compensate for weight loss as it internally attempts to control weight as a survival mechanism (Schebendach et al. 1997; Vaisman et al. 1991; Rigaud et al. 2007).

Normally the body uses glucose for energy and stores glucose for 24–48 hours. When liver glycogen is totally depleted, the body breaks down fatty acids to ketones and the body enters ketosis. The brain uses about 120 g of glucose per day. When glucose reserves are gone, the brain, skeletal muscle, cardiac muscle, and renal cortex turn to ketones for nourishment. The liver cannot use ketones for energy so protein is broken down to amino acids and the liver converts the amino acids to glucose. When glucose reserves are depleted, the body obtains protein from essentially wasting away muscles. The body adapts and tries to slow metabolism so the smallest amount of energy is used. This keeps the brain functioning. This can happen in as little as 3 days of starvation. If this process did not happen, the body would lose more than half its muscle protein leading to death within weeks.

The kidneys start to respond to the increased circulation of ketones, and the kidney turns to ammoniagenesis to maintain the acid–base homeostasis (Boag et al. 1985; Mehler and Anderson 2010). Ammonia (NH_4) titrates free H^+. If the body is deprived of vitamins and minerals, the immune system starts to shut down.

The hormonal system is affected by dropping insulin levels. Growth hormone increases breakdown of fats, and thyroid hormone levels drop causing a decrease in metabolic rate. Unfortunately, patients are frequently are treated for this starvation-induced hypothyroidism and they lose more weight (Ornstein et al. 2003; Vaisman et al. 1988; Caregaro et al. 2005).

In patients who present these metabolic changes, it is important to look for laboratory values depicting these changes. If the thyroid levels are low, thyroid stimulating hormone may be elevated sending a signal to the thyroid to work harder. Patients may be restricting fat intake yet their low-density lipoprotein and cholesterol levels may be increased as the body is trying to conserve fat. The kidney is working harder to maintain acid–base levels so the creatinine and blood urea nitrogen levels may increase indicating renal dysfunction in addition to plasma volume depletion and dehydration (Evrard et al. 2004). These levels can be restored by slow refeeding.

The body is equipped to respond to starvation since humans have had to endure periods of starvation to survive. The body adds weight first to the abdominal area to protect the internal organs much to the dismay of the patients who fear weight gain. This eventually is redistributed.

Since the brain is malnourished, the ability to make good choices or think in a rational manner is affected. Patients tend to exhibit "brain fog" which makes therapy difficult since retaining new information is difficult. The brain needs to be renourished for the recovery process to occur. This can take time and can influence length of stays in hospitals and residential centers (Davies 2015; Golden et al. 2003). The most difficult component of AN to reverse is body dysmorphia. Patients see themselves as "fat" and the idea of eating and gaining weight makes behavioral changes around food extremely difficult. This makes AN a different disease than the starvation process alone.

High levels of 5-hydroxyindoleacetic acid (serotonin) may be associated with such traits as high harm avoidance, perfectionism, exactness, and obsessive concern with symmetry. Their dysphoric mood may be due to food restriction, which lowers tryptophan levels, the precursor to serotonin. There may also be an inherent dysregulation of the emotional and reward pathways that also mediate hedonic aspects of feeding, hence the disturbed appetitive behaviors. Malnutrition can also produce alteration in many neuropeptides and monoamine function possibly to decrease energy expenditure (Forbes et al. 1984; Golden et al. 2003; Obarzanek et al. 1994; Rigaud et al. 2010; Schebendach et al. 1997).

Recent studies have looked at gut microbiota to see if increasing the diversity and abundance of the gut microbial state could relieve symptoms of AN (Keys et al. 1950; Schebendach et al. 1997; Vaisman et al. 1991). Patients often complain that it hurts to put food into their stomach. It has been shown that when normal subjects and anorexic subjects had pressure balloons inserted into the stomach, normal cues prior to mealtimes permitted a relaxation of the stomach to receive food in the normal control subjects only. The patients with AN did not have the same relaxation of the stomach adding to the discomfort accompanying feeding. This adds to their anxiety around meals. Furthermore, decreased leptin levels add to early satiety.

Anxiety is also increased with hypercortisolemia (Obarzanek et al. 1994; Volkow et al. 2010). The increase in cortisol levels in the anorexic patients result from increased cortisol pulsatility and decreased T3-regulated metabolism of cortisol. Cortisol secretion is also stimulated by hypoglycemia and hypoinsulinemia. This high cortisol level does not display the typical features of Cushing syndrome, the fatty hump between the shoulders, a rounded face, and pink or purple stretch marks, because of the client's low baseline of adipose tissue and cortisol resistance.

Women with AN are hypoestrogenic secondary to hypothalamic dysfunction. Disturbed gonadotrophic-releasing hormone leads to lower levels of gonadotrophins (follicle-stimulating hormone, luteinizing hormone) and when these are low, estrogen production is decreased (Golden et al. 2003). The absence of menstrual periods is common with this disorder with restrictive fat intake. Fertility is often restored with weight restoration. Ovarian function may parallel adrenal function.

More than 50% of adolescents with AN have evidence of osteopenia and 25% have osteoporosis (Zipfel et al. 2001). Ninety percent have evidence of reduced bone density. Malnutrition and estrogen deficiency can lead to decreased bone density. The bone metabolism is abnormal in anorexic patients due to the effects of malnutrition on osteoblastic activity as well as excessive exercise. The laboratory results will show low estrogen, low growth hormone, androgen, and T3 levels. The markers of bone formation are osteocalcin and bone alkaline phosphatase, which will be low. IGF-1 recombinant human insulin-like growth factor 1 is a hormone similar in molecular structure to insulin. It plays an important role in childhood growth and continues to have anabolic effects in adults. Giving external estrogen is not beneficial as it inhibits IGF-1. Recombinant IGF-1 promotes bone formation and reduces bone resorption (Vaisman et al. 1991). The best treatment is weight gain.

Refeeding severely anorexic patients can be difficult and requires frequent monitoring of magnesium and phosphate levels (Ornstein et al. 2003). The purpose of a slow refeeding process is to avoid rapid fluid changes in the body (Rigaud et al. 2010; Stice et al. 2008; Van Wymelbeke et al. 2004). If you feed carbohydrates to a severe anorexic, it stimulates insulin production and this can cause hemodynamic and electrolyte imbalance (intracellular influx of potassium, magnesium, and phosphorus, which is why blood levels of these electrolytes can change rapidly). Increased insulin levels can also lead to fluid retention and put more stress on the heart and lungs.

Leptin release leads to a feeling of fullness or satiety and is secreted from adipose tissue. The serum level of leptin is low in anorexic patients. Leptin works in the hypothalamus to help to regulate energy in the body along with insulin. It also is involved in menstrual recovery. Ghrelin is produced in the stomach and increases hunger and, thus, food intake (Rigaud et al. 2007). The levels are increased in anorexic patients so it suggests a decreased sensitivity to ghrelin in these patients. Ghrelin has a role in how the patients adapt to starvation with changing hormone levels to protect the patients who are in an energy-deficient state (Forman-Hoffman et al. 2006).

The body does respond to treatment and some functions return faster than others with weight restoration. Patients may have long-lasting complications such as short stature, osteoporosis, and infertility. The need for medical monitoring of these patients is obvious based on the number of bodily systems that are affected by their malnutrition. The number of people who die from AN is the highest of any mental health disorder. Knowing the physiology of AN and effectively treating a patient may involve several strategies based on which physiological changes are most life threatening and which are bringing the most satisfaction to the patient who is resistant to change.

A patient who presents for evaluation may have had an eating disorder for quite a while and his or her body may have adjusted to the decreased oral intake or the compulsive exercise. Presenting laboratory values may be marginally low or normal. The patient may be functioning at a hypometabolic rate (decreased heart rate, blood pressure, respiratory rate) and electrolytes may be normal if they have not water-loaded or used laxatives.

The anorexic patients may be using laxatives, exercising, restricting, purging, or a combination of these behaviors to keep their weight low. They may have lost their ability to have periods, have osteoporosis or osteopenia, or experience fatigue or dizziness when standing. Often a rigid or obsessive personality makes it difficult for them to ask for help or make healthy choices around food intake and exercise. They may be black-and-white thinkers, avoid risk taking, and spend a lot of time body checking and attending to internal dialogue to thoughts that keep them stuck in a cycle of restricting, exercising, or purging. They can "talk recovery" because they may have been to several treatment centers but have difficulty "walking" it. The state of starvation has become their "norm" and the thought of eating more or exercising less brings visions of "getting fat" rather than getting "healthy."

Treatment of the Anorexic Patient

There are so many factors to consider when starting individualized treatment. Medications can be adding to their insomnia, fatigue, gastrointestinal complaints, constipation, and difficulty concentrating, mimicking the same symptoms of the AN. Patients may have a fixed belief system around certain foods and insist on sticking to vegan, vegetarian, or only safe foods. The physiological changes described earlier make the refeeding process a struggle for these patients and they have frequent complaints of bloating, gas, pain, and constipation. The gas-troparesis or slowing of the stomach emptying process can take time to resolve (Schebendach et al. 1997). A smooth muscle relaxer like Bentyl combined with Erythromycin 250 mg (addresses slower gastric emptying) 30 minutes before a meal may lower the discomfort. These patients are exquisitely aware of changes in their body and sensations of discomfort. Their level of anxiety is high and the urge to medically treat this is strong. Studies have shown that due to a malnour-ished brain, the selective serotonin reuptake inhibitors (SSRIs) may not be effec-tive (American Psychiatric Association Work Group on Eating Disorders 2000). Patients have an uncanny awareness of which antidepressants or mood stabiliz-ers may cause weight gain and suggesting one of these can quickly cause the therapeutic alliance to dissolve. They are already dealing with a feeling of low self-worth and adding depression, alexithymia, anhedonia, anxiety, and distrust makes the recovery a slow process.

Methods to Identify At-Risk Anorexic Patients

Most of these patients are bright, high achievers, and their perfectionist thinking may only respond to data that is concrete such as a dexa scan revealing that their bone density is the same as someone much older. The occurrence of repeated stress fractures or emergency room visits for low potassium would be an incentive for some patients but they quickly prefer the familiar though uncomfortable physical changes of AN to changing their eating behaviors and gaining weight. The team approach is a necessity in treating these patients. The dietitian has to walk the fine line between maintaining a therapeutic relationship and insisting on changes in food consumption that the patients find difficult and scary. The shrunken, starved brain of the anorexic patients may not have the functional ability to participate in sophisticated communication and oxytocin, a hormone that is central to aspects of social communication, is reduced peripherally and in the brain (Caregaro et al. 2005; Lawson et al. 2012; Vaisman et al. 1988). Neurofunctional studies (single photon emission computed tomography) show asymmetry of blood flow to at least one area of the brain in anorexics, mostly temporal and parietal. Magnetic resonance imaging (MRI) studies show decreased volume and increased cerebrospinal fluid, suggesting starvation of the brain (Jauregui-Lobera 2011). Recovered patients showed significantly less medial prefrontal cortex activation. There is also increased activation of the medial and anterior cingulate activation in response to food stimuli. There are numerous studies showing changes in brain size and function in AN patients (Volkow et al. 2010).

The basic physiology of the brain changes in starvation making it difficult for the patients to accept the advice of the treatment team. It is known that functional MRI studies show changes in anorexic patients with body dissatisfaction over controls and stronger activation of the insula and lateral prefrontal cortex during body satisfaction rating of thin self-image (Mohr et al. 2010). Patients have a distorted view of their body, convinced that they are "fat" regardless of how little they weigh, which keeps their fear level elevated. Their ability to make good choices is lost and they struggle to make sense of what others are telling them about what they need to eat. The advice does not make sense to them. It is easy for the patients to be labeled "difficult" or noncompliant when what they perceive is their truth. It is fascinating to watch their perception change with weight restoration. They become more compliant and open to new information about their body.

The understanding of the physiology of AN, along with bulimia and BED, continues to be under investigation as newer studies utilize state-of-the-art scanning techniques. The ability to change behaviors still remains a time-consuming process involving months of treatment.

The basic physiology of the brain changes in starvation and these changes make it difficult for the patients to accept the advice of the treatment team. A combination of dysfunctions in frontal-subcortical circuits and temporal, parietal, and limbic structures may produce both the characteristic symptoms and neurocognitive deficits seen in body dysmorphic disorder. A starving brain affects the patient's ability and can change their body image distortion, self-recognition, and emotional reactions to visual stimuli. Patients have a distorted view of their body which keeps their fear level elevated. They are convinced that they are "fat" regardless of how little they weigh. Their ability to make good choices is lost. They struggle to make sense of what others are telling them about what they need to eat; it doesn't make sense to them. It is easy to label patients as "difficult" or noncompliant although what they perceive is their truth. It is fascinating to watch their perception change with weight restoration. They become more compliant and open to new information about their body.

CASE STUDY 3.1

Kelly

The patient is a 24-year-old white female with a 7-year history of restricting and purging with exercise. She presents with a chief complaint of gastroesophageal reflux disease, dizziness, and amenorrhea (1.5 years). She is 5'8" tall and weighs 110 lb. Her highest weight was 165 lb. and she is at her lowest weight currently. She restricts her intake to 600 cal/day and over-exercises by running at least four times a week. She has a history since age 7 of obsessive-compulsive disorder and is on PaxilXR 25 mg/day and Neurontin 100 mg at bedtime for restless leg syndrome. She was sexually molested at age 9 by an uncle. Her mother is obese and her father was an alcoholic. Her maternal grandmother was bulimic. She denies any substance abuse or suicidal ideation.

This patient has had episodes of low potassium (hypokalemia) and has been to the ER twice for dizziness and weakness. She does want to get pregnant at some time in the future. In her initial treatment visit, her body mass index (BMI) is 16.7. She complains of fatigue, dizziness, and feels her heart beating fast at times. The labs come back showing a low potassium level, normal amylase, low estrogen, high cholesterol, low vitamin D, and low sodium; her electrocardiogram shows a bradycardia (low heart rate of 55 bpm), and her blood pressure is low (90/60). A normal amylase level will usually indicate that the patient is not vomiting. If it came back elevated, then a lipase level would be ordered to rule out pancreatic involvement. If the lipase is normal and the amylase is high, the cause is vomiting. She is struggling to keep from moving (shaking her legs, walking when asked to sit, etc.). She has lost 15 lb. in the last month so her heart may have also decreased in size. Her provider is concerned that if refeeding occurs too quickly, the extra strain on the heart may put her in danger of heart failure. The other ions to watch are the potassium, phosphorus, and magnesium levels. The increase in glucose will stimulate insulin production and these ions move intracellularly, lowering serum levels. Low phosphate levels mean less adenosine triphosphate (ATP) for energy and can lead to muscle, respiratory, and cardiac problems. Her amylase (an enzyme in saliva would be elevated if she were purging) was normal and she had low estrogen.

Since she is a compulsive exerciser, a bone density scan will probably reveal osteoporosis (low bone mass and bone structural breakdown) or osteopenia—the beginning stages of bone loss. Since she has not had a period for over a year, the low estrogen and progesterone can add to slowing bone development. She has been restricting for some time so she will probably struggle with her refeeding schedule.

Since she has been in a starvation mode, her antidepressant (an SSRI) may not be working. Studies show that refeeding will need to happen for the medications to be effective. Starvation can shrink the cortical substance of the brain and thereby lead to increased size of the ventricles. It is sometimes difficult to tell if their cognitive difficulties are due to poor nutrition or actual

(Continued)

changes in the brain itself. When the patient is put on a refeeding schedule, it may take a few weeks to see the cognitive effects of renourishing the brain. The refeeding has to be slow to avoid any medical complications. The problem with cognitive dysfunction (sometime referred to as a brain fog) usually reverses with weight restoration and if the cognitive problems continue after weight restoration, then further neurological studies would be ordered (exam, CT or MRI, psychological testing).

BULIMIA NERVOSA

BN includes binge eating (although many patients may consider anything that enters their mouth a binge) and includes the use of compensatory behaviors to rid the body of calories. Some patients choose vomiting, compulsive exercise, laxative abuse, or a combination of these to purge calories. Each of these behaviors brings its own physiological changes.

Patients often start out by restricting the number of calories they take in but eventually following their own "rules" becomes too difficult and they engage in some compensatory behavior. Many patients will find that it is harder to purge through vomiting and may start to use exercise to burn calories. These patients may differ from anorexic patients in that they plan their exercise based on the size of their binge or what they have eaten while an anorexic patient may be restricting and still feel compelled to exercise. This obsessiveness with exercise takes on the same level of focus as their previous restricting behaviors.

The amount of exercise and calories expended start to more than compensate for the number of calories consumed. Patients may have been involved in sports during school and rather than experiencing a sense of joy, it starts to become a task or something they have to do on a daily basis to deal with their anxiety. Common warning signs of exercise addiction are in Table 3.3.

TABLE 3.3
Warning Signs of Compulsive Exercising

Exercising following a binge to compensate for calories consumed	Exercising to allow oneself to eat/consume calories	Exercising to achieve a certain weight, body shape, or weight loss goal	Maintaining an inflexible exercise schedule that cannot be altered
Missing important social or other life activities in order to exercise	Experiencing significant distress, especially guilt, when exercise is missed	Continuing to exercise despite being sick or injured	

The most important muscle that has to adapt to an increase in exercise is the heart. In untrained people, cardiac output can increase up to four times resting capacity and go from pumping 4–5 L/min at rest to 16–20 L/min during exercise, primarily through an increase in heart rate. In trained athletes, the stroke volume (amount of blood pumped with each beat) is increased by 40%–50% (Abraham et al. 2006; Boag et al. 1985; Obarzanek et al. 1994). If a trained athlete is at rest, he or she will have a slower heart rate and increased stroke volume. In time, the thickness of the left ventricular wall can increase. Changes in heart muscle occur gradually over 4–8 weeks of training. The circulatory system has to adjust to the demands of exercise by dilating the arteries in the working muscle to increase the exchanges of oxygen and removal of metabolic wastes. The nervous system stimulates the vessels to dilate. More water and protein are added to plasma volume to thin the blood and the result is an increase in total plasma volume and decrease in the relative concentration of red cells. Muscle oxygen consumption increases up to 70 times above resting values, and capillary density increases so more oxygen, nutrients, and hormones can be delivered to the muscles, causing an increase in size (Golden et al. 2003). This is the scenario in someone who is being trained properly and is taking in a healthy amount of calories.

Most of the time, patients with AN who are over-exercising or those patients who are purging with both vomiting and exercise put themselves at risk for cardiac problems. The heart needs healthy muscle to adapt to increased stroke volume. Patients who have depleted their carbohydrate stores and have used muscles to provide fatty acids for energy have muscle wasting and cannot meet the extra stress of exercise. Patients will complain of fatigue, dizziness, fainting, and passing out during their exercise periods. They usually have depleted their fat stores and have little reserve to provide the extra energy needed while exercising. Most people will slow down or stop during pain accompanying exercise. If the patients are unable to (based on the compulsion), stress fractures can occur (microfractures of the bone due to overuse). Previously, it was noted that patients who have restricted caloric intake also have thinner bones making stress fractures a real concern for the bulimic patients who are purging with exercise and restricting at the same time.

There may be severe consequences with those patients that exercise compulsively. They may find their exercise routine takes time away from previously satisfying social relationships. It may even escalate and take time away from their work or school performance. Many patients prefer to isolate when exercising and this means that most of their free time is allotted to their routines. Excessive exercising can also lead to dehydration, insomnia, and the release of free radicals that have been linked to cellular mutations (Vaisman et al. 1991; Obarzanek et al. 1994; Van Wymelbeke et al. 2004). Females may stop menstruation and develop amenorrhea for months or years. Many patients are unaware of the results of over-exercising and have had to be hospitalized to finally get treatment for their purging with exercise.

Purging may also occur through vomiting. Some patients have a strong gag reflex and have to induce it with their finger or a toothbrush. They talk about liking the empty feeling that accompanies it. Other patients can "spontaneously vomit" and may do so several times a day. The regurgitation of gastric contents results in the physical problems listed in Table 3.4.

TABLE 3.4
Physical Complications of Purging by Vomiting

Poor skin turgor	Russell's sign (excoriations on the back of the hand below the index finger)	Erosion of dental enamel
Blood-streaked vomitus	Esophageal changes (precancerous)	Parotid gland swelling (occurs 2–3 days after cessation of vomiting)

Since the level of shame and guilt can be so high for these patients, they usually present with gastrointestinal complaints such as acid reflux or sore throat. Patients do not realize that changes in blood pressure occur with vomiting. When pressure readings were taken in the middle cerebral arteries, there could be as much as a 29% increase in blood pressure (Yager et al. 2006). This causes autoregulatory responses, and can easily result in a stroke. Repeated changes in cerebral vessel pressure could lead to wearing down of the vessels. The effects of electrolyte imbalance due to purging could cause the heart to arrest, leading to the brain not getting the oxygen it needs. Electrolytes are lost through chronic vomiting and low potassium can cause abnormal heart rhythms, muscle weakness, constipation, and if prolonged can damage the kidneys. Loss of calcium can cause spasms of the legs or arms, tingling in both hands and feet, irritability, depression, confusion, or serious disorientation. Low sodium can cause similar symptoms such as fatigue, headache, even coma, or unconsciousness. Sudden drops in sodium can cause your brain to swell leading to coma or death. Patients who water load by drinking large volumes of water can also cause their sodium levels to drop (Rigaud et al. 2010).

The repeated washing of the esophagus and teeth with gastric fluid can lead to esophageal varices (rupture of the tiny blood vessels) or to loss of dental enamel. The loss of enamel can make the teeth sensitive to hot or cold foods or liquids. Dental caries are common and many patients have had repeated dental work done because of their purging. It is also common to see swelling of the parotid glands 2–3 days after the cessation of purging. There is also enlargement of the salivary glands in some patients. If patients are drinking large amounts of alcohol and vomiting, the risk of esophageal damage is greater. If patients have an elevated amylase level but normal lipase level, it is an indication that the salivary glands and not the pancreas are the source of the amylase production.

If the stomach contents are spontaneously emptied by vomiting or stay low due to restriction, the patients may experience delayed gastric emptying that can lead to a bloated uncomfortable feeling. They may also have caused the GI tract to slow down, which may result in constipation. This may be the one thing that brings them in for treatment.

Other patients may use laxatives as a way to achieve a feeling of "emptiness" or flatten their stomachs. A major concern of someone abusing laxatives is a "cathartic colon," which is colon nerve damage caused by prolonged use. This can be life-threatening, which is why most patients are taken off laxatives in treatment.

Treatment usually involves a substance (polyethylene glycol or lactulose) that osmotically draws fluid into the colon (Mehler and Anderson 1999, 2010). This can aid in stimulating a bowel movement. The bulimic patients who have been on laxatives have difficulty with fluid movement after stopping the laxatives. Laxatives remove water from the colon as well as food residue. The weight loss is temporary and restored with fluid rehydration. The dehydration can lead to tremors, weakness, blurry vision, fainting spells, kidney damage, and in some cases, death. The laxatives also stimulate nerve endings in the gut to the point they no longer respond to stimulation and the patients cannot have a bowel movement normally. Patients are also more open to infection because laxatives and enemas strip away the protective mucus in the colon.

A metabolic alkalosis (low chloride, low potassium, low bicarbonate, low sodium) or a metabolic acidosis (severe diarrhea) usually indicates laxative abuse and needs to be treated (Mehler and Anderson 1999, 2010; Moukaddem et al. 1997; Rigaud et al. 2007). Dehydration also leads to the production of aldosterone that acts on the kidneys to aid in conservation of sodium, secretion of potassium, water retention, and stabilizes blood pressure. Slow infusion with saline can stop aldosterone production. If too much fluid is given too quickly, a person can develop edema and the extra fluid can space into the lungs or abdomen. Patients have had to have their lungs tapped to get rid of the extra fluid. Table 3.5 shows the effects of purging on electrolyte concentrations.

The EKG can aid in determining an electrolyte abnormality. Low potassium can cause T-wave flattening, U-waves, and ST segment depression. Low magnesium and low calcium can cause prolonged Q-T interval and nonspecific T-wave changes (Mehler and Anderson 1999, 2010).

BINGE-EATING DISORDER

Binge-eating disorder has a variety of physiological changes that occur when an excess of calories are consumed in a short amount of time. This differs from simply overeating because of a co-occurring sense of loss of control around the eating behavior. People with BED tend to eat rapidly, eat when not hungry, and will continue to eat until uncomfortably full. Most patients eat alone and express disgust, guilt, shame, or embarrassment after bingeing. There are no compensatory behaviors after consuming their food. While the frequency of binge eating can vary, the frequency of at least once a week for 3 months meets criteria for the *Diagnostic*

TABLE 3.5
Medical Complications of Purging

Purge Type	Sodium	Potassium	Chloride	Bicarbonate	pH
Vomiting	High, low	Low	Low	High	High
Laxatives	High, low	Low	Low, high	Low	High, low
Diuretics	High, low	Low	Low	High	High

CASE STUDY 3.2

Andrea

Andrea is a 53-year-old female who is purging by vomiting three to seven times a day and using 20–30 Dulcolax laxatives/day. She binges daily and usually consumes about 10,000 cal/day. She is 5′2″ tall and weighs 160 lb. Her lowest weight was 92 lb. and her highest weight was 202 lb. She has had three initial treatments at the in-patient level of care and relapsed quickly after discharge each time. Her medications include Luvox 200 mg at bedtime, Trazodone 200 mg at bedtime, and Xanax 2 mg three times a day. She has had a breast reduction and is postmenopausal without hormone replacement therapy.

PRIOR TREATMENTS AT THE IN-PATIENT/RESIDENTIAL LEVEL OF CARE

A urinalysis would show if her urine was concentrated or diluted (based on the specific gravity). Since she is losing fluids by vomiting and having diarrhea, it would be important to see if her kidneys are able to compensate and handle the fluid loss. It would be necessary to stop the use of Dulcolax and be ready to see water retention. Since she has been using laxatives, her colon would not be functioning to regulate fluids in a normal manner.

The first orders would be laboratory values to look at her serum electrolytes (expect low potassium, changes in sodium, chloride, PH, bicarbonate). She would need stabilization of her electrolytes. She would also have a urinalysis to provide the specific gravity of her urine to determine how concentrated her urine is and how the kidneys are compensating. She is losing fluids by vomiting and diarrhea. She would be taken off the Dulcolax and carefully monitored for fluid retention. The first priority would be to correct the metabolic alkalosis caused by dehydration, since dehydration stimulates aldosterone production that can cause renal potassium loss. Intravenous fluid replacement with sodium-containing solutions will stop the aldosterone production. Replacement of sodium is also crucial but in a safe, monitored environment to avoid neurological complications. In some severe cases, an aldosterone antagonist like spironolactone will be given.

The replacement of fluids would be slow (50 cc/hour) to avoid fluid overload. An EKG would show changes due to alterations in electrolyte levels. The first 48 hours are especially important due to the patient's possible cardiac weakness and the possibility of edema of the hands, feet, and face. If too much fluid is retained, the fluid can flow into areas such as the lungs and abdomen. This would sometimes require removal of excess fluid from these areas. The cessation of laxatives is extremely hard for the patient and the GI symptoms of constipation, bloating, abdominal pain, and discomfort can be overwhelming. These complaints are important and an abdominal x-ray can show the amount of stool in the large intestine. The time for the stabilization is individually determined based on the amount and length of time of laxative abuse. The colon needs time to function normally and the substitution of a nonstimulant laxative to avoid further nerve damage in the colon is often needed.

(Continued)

CASE STUDY 3.2 *(CONTINUED)*

Since this patient has been vomiting, it is important to look for any blood in the vomitus possibly indicating damage to esophageal vessel. The patient may have difficulty with swallowing, sore throat, enlarged parotid glands (days after cessation of vomiting), and acid reflux. Medication can help to reduce gastric acid production. The body takes time to return to normal functioning and the process may take weeks.

and Statistical Manual of Mental Disorders, Fifth Edition (DSM-5; American Psychiatric Association 2013).

People who suffer from BED may or may not be classified as obese, and those who are obese do not necessarily have BED. Psychologically, women who are obese and meet criteria for BED score higher on the neuroticism scale and higher on symptom scales measuring depression, anxiety/phobia, and neurovegetative symptoms (Abraham et al. 2006; Bulik et al. 2002; Van Wymelbeke et al. 2004).

The major focus of BED is a feeling of loss of control over their eating. Patients will plan a binge and often not be able to stop once they have obtained the binge foods. Someone who has BED may have the following medical issues: metabolic syndrome, reduced high-density lipoproteins, hypertriglyceridemia, acute or chronic gastritis, GERD, type II diabetes mellitus, insulin resistance, insulin suppression, arthritis, osteoarthritis, edema, obstructive sleep apnea, urinary incontinence, irritable bowel syndrome, cancer (various forms), heart disease due to elevated triglyceride levels, hypertension, high blood pressure, high cholesterol, blunted cortisol response, menstrual dysfunction, infertility, gall bladder disease, liver disease, and kidney disease (Mitchell 2016).

Many of these medical complications are the same health problems associated with clinical obesity. The psychological focus of someone who has BED will differ from someone who is obese without BED. The patient with BED may change their lifestyles to make time for binges. They may avoid mealtimes or social situations involving food for fear of losing control in a public setting. A numb feeling may accompany bingeing; like being on autopilot. They may feel guilty, lie about what they have eaten, or make excuses to hide their behavior. They may feel that eating is the only way to relieve stress. Their binging may be a maladaptive form of coping or an attempt to fill a void inside. There are people who are overweight for various reasons (hormonal, genetic, social, etc.) who do not experience these feelings.

Studies show that metabolic syndrome occurs in about 50% of patients with BED. Those that develop metabolic syndrome (hypertriglyceridemia, reduced HDLs, hypertension, and insulin resistance) tend to have an excess of visceral fat (apple shaped as opposed to pear shaped; Golden et al. 2003; Obarzanek et al. 1994; Rigaud et al. 2007). This visceral blood supply goes to the liver and contributes to a higher level of liver synthesis of plasma lipids. Patients are measured with skinfold thickness techniques, underwater weighing, BMI, and waist-to-hip ratios. The genetics for BED are different from those who suffer from obesity. There are obese people who do not have BED and there are normal weight individuals who binge. The average caloric consumption per binge can range from 1000 cal to 5000 kcal. Patients often express anxiety, depression, or other mood disorder symptoms.

A body at rest only needs a limited amount of food to meet its energy needs; this is known as the basal metabolic rate. When a person binges, the excess carbohydrates are stored in the liver and muscle as glycogen (Schmidt 2016). The excess fats are stored in adipose tissue as triglycerides and can lead to feeling very full and slower digestion. This can cause stomach distention. There can also be an increase in tissue proteins.

Bingeing can cause insulin produced by the pancreas to increase in the blood. Insulin is responsible for removing excess glucose from the blood into the cells to be used for energy or converted to fat for storage. It can also inhibit glycogen, which is a hormone, that signals us when we are full. If the insulin is not working in that capacity (insulin resistance), it interferes with our ability to regulate appetite. Glucagon causes a release of stored sugar into the blood to be used for energy. If insulin fails to cause the excess glucose to enter the cells, it stays in the blood causing an elevated blood glucose level. If the insulin is released too quickly, the result can be a rapid decrease in blood sugar levels. This leaves the blood glucose supply to the brain to lower and a coma can result. High insulin and low blood sugar can also suppress serotonin that normally decreases carbohydrate cravings. The suppression of serotonin can lead to a higher desire for fats and sweets (Mitchell 2016). The excess calories from these foods will be stored as fat in adipose cells. The frequency of bingeing can cause variations in blood sugar levels.

People who ignore hunger or suppress emotional needs take in little food, leading to an excess of gastric acid. The gastric acid, usually involved in breaking down food, is now available to irritate and erode the lining of the empty stomach. People may eat more sweets to keep the stomach full, causing more gastric secretion of stomach acid. The amount of stomach acid can affect protein digestion and alter the protective barrier responsible for stopping bacterial overgrowth.

Obese women who also have a diagnosis of BED score higher on neuroticism and symptom scales measuring depression, anxiety/phobia, and neurovegetative symptoms. They also have similar medical problems to the obese population who do not have BED (Bulik 2005; Bulik et al. 1996, 1997, 2012). These patients also suffer from psychological distress and turn to lying about food eaten, feel numb while binging, experience embarrassment over how much they are eating, and suffer from tension relieved only by eating. The lack of control and the intensity of the behavior are typical of BED. It is a disease that also takes a team (physician, psychiatrist, therapist, and dietitian) to treat and support the patient during recovery.

CASE STUDY 3.3

Ann

Ann has been a binge eater for most of her teens. She is now 20 and has been diagnosed with metabolic syndrome and wants to get healthy. She is 5'4" tall and weighs 250 lb. She was heavy as a child but gained 60 lb. in the last 3 years. She is afraid of what might happen if she does not change her eating habits. She is shy with other people and has never been in a relationship. She is having difficulty maintaining a healthy blood sugar level and is now on metformin with a possibility of having to go to insulin to regulate her glucose levels. She avoids exercise because she has chronic knee and hip pain. Her laboratory results show an elevated cholesterol level, elevated blood glucose level, and decreased HDLs. Her blood pressure is up and she has recently started on an antihypertensive medication. She has the typical "apple" shape with increased abdominal girth. She is undergoing insulin studies. She becomes short of breath easily with exertion and has been suffering from a co-occurring depression for years. She describes feeling a lack of control when she binges and has a lot of shame and guilt. She has tried fad diets and has lost up to 50 lb. but has not been able to stick to one and regains the weight quickly. She meets criteria for BED since she binges at least once per week, feels a lack of control over her binges, and has a lot of shame and guilt around her behaviors.

Ann's laboratory values are consistent with her diagnosis of metabolic syndrome. She has been storing the additional calories in adipose tissue. One problem with expanded adipose tissue is that it is relatively metabolically inert compared to the nonobese individual. The high fat content of her binges causes an excessive release of fatty acids and may induce insulin resistance or interfere with release of insulin from the pancreas. The overabundance of fat in muscle cells can be strongly associated with impaired glucose uptake and oxidation by both insulin-dependent and noninsulin-dependent mechanisms. The use of a hemoglobin A1c can help the providers to follow her control around her blood glucose levels over time. A homeostatic model assessment for insulin resistance (HOMA-IR) and quantitative insulin sensitivity check index (QUICKI) are the widely used indices for assessing insulin resistance in practice. The input of an endocrinologist can help the team to determine the best way to follow the patient's medical status during treatment. Some patients may be able to work with a primary care physician who feels comfortable ordering these tests (Olatunbosum 2015).

Ann would benefit from a BED program that would address her medical issues and work with her to change her relationship with food. She has been able to lose weight but has always gained it back. She has low self-esteem and has not been able to socially engage with others. She has used food to self-soothe. She can benefit from therapy, which can give her options to deal with the feelings that lead to bingeing (dialectical behavior therapy [DBT], cognitive-behavioral therapy [CBT], etc.). She would also need a support system so she can talk about her fears and the

(Continued)

consequences she has had to face due to her eating disorder. The medical field is not known for their compassion in dealing with the medical issues caused by overeating. It would be important to find a team of providers who can differentiate her from her disease and offer a safe environment to heal. This team would include not only a therapist and nutritionist, but also a medical provider who is comfortable ordering a hemoglobin A1C to monitor blood sugar levels over time. The medical provider should also be willing to listen to GI complaints caused by bingeing and help her to feel comfortable discussing her issues.

CONCLUSION

Neurophysiological complications of eating disorders greatly impact patients' ability to function cognitively, physically, and socially. When patients cannot think rationally, they typically make unwise decisions about their health care. When they cannot function physically, they have difficulty in finding the energy to follow through with health-care recommendations. It is critical for providers to address and resolve the physical complications of eating disorders, patiently working through the logistical and interpersonal barriers to providing excellent medical and nutritional services.

REFERENCES

Abraham, SF, Hart S, Luscombe G, and Russell J. Fluid intake, personality and behaviour in patients with eating disorders. *Eating and Weight Disorders* 11, no. 1 (2006): 30–34.

American Psychiatric Association. *Diagnostic and Statistical Manual of Mental Disorders* (5th ed.). Washington, DC: Author, 2013.

American Psychiatric Association Work Group on Eating Disorders. Practice guideline for the treatment of patients with eating disorders (revision). *American Journal of Psychiatry* 157, no. 1S (2000): 1–39.

Birmingham, CL, Hlynsky J, Whiteside L, and Geller J. Caloric requirement for refeeding inpatients with anorexia nervosa: The contribution of anxiety exercise, and cigarette smoking. *Eating and Weight Disorders* 10, no. 1 (2005): e6–e9.

Boag, F, Weerakoon J, Ginsburg J, Havard CW, and Dandona P. Diminished creatinine clearance in anorexia nervosa: Reversal with weight gain. *Journal of Clinical Pathology* 38, no. 1 (1985): 60–63.

Bulik, CM. Exploring the gene–environment nexus in eating disorders. *Journal of Psychiatry and Neuroscience* 30, no. 5 (2005): 335.

Bulik, CM, Baucom DH, and Kirby SJ. Treating anorexia nervosa in the couple context. *Journal of Cognitive Psychotherapy* 26, no. 1 (2012): 19–33.

Bulik, CM, Sullivan PF, Carter, FA, and Joyce PR. Lifetime anxiety disorders in women with bulimia nervosa. *Comprehensive Psychiatry* 37, no. 5 (1996): 368–374.

Bulik, CM, Sullivan PF, Fear JL, and Joyce PR. Eating disorders and antecedent anxiety disorders: A controlled study. *Acta Psychiatrica Scandinavica* 96, no. 2 (1997): 101–107.

Bulik, CM, Sullivan PF, and Kendler KS. Medical and psychiatric morbidity in obese women with and without binge eating. *International Journal of Eating Disorders* 32, no. 1 (2002): 72–78.

Caregaro, L, Di Pascoli L, Favaro A, Nardi M, and Santonastaso P. Sodium depletion and hemoconcentration: Overlooked complications in patients with anorexia nervosa. *Nutrition* 21, no. 4 (2005): 438–445.

Davies, M. Anorexia nervosa may be partly related to an imbalance of the gut neurobiology. *Daily Mail.* 6 October 2015. Available at https://www.sott.net/article/303961-Anorexia-nervosa-may-be-partly-related-to-an-imbalance-of-the-gut-microbiota

Evrard, F, da Cunha MP, Lambert M, and Devuyst O. Impaired osmoregulation in anorexia nervosa: A case-control study. *Nephrology Dialysis Transplantation* 19, no. 12 (2004): 3034–3039.

Forbes, GB, Kreipe RE, Lipinski BA, and Hodgman CH. Body composition changes during recovery from anorexia nervosa: Comparison of two dietary regimes. *American Journal of Clinical Nutrition* 40, no. 6 (1984): 1137–1145.

Forman-Hoffman, VL, Ruffin T, and Schultz SK. Basal metabolic rate in anorexia nervosa patients: Using appropriate predictive equations during the refeeding process. *Annals of Clinical Psychiatry* 18, no. 2 (2006): 123–127.

Golden, NH, Katzman DK, Kreipe RE, Stevens SL, Sawyer SM, Rees J, Nicholls D, and Rome ES. Eating disorders in adolescents: Position paper of the Society for Adolescent Medicine. *Journal of Adolescent Health* 33, no. 6 (2003): 496–503.

Jauregui-Lobera, I. Neuroimaging in eating disorder. *Journal of Neuropsychiatric Disease and Treatment* 7 (2011): 577–584.

Keys, A, Brozek K, Henschel A, Mickelsen O, and Taylor HL. *The Biology of Human Starvation.* Minneapolis, MN: University of Minnesota Press, 1950.

Lawson, EA, Holsen LM, Santin M, Meenaghan E, Eddy KT, Becker AE, Herzog DB, Goldstein JM, and Klibanski A. Oxytocin secretion associated with severity of disorder eating psychopathology and insular cortex hypoactivation in anorexia nervosa. *Journal of Clinical Endocrinology and Metabolism* 97, no. 10 (2012): E1898–E1908.

Mehler, PS, and Anderson A. *Eating Disorders: A Guide to Medical Care and Complications* (2nd ed.). Baltimore, MD: Johns Hopkins Press, 2010.

Mitchell, JE. Medical comorbidity and medical complications associated with binge-eating disorder. *International Journal of Eating Disorders* 49, no. 3 (2016): 319–323.

Mohr, HM, Zimmermann J, Röder C, Lenz C, Overbeck G, and Grabhorn R. Separating two components of body image in anorexia nervosa using fMRI. *Psychological Medicine* 40, no. 9 (2010): 1519–1529.

Moukaddem, M, Boulier A, Apfelbaum M, and Rigaud D. Increase in diet-induced thermogenesis at the start of refeeding in severely malnourished anorexia nervosa patients. *American Journal of Clinical Nutrition* 66, no. 1 (1997): 133–140.

Obarzanek, E, Lesem MD, and Jimerson DC. Resting metabolic rate of anorexia nervosa patients during weight gain. *American Journal of Clinical Nutrition* 60, no. 5 (1994): 666–675.

Ornstein, RM, Golden NH, and Jacobson MS. Hypophosphatemia during nutritional rehabilitation in anorexia nervosa: Implications for refeeding and monitoring. *Journal of Adolescent Health* 32, no. 1 (2003): 83–88.

Rigaud, D, Boulier A, Tallonneau I, Brindisi MC, and Rozen R. Body fluid retention and body weight change in anorexia nervosa patients during refeeding. *Clinical Nutrition* 29, no. 6 (2010): 749–755.

Rigaud, D, Verges B, Colas-Linhart N, Rigaud D, Verges B, Colas-Linhart N, Petiet A, Moukkaddem M, Van Wymelbeke V, and Brondel L. Hormonal and psychological factors linked to the increased thermic effect of food in malnourished fasting anorexia nervosa. *Journal of Clinical Endocrinology and Metabolism* 92, no. 5 (2007): 1623–1629.

Schebendach, JE, Golden NH, Jacobson MS, Hertz S, and Shenker IR. The metabolic responses to starvation and refeeding in adolescents with anorexia nervosa. *Annals of New York Academy of Science* 817 (1997): 110–119.

Schmidt, U, Adan R, Böhm I, Campbell IC, Dingemans A, Ehrlich S, Elzakkers I, Favaro A, Giel K, Harrison A, Himmerich H, Hoek HW, Herpertz-Dahlmann B, Kas MJ, Seitz J, Smeets P, Sternheim L, Tenconi E, van Elburg A, van Furth E, and Zipfel S. Eating disorders: The big issue. *Lancet Psychiatry* 3, no. 4 (2016): 313–315.

Stice, E, Spoor S, and Bohon C. Relation of reward from food intake and anticipated food intake to obesity: A functional magnetic resonance imaging study. *Journal of Abnormal Psychology* 117, no. 4 (2008 Nov): 924–935.

Vaisman, N, Corey M, Rossi MF, Goldberg E, and Pencharz P. Changes in body composition during refeeding of patients with anorexia nervosa. *Journal of Pediatrics* 113, no. 5 (1988): 925–929.

Vaisman, N, Rossi MF, Corey M, Clarke R, Goldberg E, and Pencharz PB. Effect of refeeding on the energy metabolism of adolescent girls who have anorexia nervosa. *European Journal of Clinical Nutrition* 45, no. 11 (1991): 527–537.

Vaisman, N, Rossi MF, Goldberg E, Dibden LJ, Wykes LJ, and Pencharz PB. Energy expenditure and body composition in patients with anorexia nervosa. *Journal of Pediatrics* 113, no. 5 (1988): 919–924.

Van Wymelbeke, V, Brondel L, Marcel Brun J, and Rigaud D. Factors associated with the increase in resting energy expenditure during refeeding in malnourished anorexia nervosa patients. *American Journal of Clinical Nutrition* 80, no. 6 (2004): 1469–1477.

Volkow, ND, Wang GJ, Fowler JS, Tomasi D, Telang F, and Baler R. Addiction: Decreased reward sensitivity and increased expectation sensitivity conspire to overwhelm the brain's control circuit. *Bioessays* 32, no. 9 (2010): 748–755.

Yager, J, Devlin MJ, Halmi KA, Herzog DB, Mitchell JE, Powers P, and Zerbe KJ. Treatment of patients with eating disorders, third edition. American Psychiatric Association. *American Journal of Psychiatry* 163, no. S7 (2006): 4–54.

Zipfel, S, Seibel MJ, Löwe B, Beumont PJ, Kasperk C, and Herzog W. Osteoporosis in eating disorders a follow-up study of patients with anorexia and bulimia. *Journal of Clinical Endocrinology and Metabolism* 86, no. 11 (2001): 5227–5233.

4 The Treatment of Eating Disorders

Jonna Fries, PsyD and Veronica Sullivan, PhD

CONTENTS

LEARNING OBJECTIVES

After reading this chapter, the reader should be able to do the following:

- Understand the complexity of selecting individualized eating disorder treatment
- Be familiar with the empirically validated treatments for anorexia nervosa, bulimia nervosa, and binge-eating disorder
- Recognize the process used by the American Psychological Association, Division 12 and National Institute for Clinical Excellence guidelines for validating various eating disorder treatment modalities
- Explain the rationales and theoretical bases, including mechanisms of change, for a number of eating disorder treatments
- Identify some of the emerging and alternative methods of treating eating disorders

NO ONE SIZE FITS ALL

This chapter presents the most evidenced-based, foundational, and commonly practiced therapeutic approaches to anorexia nervosa (AN), bulimia nervosa (BN), and binge eating disorder (BED). In an ideal world, the treatment of eating disorders (EDs) would be the result of an incisive decision-making process. From a menu of all known options, each of them evidenced-based, therapists would carefully select an integrative plan to effectively address the ED and all comorbidities and underlying problems for each client. However, the treatment of EDs is dependent on a number of complex and fluctuating systemic limitations and individual factors including cost of research, dissemination of information about effective treatments, training availability to therapists, cost of training therapists, symptom presentation and changes in symptoms, insurance restrictions or being uninsured, cost of treatments, inpatient or outpatient settings, session limits at specific sites, cooperation of others with treatment recommendations (in group and in family modalities), translation of treatment from manualized research protocols to primary care settings, and client preferences. Recovery is, in turn, dependent on these and more factors including age, diagnosis, genetics and neurophysiology, symptoms and changes in symptoms, motivation, finances, time available to focus on treatment, and more. The complexities of these moving parts make the treatment of EDs a challenge even for the most experienced and heavily resourced therapists.

Eating disorders are typically treated in an eclectic or integrated manner (see Appendix 4.1 for an example of an integrative thought record). Eclectic refers to the astute selection of a theoretically based intervention, implemented to address a specific problem maintaining the disorder, regardless of the overarching theoretical orientation of the provider. Integration is an organic combination of one's collective knowledge that results in a new and unique approach (Goldenberg and Goldenberg 2013). It was found that 40% of community therapists used intentionally integrated approaches or identified as eclectic practitioners (Thompson-Brenner and Westen 2005). As an example of eclectic and multidisciplinary treatment with long-lasting reduction of ED symptoms, Rogers Memorial Hospital's Residential Eating Disorders Center conducted a study on males with EDs. They implemented effective treatments that included cognitive-behavioral (CBT), interpersonal, psychodynamic, experiential, educational, pharmacological, nutritional, and family therapies to target different aspects of EDs (Weltzin et al. 2007).

While this chapter broadly reviews a number of strongly empirically validated treatment approaches including CBT, interpersonal psychotherapy (IPT), and family-based therapy (FBT) or Maudsley therapy, it also covers other treatment approaches that have less empirical validation yet are frequently used by treatment providers including dialectical behavior therapy (DBT), psychodynamic approaches, as well as group therapy. Emerging and alternative treatments for EDs are also discussed since many therapists and treatment centers are now eclectically implementing a newer generation of treatments such as EMDR, Somatic Experiencing, equine therapy, neurofeedback, yoga, and use of technology and social media, with innovative treatments continuously emerging.

It is important to note that in addressing EDs, there are many aspects of recovery to consider including ability to function at work or in school, quality of relationships, perceptions of and relationship with self and one's body, and physical health including weight gain or loss. Improvements in one area are not necessarily matched in other domains, and generous time allotted to the process of recovery is often essential. An average length of treatment before recovery has been found in one community study to be 6 months (Thompson-Brenner et al. 2010) though the range may vary considerably based on the numerous factors noted above.

EMPIRICALLY VALIDATED TREATMENTS

One might ask, why even consider treatments that are not evidenced based? Carolyn Costin, an internationally renowned expert in the field of EDs addressed this in a conversation with one of the authors (Costin 2012). Costin considers it imperative to be steeped in evidenced-based treatments (EBTs) such as CBT and DBT, particularly for symptom abatement, and considers IPT and psychodynamic approaches pragmatic in resolving the underlying issues that maintain the ED, a key factor in preventing relapse. Being strongly grounded in these EBTs, including FBT in the treatment of anorexia, allows for the resolution of many symptoms, particularly if a client has not previously been exposed to the approach, or if the approach has not yet been given a fair trial. However, it is well known that there are many treatment-resistant ED cases, and that many clients have been through several trials of evidenced-based approaches that have not resolved symptoms. Costin considers adjunctive therapies, such as EMDR for trauma, mindfulness training, and art, dance, psychodrama, and somatic therapies as important aspects of treatment and recovery. In another example of the use of adjunctive therapies, Jeanne Rust, founder and CEO of an ED treatment center, includes neuro feedback, somatic therapies, and the Emotional Freedom Technique in the successful treatment of EDs (Rust and Beck 2012).

It is advised that treatment providers refrain from the assumption that untested interventions are ineffective. Interventions that have not been evaluated with scientific rigor may still be effective (American Psychological Association Presidential

Task Force on Evidence-Based Practice 2006; Kazdin 2008). Not all psychologists agree on which treatments are supported by research and many acknowledge that there is a healthy debate regarding the definition of research support and which treatments are empirically validated (Beutler 1998; Norcross 1999; Spring et al. 2005; Wampold 2001).

One cause for concern in evaluating the effectiveness of empirically validated treatments of EDs is dropout rates in controlled studies. Randomized controlled trials include many safeguards that make them the most widely accepted practice of testing interventions. In the treatment of EDs, attrition, or dropout, rates are very high. The results of randomized controlled trials typically do not fully address the reason for attrition. Attrition in different phases of treatment tends to be attributed to different causes. Early dropout may be related to individual psychopathology, no improvement with treatment, or perception that the treatment is too difficult. Dropout after treatment and before follow-up is sometimes attributed to relapse and subsequent shame. Attrition rates in ED trials have been reported as ranging from 0% to 78.6%, thus making it difficult to determine if the treatment would be considered effective had those who dropped out remained in the study. However, these difficulties are typically not factored into reported results (Stein et al. 2011).

TREATMENT GUIDANCE

Those in the business of primarily treating EDs will be familiar with these important resources guiding treatment: The APA's Division 12 Presidential Task Force on Evidence-Based Practice (American Psychological Association Presidential Task Force on Evidence-Based Practice 2006) along with APA's Division 12 website (American Psychological Association, Division 12 2016), and the National Institute for Health and Care Excellence (NICE) guidelines (National Collaborating Centre for Mental Health 2004).

In an effort to support evidenced-based psychological treatment, APA Division 12 formed the Task Force on Promotion and Dissemination of Psychological Procedures to establish and promote empirically supported treatments (ESTs) (American Psychological Association Presidential Task Force on Evidence-Based Practice 2006). The sought-after label of "empirically supported" is bestowed after a rigorous process of research that provides evidence that the treatment is efficacious, meaning it has significant results in a research setting, and also effective, meaning it has significant results in settings outside a well-controlled research environment.

APA Division 12 labels a treatment as having strong research support if it meets criteria for *well-established treatment*, meaning a number of well-designed studies conducted by independent investigators similarly supported a treatment's efficacy (Chambless and Hollon 1998). APA Division 12 labels a treatment as having modest research support if it were to meet Chambless et al.'s criteria for *probably efficacious treatment*, meaning one well-designed or two or more adequately designed studies support a treatment's efficacy. Treatments labeled as having strong or modest research support must also be found to be efficacious in randomized control trials. Therapies recommended by APA Division 12 for AN are FBT and CBT; for

BN are CBT, IPT, FBT, and the Healthy-Weight Program; and for BED, cognitive-behavioral therapy adapted for bulimia nervosa (CBT-BN) and IPT, as illustrated in Table 4.1.

The NICE guidelines score treatments based on quality of care and value for resources spent on treatments (National Collaborating Centre for Mental Health 2004). Approaches are given a score of A, B, or C depending on the level of evidence with A representing the most rigorous evidence and C representing less rigorous evidence. Treatments that are assigned a grade of A are limited to the gold standard in mental health treatment research; that is, either at least one randomized controlled trial that shows good quality and consistency in addressing the stated problem, or a meta-analysis of randomized controlled trials with similarly stringent standards of quality and consistency in addressing the treatment problem. Treatments that area assigned a grade of B include well-designed trials without randomization or a well-designed quasi-experimental design. Also assigned a grade of B are correlation studies, comparative studies, retroactive, or descriptive studies. Treatments assigned a

TABLE 4.1
Empirically Validated Treatments According to APA Division 12 Guidelines

Eating Disorder	Empirically Validated Psychological Treatments and Other Psychological Treatment Recommendations	Strong Research Support	Modest Research Support	Controversial Research Support
Anorexia Nervosa	Cognitive-behavioral therapy	–	X (for posthospitalization relapse prevention)	X (for acute weight gain)
	Family-based treatment	X (for adolescents)	–	–
Bulimia Nervosa	Cognitive-behavioral therapy	X	–	–
	Interpersonal psychotherapy	X	–	–
	Family-based treatment	–	X	–
	Healthy-Weight Program	–	–	X
Binge-Eating Disorder	Cognitive-behavioral therapy	X	–	–
	Interpersonal psychotherapy	X	–	–

grade of C include those based on expert opinion or committee reports, or therapies extrapolated from A or B studies. C grades indicate that good quality studies are absent or not easily available. Therapies recommended by NICE for AN are cognitive analytic, CBT, IPT, family interventions, and focal psychodynamic, all with a grade of C; for BN, the therapies recommended are evidenced based self-help with a grade of B, CBT-BN with a grade of A, and, as an alternative to CBT, IPT with a grade of B; and recommended for BED, evidence-based self-help with a grade of B, CBT-BN with a grade of A, and, for persistent BED, IPT, or DBT, both with a grade of B, as illustrated in Table 4.2 (National Collaborating Centre for Mental Health 2004).

TABLE 4.2

Empirically Validated Psychological Interventions According to National Institute for Clinical Excellence

Eating Disorder	Empirically Validated Psychological Treatments and Other Psychological Treatment Recommendations	Grade A	Grade B	Grade B
Anorexia Nervosa	Cognitive-analytic therapy Cognitive-behavioral therapy	–	–	X
	Focal dynamic therapy	–	–	X
	Family interventions	–	–	X
		–	–	X(focused on ED explicitly)
	Consider therapist and patient preferences	–	–	X
Bulimia Nervosa	Evidence based self-help program	–	X(offer professional support toward patient's self-help program	–
	Interpersonal psychotherapy	–	X(as an alternative to CBT; inform patients that results will likely take 8–12 months)	–
	Cognitive-behavioral therapy for bulimia nervosa	X(for adults with BN; 16–20 sessions for 4–5 months)	–	–
	Treatments other than CBT	–	X(offer when patients do not respond to CBT or do not want CBT)	–

(Continued)

TABLE 4.2 (CONTINUED)
Empirically Validated Psychological Interventions According to National Institute for Clinical Excellence

Eating Disorder	Empirically Validated Psychological Treatments and Other Psychological Treatment Recommendations	Grade A	Grade B	Grade B
Binge-Eating Disorder	Evidence based self-help program	–	X	–
	Cognitive-behavioral therapy adapted for BED	X(for adults)	–	–
	Interpersonal psychotherapy			
	Dialectical behavior therapy	–	X(for adults with persistent BED)	–
	Inform patients that psychological interventions have limited effect on body weight	–	X(for adults with persistent BED)	–
		X	–	–

COGNITIVE-BEHAVIORAL THERAPY (CBT)

CBT is an empirically validated treatment for both BN and BED, with modest support for post-hospitalization relapse prevention for AN (American Psychological Association, Division 12 1995; Chambless and Hollon 1998). Perhaps it is not surprising that CBT is an empirically validated treatment given that "eating disorders are essentially 'cognitive disorders'" and that they "share a distinctive 'core psychopathology' that is cognitive in nature" (Fairburn 2008). CBT is often thought to be the benchmark for ED treatment both because of its effectiveness and because it tends to work quickly when compared to other treatment protocols (Fairburn et al. 2015; Poulsen et al. 2014; Zipfel et al. 2014). An enhanced version of CBT, known as CBT-E, has recently emerged. It aims to be transdiagnostic in its scope as an emerging treatment for BN, AN, BED and what was formerly referred to as eating disorder not otherwise specified (EDNOS) and is now known as other specified feeding and eating disorder (OSFED; Zipfel et al. 2014; Fairburn et al. 2003; American Psychiatric Association 2013).

COGNITIVE-BEHAVIORAL THERAPY ADAPTED FOR BULIMIA NERVOSA

Cognitive-Behavioral Therapy-Bulimia Nervosa was first described in 1981 (Fairburn 1981); since then, manual-based CBT-BN has become the gold standard empirically validated treatment for BN (Fairburn et al. 1993). Individual CBT-BN treatment typically lasts for 16–20 weekly sessions over 4–5 months and aims to address cognitive distortions about body shape and weight and replace dysfunctional rule-based dieting with regular, flexible eating behaviors. There are three phases of treatment: phase one goals are to adopt a plan of regular eating; phase two goals are related to overall moderation of food intake without restrictive rules and modification of maladaptive thought patterns that perpetuate the ED; and phase three goals are consolidation of learning and relapse prevention planning (Fairburn et al. 1993). CBT-BN has been shown to be more effective than antidepressants in producing complete cessation of binge eating and purging, with total elimination of these behaviors in roughly 30%–50% of all treatment cases (Wilson et al. 2007).

COGNITIVE-BEHAVIORAL THERAPY FOR BINGE EATING DISORDER

While there are significantly fewer clinical studies on the treatment of BED compared to BN, CBT is also considered the recommended treatment for BED, with recommendations from both the APA Task Force (American Psychological Association Presidential Task Force on Evidence-Based Practice 2006) and a grade of A from NICE (National Collaborating Centre for Mental Health 2004). While this version of CBT for BED is slightly longer (22 sessions in 24 weeks) than that for BN, the treatment is identical. CBT adapted for BED follows the same model and structure of the manualized treatment for CBT-BN by Fairburn and colleagues (National Collaborating Centre for Mental Health 2004), with the recognition that sufferers of BED tend to have far less restrictive eating than those with BN (Masheb and Grilo 2000), and are thus far more likely to be overweight or obese. CBT has been selected as an empirically validated treatment for BED due to its relatively high remission rate, with over 50% of treatment cases in remission from binge eating at the end of treatment and significant improvement in BED core symptoms and associated psychopathology even when studied at 4 years posttreatment (Wilson et al. 2007; Fischer et al. 2014).

COGNITIVE-BEHAVIORAL THERAPY FOR ANOREXIA

While CBT is the most frequently tested individual treatment for AN, results have been inconclusive, partially due to a lack of standardization as well as attrition in study samples, an all too common challenge to identifying EBTs for AN (Fischer et al. 2014). However, a recent review of 16 studies concluded that AN patients treated with various formats of CBT do tend to show improvement on physical and psychological outcomes overall (Galsworthy-Francis and Allan 2014). Though CBT for AN did not appear to be superior to other types of treatment on key outcome measures such as body mass index (BMI), ED symptoms, and broader psychopathology, it did show promise in reducing dropout rates compared to other treatments..

The initial CBT treatment framework for AN was originally described by Garner and Vitousek (Garner and Bemis 1982, 1985) and shares many of the same features of the treatment for BN as originally outlined by Fairburn (1985). The main difference in working with patients with AN is the need to address motivational differences as well as immediacy of health risks associated with semistarvation and need for weight gain (Garner et al. 1997). Typically, individual CBT treatment for anorexia is fairly long term with 1–2 years of treatment recommended for patients who begin treatment at low weight and approximately 1 year for those who are weight restored.

COGNITIVE-BEHAVIORAL THERAPY-ENHANCED: A TRANSDIAGNOSTIC TREATMENT

Recently, CBT-E (Fairburn 2008; Fairburn et al. 2003) has been introduced in which a single treatment aims to be suitable across EDs. This was created based on the fact that about half of the individuals who present for treatment fail to meet full criteria for AN or BN and thus received the diagnosis of EDNOS or OSFED. As a subclinical category, the diagnosis of OSFED may convey a less severe presentation of an ED but this should not be assumed Furthermore, symptom presentation often shifts, with approximately half of those with AN experiencing a shift to BN or OSFED, and a number of BN patients shifting to OSFED in absence of full remission. Prior to the emergence of CBT-E, there was no recommended treatment for OSFED.

CBT-E was developed based on the notion that all EDs share a similar basis of psychopathology; therefore, CBT-E is a treatment for transdiagnostic ED psychopathology rather than any specific ED diagnosis, and can be used to treat OSFED as well as AN and BN (and presumably BED) by tailoring the treatment for each unique individual (Fairburn et al. 2003). Cooper and Fairburn (2011) proposed that in addition to maladaptive core processes (i.e., thought and behavior patterns developed in response to challenging life events) maintaining ED pathology, there are four additional maintaining mechanisms that in certain patients prevent change. These include clinical perfectionism, mood intolerance, core low self-esteem, and interpersonal difficulties.

There are various forms of CBT-E: the focused version (CBT-Ef) is considered the default treatment and concentrates on core ED psychopathology; it is suitable for the majority of patients and also incorporates addressing mood intolerance. The broad version (CBT-Eb) has additional treatment modules that address clinical perfectionism, core low self-esteem, and interpersonal difficulties. There are also two intensities, with a 20-session version for patients with a BMI over 17.5 and a more intensive 40-session version for patients who are underweight (BMI between 15.0 and 17.5), as well as versions for patients under age 18 and a group version (see Fairburn, 2008 for full treatment details). Though further research is needed to determine the efficacy of CBT-E across various treatment populations, preliminary evidence by the developer has been promising (Fairburn et al. 2009, 2015). It is important to note that while CBT-E is a comprehensive treatment to address the commonly experienced cognitive underpinnings of EDs, many will require a treatment team including a physician and a nutritionist to provide the best possible care.

FAMILY-BASED THERAPY (FBT): THE MAUDSLEY METHOD

One of the first pioneers to include families in the treatment of EDs was Salvador Minuchin, who believed that individual behavior change could be made by addressing dysfunctional family patterns (Minuchin et al. 1978). Modeled after Minuchin's work, Dare and colleagues developed what is still commonly referred to as the Maudsley method or Maudsley approach at the Maudsley Hospital in London in the 1980s (Dare 1985). This method was then manualized for treatment of AN in 2001 by Lock and colleagues who named it *family-based treatment* (Lock et al. 2001). Today the names are often used interchangeably. By manualizing the FBT approach, it could be more consistently studied across varying treatment sites and with diverse populations.

Research indicates that FBT is the most promising treatment for adolescents with AN (Bulik et al. 2007; Hurst et al. 2012; Treasure et al. 2010). Unfortunately, little research exists examining the Maudsley model in adults with AN, though encouraging results from a recent study suggests that MANTRA (Maudsley Model for Treatment of Adults with Anorexia Nervosa), a new outpatient treatment for adults with AN, may be worth further investigation (Wade et al. 2011). Also, very little research on FBT for BN in adolescents has been published and the few publications have been contradictory, suggesting more research is needed to determine if this may also be an effective treatment for BN (Lock 2011). One recent study suggested that FBT may have promising effects among adolescents with bulimia, demonstrating that FBT was superior to CBT for adolescents with BN in promoting abstinence from binge eating and purging at a 6-month follow-up and comparable to CBT at 12-month follow-up (Le Grange et al. 2015). A meta-analysis examining the efficacy of FBT compared to individual therapy for adolescents with either AN or BN suggested that FBT was not significantly different than individual therapy at end of treatment, but was superior when follow-up data at 6–12 months was analyzed (Couturier et al. 2013). However, only three studies were included in the meta-analysis given strict inclusion criteria. No studies have examined the use of FBT with BED to the authors' knowledge, which is likely due to the relatively new clinical recognition of this disorder.

Family based therapy is unique in that it considers the family unit a key component in the patient's recovery. It incorporates a number of different family therapy approaches including Milan systemic, strategic, structural, and narrative therapy (Lock et al. 2001). FBT is an intensive outpatient treatment that is conducted in three phases, generally within 20–24 treatment sessions over a period of approximately 12 months.

In Phase 1 of treatment, which generally lasts for 10 weeks, the goal is weight restoration and a return to normal eating patterns. This phase is intended to replicate the initial phase of treatment in inpatient settings and the therapist works closely with parents to help the patient restore weight through refeeding and limits on physical activity (Lock et al. 2001). Eating-disordered behavior is viewed as external to the patient and thus outside of their control. In FBT's initial stages, the parents actively take control of the patient's (usually an adolescent) eating-disordered behaviors. A family meal is held in the presence of the therapist so that he or she may observe typical family eating patterns and assist the parents in most effectively encouraging the weight-restoration process; parents are coached to support rather than criticize the patient throughout this process. Psychoeducation about the dangers of malnutrition is also provided during this first phase. The aim of Phase 2 is negotiating a new pattern of family relationships. This begins when the patient accepts the family's support and takes in increased food intake without conflict which leads to a steady weight gain. During this phase, parents are encouraged to give some of the control back to the patient, for example, allowing them to have more autonomy over what he or she eats. Parents may allow some meals to be unsupervised and may have less control over the patient's activities. Therapy sessions continue to address working toward a healthy weight and overall reduction in ED symptoms (Lock et al. 2001). Phase 2 typically lasts for 7 weeks.

Phase 3, which typically lasts about 3 weeks, focuses on establishing healthy adolescent identity and also addresses termination. This phase begins when the patient is able to maintain weight above 95% of ideal weight and is able to refrain from restricting in multiple settings (e.g., while outside of the family home; Lock et al. 2001; Treasure et al. 2007). Treatment addresses the effect that the ED has had on the adolescent's development and aims to restore healthy adolescent identity. Both the therapist and the family support the adolescent in gaining greater independence while establishing healthy boundaries within the family. Termination issues are also addressed as the entire family reflects on their progress through treatment and prepares to handle future problems without the therapist's guidance.

Hurst et al. (2012) identified a number of challenges they have encountered as counselors working with this treatment model. The first challenge they have observed has been fatigue for the family, given the serious nature of AN, and the typically extensive length of the illness. The authors of the study recommend that therapists validate these feelings while balancing the need for parents to stay motivated and hopeful.

The second challenge acknowledged is when older adolescents have already begun moving toward individuation prior to the onset of AN; in most cases, the adolescent then regresses developmentally, which may be confusing as both the child and the parents renegotiate their roles. In this case, Hurst et al. (2012) recommend the counselor remind parents that this is only a temporary change in roles, and that the previous developmental course will resume in later phases of treatment.

The third challenge named by Hurst et al. (2012), and perhaps the most difficult, is the struggle when there is slow or no weight gain during Phase 1. It is essential that the therapist work with the family to develop hypotheses for why this may be occurring. Due to the secretive and covert behaviors often used by anorexic patients who may be resistant to recovery, the family may need to take a more active role to detect and prevent these behaviors.

In the fourth challenge, the authors assert that Maudsley treatment can be challenging with single-parent families, resulting in increase in parental burnout and extension of time needed in treatment. The therapist should be mindful about taking on a co-parenting role and should aim to help the single parent bring in additional support from other friends or family members during this difficult process (Hurst et al. 2012).

INTERPERSONAL PSYCHOTHERAPY

Initially developed as a time-limited treatment for depression, IPT has been shown to be efficacious in addressing many disorders that are accompanied by depressive symptoms. Manualized in 1984, it has been extensively tested by the National Institute of Mental Health. IPT is recommended by NICE (National Collaborating Centre for Mental Health 2004) for AN with a grade of C, for BN with a grade of B, and for persistent BED with a grade of B (see Birchall 1999 for an excellent review). It is considered an empirically validated treatment with strong research support for both BN and BED by APA Division 12.

Interpersonal psychotherapy was modified for those with BN from IPT's original protocol for depression. CBT interventions were carefully removed in order to make comparisons to CBT in a clinical trial. Interpersonal psychotherapy was found to result in similar improvements as CBT in follow-up measures; however, CBT alleviated BN symptoms more rapidly than the modified version of IPT, resulting in less favorable short-term outcomes for IPT. Thus, some cognitive and psychoeducational interventions have been reinserted into IPT for its use for BN (IPT-BN), resulting in shorter term improvements (Arcelus et al. 2009).

The NICE guidelines consider IPT-BN an alternative to CBT for BN, but caution that recovery may take longer, typically 8–12 months (National Collaborating Centre for Mental Health 2004). A benefit of IPT-BN is that it can be easily taught to competent therapists (Tanofsky-Kraff et al. 2010). Interpersonal psychotherapy has been shown to be effective for reducing binge episodes in obese adults and for weight maintenance in adolescent girls at high risk of weight increase, and therefore has been found to be an effective treatment for those with BED in addition to BN (Wilfley et al. 2002). It was found that some patients with more severe self-esteem deficits had more difficulty improving with IPT. In these cases it is suggested that increased attention be paid to improving selfesteem and the more rigidly held dysfunctional beliefs related to body image (Arcelus et al. 2009).

IPT-BN is implemented in 45-minute sessions held once weekly for 12–16 weeks, with a beginning, middle, and end stage. Initially, the therapist assesses relationship patterns, satisfaction in the interpersonal arena, capacity for intimacy, and the issues involved in current relationships. The therapist's task is to identify and focus on the interpersonal difficulties that contribute to the maintenance of the BN, and to provide psychoeducation about the ED, diet, and comorbid disorders. A food journal may be used to gain insight into the relationship between interpersonal issues and food-related behaviors and cognitions. Through this process, one of the following four overarching interpersonal contexts emerges as the focus of treatment: interpersonal role disputes in which the client is struggling with a significant other, interpersonal role transitions in which the client is experiencing a major life change, complicated bereavement, or interpersonal deficits, which is a classification meant to capture interpersonal struggles that do not neatly fall into the three other types (e.g., interpersonal sensitivity). The categorical goals of the four treatment foci are, respectively, addressing an interpersonal dispute, resolving problems associated with transitioning into a new role, mourning the loss of a significant person, and improving social efficacy. The therapist elicits the patient's agreement on the treatment focus. Throughout treatment, the therapist links symptoms to the interpersonal focus and thereby destigmatizes the symptoms, in part by assigning the sick role to the patient, a designation that instills a container for the illness, and motivates the patient to move out of the sick role.

The designated area of focus is worked through in the middle sessions. In all four categories, the therapist tracks interpersonal issues arising in the therapeutic dyad and intervenes with clarification and exploration, provides interpersonal skills including expression of emotion, teaches communication analysis techniques and skills, and encourages appropriate social risk taking.

In the end stage, the therapist reviews treatment progress and skill acquisition with the patient and encourages the patient to take on an increasingly autonomous role in implementing skills. Termination is processed as an interpersonal event as a model for direct and meaningful interpersonal process, drawing attention to the complex issues that are embedded in relationships and endings. IPT therapy may be titrated in the end phase with monthly check-ins tapering off to biannual or as needed sessions. The time limited frame is thought to inspire the client to progress (Arcelus et al. 2009; Markowitz and Weissman 2012).

PSYCHODYNAMIC PSYCHOTHERAPY

Psychodynamic psychotherapy for EDs is practiced widely in the community, with brief treatments lasting as little as 6 weeks to open-ended treatment, with an average session number falling between 25 and 30 over the course of a year (Thompson-Brenner and Westen 2010). Psychodynamic psychotherapy is usually accomplished in less frequent meetings than psychoanalysis, meeting one to two times per week. Psychodynamic psychotherapy is said to have several features that may distinguish it from other therapies. Self-exploration is a goal of psychodynamic psychotherapies, and this endeavor is often worked through using the therapeutic relationship between the therapist and client as a reflection of the client's intrapsychic patterns. Throughout therapy, the therapist calls attention to the client's defenses. Psychodynamic psychotherapy is typically unstructured; it seeks to identify recurrent themes, tracks connections between feelings and perceptions to past experiences, and makes salient the emotions considered by the client to be unacceptable (Shedler 2010).

Blagys and Hilsenroth (2000) distinguished foci of psychodynamic psychotherapies as compared with CBT. In psychodynamic treatment, and generally not a primary focus in CBT, there is a focus on affect and emotional expression. Therapists guide clients in exploring avoidance or behaviors interfering with therapy goals. Treatment aims to uncover the impact of past relationships on behavioral, cognitive, emotional, experiential, relational patterns, and interpersonal experiences while placing an emphasis on the therapeutic relationship. Throughout, therapists continue to discuss wishes, dreams, or fantasies.

FOCAL PSYCHODYNAMIC PSYCHOTHERAPY

Focal psychodynamic psychotherapy, a specific type of psychodynamic psychotherapy recommended by NICE with a grade C for those with AN (National Collaborating Centre for Mental Health 2004) is nondirective and time limited (1 year with weekly sessions). Therapists refrain from giving advice about eating behaviors, but instead, discuss the meaning of these symptoms in the context of the client's personal and family history and the impact of the symptoms on current relationships. Like most dynamic therapies, focal psychodynamic focuses on the client's relationship with the therapist and, like many approaches to resolving EDs, focal psychodynamic makes salient the manner in which symptoms interfere with treatment progress (Dare et al. 2001).

COGNITIVE-ANALYTIC THERAPY

Cognitive analytic therapy, also recommended by NICE with a grade C for those with AN (National Collaborating Centre for Mental Health 2004), is a blend of cognitive therapy and psychoanalytic psychotherapy. Target problems are identified, along with the target problematic procedures that maintain the negative affect, symptoms, interpersonal difficulties, negative body image, and so on. Similarly, reciprocal roles and reciprocal-role procedures explore the influence of early relational experiences on current relationship with self and other. Clients are guided in a project of diagramming these evolving experiences of self and anorexia. The relationship between the therapist and the client, as well as the client's family and significant other relationships are explored. Collaboratively bringing to the client's awareness the internalization of meaningful social experiences, and the articulation of these in therapy, serves to enhance the client's capacity for understanding self in relation to others. The therapist functions in a reparative relational role, while refraining from colluding with the AN (Bell 1999; Dare et al. 2001; Ryle and Kerr 2003).

EFFICACY OF PSYCHODYNAMIC PSYCHOTHERAPIES FOR EDS

Few studies have been conducted to measure the efficacy of psychodynamic psychotherapy implemented in the treatment of EDs. Generally, research has shown psychodynamic psychotherapies have been found to have similar effect sizes as other EBTs (Shedler 2010). Fonagy et al. (2005) reviewed brief psychodynamic psychotherapy treatment studies and concluded that it was found to be as effective as strategic family therapy and behavioral therapy for those with anorexia, with less favorable outcomes for bulimia.

As previously discussed, integration of therapies is thought to strengthen treatment by simultaneously targeting multiple aspects of a disorder. Psychodynamic therapy, when combined with behavioral strategies, was found in one study of those with BN and BED, to be as effective as CBT and more effective than IPT in rapidity of symptom relief (Murphy et al. 2005). Similarly, Heenan (2005) recommends combining CBT interventions along with feminist psychodynamic work for those diagnosed with OSFED.

PSYCHODYNAMIC TREATMENT OF EDS: IN THE TREATMENT ROOM

At times, it may appear that psychodynamic theory and delivery of interventions are so tightly woven that they appear to be one and the same. Silver and White (2011), respectively, a psychoanalyst and patient, co-wrote an article describing Silver's analytic treatment of White's AN psychosis, integrating theory, treatment, and patient experiences, with the patient as astute a theorist as the analyst. In the dynamic conceptualization of body and mind, there is great entanglement as well. Orbach (1978), a psychoanalytic practitioner who greatly influenced a generation of consumers and practitioners in the conceptualization and treatment of body image, considered overeating as an attempt to meet one's emotional needs through the vehicles of food and body image, and as a means of expressing the inexpressible. Women who overeat, Orbach theorizes, express a desire to rebel against the demand to be seen as the perfect female, reject the cultural ideal of vanity, regain power through avoiding sexual objectification, replenish the consistently emptying maternal supply of emotional strength, avoid being placed in competition, and draw on food and fat to assist in individuating (Orbach 1978). People who overeat may also take pleasure in the autonomous power to reject or accept objects, and this may occur in the arena of food and body image (Heenan 2005). Heenan conceptualizes that in those with EDs, the body mediates between the conscious and unconscious minds and that this takes place within two worlds: the internal and the interpersonal. The identification of these dynamic processes in therapy is a goal of therapy.

COMMUNICATING THROUGH FOOD BEHAVIORS

Much of the focus of psychodynamic therapies in the treatment of EDs is on the symbolic communication of the unacceptable through food behaviors and via the body, rather than using the symbols of verbal language to communicate. The process of eating is considered an introjection of the representation of the past relationship between the client as an infant and the primary caregiver. Drawing from object relations theory, food is connected symbolically and physiologically to the mother; thus, food becomes a transitional object that is readily available. In navigating the developmental task of individuation, one projects feelings about self and other onto transitional objects such as food; this is in an attempt to manage one's feelings, impulses, wishes, and fantasies. This process may be used maladaptively when the mother is unavailable emotionally, energetically, or physically, and the client uses food to communicate loss, rage, or disappointment. A goal of treatment, from this perspective, is to make salient these hidden conflicting motivators and to work toward acceptance of their existence (Sugarman 1991).

COMMUNICATING THROUGH THE BODY

One who has BN may be thought of as unable to communicate verbally one's needs, wishes, and affect, and thus communicates somatically. Complicating adaptive maturation during adolescence is a problematic relationship with the primary caregiver, typically the mother. Rebelling or conforming to what one unconsciously believes is the mother's imagined ideal body, the adolescent expresses somatically an anxious attempt to reject or to adhere to the mother's ideal. The body is thought of as separate from self so that needs, wishes, and affect are not communicated as representational of an integrated whole self. Instead, that which seems unacceptable is communicated somatically, outside of one's awareness. In psychodynamic treatment, a value held is for verbal and insightful, rather than somatic and unconscious, communication. In treatment, the gradual reduction of difference between ideal and actual-unacceptable somatic self-representation leads to more authentic self-representation.

DIALECTICAL BEHAVIOR THERAPY (DBT)

Dialectical behavioral therapy was initially developed by Marsha Linehan for difficult to treat, suicidal patients with borderline personality disorder and other comorbidities in response to obstacles experienced when treating this population with CBT. This challenging population is known to display behaviors both in session and outside of sessions that interfere with treatment success, and DBT was designed to directly intervene on these barriers. The obstacles included suicidality, chaotic and threatening behaviors, severely unregulated emotions, and the necessity to address these in order to teach distress tolerance and behavioral skills. The use of DBT has since been broadened to use with a variety of populations and disorders, including EDs, and has been found to be particularly effective with those who engage in binge eating. DBT modified for those with persistent BED has been awarded a B grade by NICE (National Collaborating Centre for Mental Health 2004).

A recent meta-analysis of eight studies examined to what degree DBT is effective in reducing frequency of ED episodes (Lenz et al. 2014). Both between-groups and single-group studies demonstrated large effect sizes suggesting that DBT may be efficacious in reducing episodes among women diagnosed with EDs. In another study, it was found that DBT skills allowed participants to resist the urge to binge when experiencing distressing emotions. In an initial uncontrolled study of those with BED, DBT (adapted for BED) was effective in retaining all participants and in 82% of participants, binge eating was absent at the end of treatment. In a later controlled study (DBT adapted for BED vs. waitlist), 90% were abstinent from binge eating at the end of the study. Researchers suggested that DBT might be a better treatment choice for those with BED with higher levels of negative affect while CBT might be a better choice for those with higher levels of dietary restraint (Telch et al. 2001).

THEORETICAL CONSTRUCTS OF DBT

Underlying principles of DBT include dialectics (defined below), a balance of behavioral theory, and Zen eastern philosophies of acceptance, presence, and mindfulness, as well as validating clients' experiences and teaching the client to validate self. Mindfulness is concerned with cultivating the ability to maintain a nonjudgmental awareness of self, other, and world in the present moment. The term dialectical is explained as reasoning that seeks to resolve the conflict of two contradictory ideas. The dialectic in DBT focuses on resolving the conflict between acceptance of self and the desire or need to change; that is, the Zen practice of acceptance of current circumstantial and internal difficulties and the simultaneous behavioral goal of change. This conflict is understood to be the primary difficulty when treating this challenging population with CBT. In CBT treatment with this population, it was found that clients became enraged or otherwise emotionally dysregulated when faced with a treatment that primarily focuses on change.

Through a balanced view of acceptance and change, DBT's dialectics offers a theoretical grounding and process for mediating the client's commonly occurring dysregulated emotional and behavioral reaction to the goal of change. This may be accomplished in session by consistently moving toward change while interjecting an acknowledgment of challenges; this provides the scaffolding for the client to accept the current state of challenges, and it is validating, which allows the client to develop a positive and continuously adaptive self-concept, both of which support the client in moving past barriers to change.

There is an acknowledgment and integration of emotional thinking and rational thinking, leading to Wise Mind, a DBT construct, which may be understood as inner wisdom. DBT is based on the assumption that the most important etiological factor in the development of borderline personality disorder is the impact of an invalidating environment on a child who is biologically predisposed to impulsivity, sensitivity, emotional reactivity, and who has difficulty in regulating emotions. When the child becomes emotional, rather than receiving a validating response from caregivers, the child receives communication invalidating an internal experience. The child does not learn to manage distressing emotions or the factors contributing to and conse- quent to these emotions. Experiencing their environment as invalidating is common for those with EDs.

Assumptions Regarding Clients and Therapists in DBT

There are several assumptions about clients that are made in DBT, including that clients are doing as well as they can, that they want to improve, that they must learn new behaviors, that they can succeed in treatment, that they need to be in a process of problem resolution regardless of how the difficulty was initiated, that there is room for improvement, and that, for some, life is unbearable without change. Assumptions are also drawn regarding DBT counselors including that helping clients change is a compassionate and kind endeavor, that counselors must be clear and precise, that the therapeutic relationship is egalitarian, that counselors and clients are both chal- lenged by universal principles, that counselors need support in their work, that coun- selors can fail, and that DBT can fail.

Stages and Modalities of DBT Treatment

DBT includes four stages of treatment. Stage I addresses severe and complex prob- lems, focusing on reduction of suicidal or other life-threatening behaviors, behaviors that interfere with therapy, and behaviors that severely and negatively impact qual- ity of life. Stage II helps the client experience emotions without the internalized invalidating and hence traumatizing response. Stage III deepens insights gained and increases the client's sense of connectedness while continuing to address problems in living, which serve as obstacles to well-being. To increase the client's capacity for joy and sense of freedom, Stage IV addresses a common end-stage of treatment perception of incompleteness.

DBT is conducted in multiple modalities including individual psychotherapy, skill training groups, coaching by telephone, and use of a therapist consultation team. The therapy is structured to achieve the client's goals. Clients are taught emotion regulation skills, skills to reduce maladaptive emotional responses, and dysfunctional impulsivity. They are taught how to self-soothe and to survive crises resiliently. Clients are also taught assertiveness skills that are consistent with maintaining relationships while also cultivating self-respect (Neacsiu et al. 2012).

GROUP TREATMENT

While not an empirically validated treatment according to APA Division 12 or NICE Guidelines, group therapy is commonly used in ED treatment and can be quite beneficial. Many of the therapeutic factors of group therapy, such as instillation of hope, developing social skills, imparting of information, cohesion, and catharsis (Yalom 1995) may be particularly helpful in this population because of the social isolation, distorted thinking, and feelings of uniqueness that eating-disordered patients often experience. While group treatment has been found to be efficacious with both BN and BED patients, there is a lack of empirical data to support the efficacy of group treatment with AN patients. In fact, "treatment studies since the 1980s have focused almost exclusively on bulimic patients" (Polivy and Federoff 1997). Therefore, while group treatment can be recommended for both BN and BED, the benefits of group treatment for clients with AN are more uncertain.

The majority of studies on group therapy have been done with patients with BN, and consensus across studies shows that there is no advantage of individual treatment over group treatment for BN, both having about a 40% posttherapy abstinence rate (Nevonen and Broberg 2006; Polivy and Federoff 1997; Tasca and Bone 2007). A meta-analysis of 40 studies of group therapy for BN suggests a moderate effect size of +0.75 at posttreatment suggesting that group therapy is a beneficial treatment modality for EDs (Fettes and Peters 1992). Group therapy has also been found to be effective in reducing binge eating in those with BED (Hepworth 2011; Ricca et al. 2010; Wilfley et al. 2002), with a similar response compared to individual treatment on outcome measures (Ricca et al. 2010). As stated above, group therapy as a treatment for AN is somewhat more controversial both because there is a dearth of research on its efficacy and because there are some indicators that group therapy may actually detract from recovery by creating a competitive environment and one in which tips and tricks can be exchanged. However, there have been some studies reporting it may be efficacious, as detailed below.

Types of Group Therapies

A number of types of group therapy are generally offered for those with EDs, including CBT, IPT, psychodynamic, behavioral, psychoeducational, addiction model (e.g., Overeaters Anonymous), intensive short-term therapies, mindfulness-based groups, and single-issue approaches (targeting one aspect, such as body image or nutrition counseling). Specifics of the various group treatment modalities vary considerably. For example, group therapy using CBT has largely been adapted from Fairburn's model for individual treatment (Fairburn et al. 1993) and consists of 20 group sessions over 22 weeks with three distinct phases. The first phase (sessions 1–7) relies on daily self-monitoring to promote eating behavior normalization with the goal of developing a pattern of moderate and consistent restraint. The second phase (sessions 8–14) relies on cognitive interventions and problem-solving to manage the negative thoughts that predispose binge eating. The third phase (sessions 15–20) is focused on relapse prevention.

Interpersonal psychotherapy for group (IPT-G) was published in manualized form in 2000 (Wilfley et al. 2000). Rather than addressing ED symptoms, IPT-G emphasizes identifying and modifying current interpersonal difficulties and life stressors. Similar to CBT, IPT-G generally lasts 20 sessions and is divided into three stages, beginning with an initial screening and pregroup meeting (Wilfley et al. 2000). Unlike CBT, IPT-G leaders provide information to group members in writing throughout the process, such as documenting treatment goals at the beginning of treatment and progress toward goals after each session. In a study comparing group CBT and group IPT for women with non-purging bulimia, both groups showed significant improvement in reducing their binge eating compared to those assigned to waitlist condition and recovered at equivalent rates both posttreatment and at 1-year follow-up (Wilfley et al. 1993, 2002).

The addiction model guides groups such as Overeaters Anonymous, a selfhelp group initially created for members who engaged in overeating but which grew to be inclusive of EDs such as BN, AN, and what is now called OSFED (Suler and Bartholomew 1986). Foundational to the 12-Step addiction model, Overeaters Anonymous members are taught to accept their limitations and their powerlessness over food and eating (Ronel and Libman 2003), relinquishing control over food to a transcendent or higher power, and taking action toward change (Schiff 2000). Several elements of Overeaters Anonymous have been found to be helpful toward symptom abatement including regular meeting attendance and daily contact with a sponsor (Malenbaum et al. 1988; Wasson and Jackson 2004). The addiction model has been criticized for ignoring the psychosocial factors underlying EDs, such as the role of dietary restraint and abnormal attitudes about body weight and shape as well as ignoring the difference among the various EDs (Polivy and Federoff 1997; Wilson 1991).

The addiction model typically recommends restricting types and amounts of foods. Restricting, known as dietary restraint, is a phenomenon in which certain foods are labeled as "bad" and "good," with "bad" foods not permitted to the dieter. It is thought that the presence of a food rule (e.g., "sugar is bad; no sugar allowed") brings the mind's focus to that food, creating a drive to eat that specific food. When the drive is compiled with guilt for breaking a diet rule, the dieter is likely to binge on that food. Dietary restraint is often cited as a reason for binge eating.

The addiction model has also been criticized due to its characterization of addiction as a permanent condition, rather than a disorder from which complete remission is possible. While abundant evidence is emerging that disordered eating mirrors drug abuse in many neurophysiological pathways (see Smith and Robbins, 2013 for an excellent review), addiction models that fail to incorporate psychosocial factors will likely continue to be challenged by those who work as providers treating those with EDs. Evidence has been challenging to gather from 12- Step programs with the protections of anonymity acting as a barrier to researchers' ability to access participants for study purposes. Treatment providers vary widely in their comfort in recommending Overeaters Anonymous, with some basing their own treatment on the 12-Step model, some using Overeaters Anonymous as an adjunctive referral (particularly when clients have few or no resources), and some being vehemently opposed.

It has been asserted that the negative aspects of group therapy are rarely taken into account and that group treatment may be particularly harmful for patients with AN (Vandereycken 2011). For example, groups and specialized in-patient treatment in general can lead to patients over-identifying with having an ED, and, thus, become reluctant to let go of this identity or develop competitiveness, for example, to be the best or most "successful anorexic." In mixed groups of clients with AN and clients with BN, those with BN have reported feeling intimidated by very thin clients with AN and also reported feeling more disgusted with themselves based on this comparison (Enright et al. 1985). However, a number of ED treatment centers continue to use group therapy for patients with AN and some past studies have shown groups to be beneficial with this population (Inbody and Ellis 1983; Piazza et al. 1983; Yellowlees 1988; Piazza and Stenier-Adair 1986). Given the oftenperfectionistic and competitive personality typical of those with AN, combined with the fact that those with AN tend to be resistant to treatment (Garner et al. 1997), it is still questionable whether group therapy is the most efficacious avenue for treatment, but more rigorous and current research is needed before this can determined.

No singular therapeutic approach to the treatment of EDs in group therapy has been found to be consistently superior to another. Group treatment may be a better fit for some patients than individual treatment and is likely t be more cost effective and efficient due to the consolidation of resources.

EMERGING AND ALTERNATIVE TREATMENTS

It is important to stay at the forefront of emerging and alternative treatments, especially as a more technologically savvy population seeks treatment. A brief overview of yoga and technology, two of the more commonly used emerging treatments, are outlined below. Other therapies are also gaining research support as providers look to "think outside the box" of traditional modalities for EDs, including compassion-focused therapy (CFT), EMDR, mindfulness meditation, and drama therapy in addition to many others (Gale et al. 2014; Kelly et al. 2014; Halvgaard 2015; Katterman et al., 201Wood and Schneider 2015; Shapiro 2009).

Yoga

Yoga is an ancient practice that has seen such a dramatic increase in popularity over the last several years that it is now considered a part of the mainstream culture. The practice of yoga has long been used to increase mindfulness and relaxation. It focuses on the mind–body connection in a way that traditional exercise does not. Recently, clinicians at ED treatment programs have begun to successfully incorporate yoga into their treatment plan as an effective adjunct tool to more conventional therapies (Boudette 2006; Douglass 2009; Wyer 2001). For now, evidence of the benefits of yoga in ED treatment are primarily anecdotal with only a few research studies supporting the efficacy of yoga (McIver et al. 2009; Scime and Cook-Cottone 2008) and at least one showing that while yoga was not effective in changing ED behaviors or thoughts, it was not harmful (Mitchell et al. 2007). Daubenmier (2005) showed that those practicing yoga had less self-objectification and greater body satisfaction compared to those who did aerobics or did neither aerobics or yoga, and that yoga practitioners demonstrated fewer disordered eating attitudes compared to aerobic exercisers.

It is important to note that this is not a treatment that is appropriate for everyone seeking ED treatment. For example, a referral to yoga for a patient who has used exercise destructively or is extremely resistant to exercise would likely not be appropriate (Boudette 2006). Douglass asserts that it is also important that yoga is used by a patient to increase awareness and self-care, rather than misused as an additional way to discipline or control the body, or to expel calories. For this reason, a slower, mindfulness-based yoga practice is recommended to those in recovery rather than the more vigorous types of power yoga often practiced in a heated room (Douglass 2009). In a more recent article, Douglass also provides a number of suggestions for residential and clinical programs about what to take into account when hiring a yoga teacher. These include extensive training in EDs, a willingness to receive clinical supervision, and a collaborative attitude as part of the treatment team (Douglass 2011).

TECHNOLOGY

In these rapidly changing times, perhaps it comes as no surprise that technologybased interventions are emerging as a promising method of treatment delivery in the ED field. A number of treatment modalities have been used, including e-mail (Yager 2003), the internet (Fichter et al. 2012; Paxton et al. 2007), mobile device applications or "apps" (Boh et al. 2016), and even text messaging (Bauer et al. 2012, 2003). A number of recent meta-analyses and reviews have demonstrated that electronic treatment modalities, sometimes called e-therapy, are generally effective and well-received (Aardoom et al. 2013; Bauer and Moessner 2013; Dölemeyer et al. 2013). However, a recent review that focused on the more stringent NICE guidelines for research on e-therapy was less decidedly positive, concluding that the evidence base is still too small and effect sizes too mild to make firm conclusions; the authors encourage better research methods and more research attention on etherapy going forward (Loucas et al. 2014). While using technology may have its own set of drawbacks, including absence of nonverbal cues and need for safeguards regarding confidentiality, security, and risk assessment, it also has the potential to greatly increase access and adherence to treatment.

Paxton et al. (2007) reported results from a study of an eight-session, therapist-led, small group addressing body dissatisfaction and disordered eating in adult women compared face-to-face and internet modalities using a manualized CBT group intervention. Results showed that both delivery approaches achieved positive outcomes. While the gains were larger at the end of treatment for the face-to-face group than those in the internet group, at 6-month follow-up there were equivalent gains for both intervention groups. The authors suggest that, from the therapist's perspective, it is harder to assess when a response is required as it can be difficult to determine in the absence of nonverbal cues if a participant is thinking, typing, in need of support, or not concentrating. The authors suggest that in order to minimize these concerns, therapists may be more explicit in checking thoughts and feelings of participants as well as use more emotionally expressive language than might be typical in face-toface interaction.

Some benefits to this internet treatment modality include the means to extend treatment over a wide geographic area (including rural areas that may not have accessible treatment providers) and an ability to offer treatment to those who may otherwise avoid face-to-face treatment because of shame or stigma.

Bauer et al. (2003, 2012) have examined the use of text messaging as a means to support patients after discharge from inpatient treatment. Participants were adult women with either full or subthreshold bulimia. The intervention consisted of weekly texting interaction between patient and provider for 16 weeks following discharge from the hospital. Patients would report on three key bulimic symptoms (body dissatisfaction, frequency of binges, and frequency of compensatory behavior); feedback from providers was formulated to signal social support and show care, reinforce symptom improvement, and remind patients of CBT strategies they had learned while in treatment. At the end of 16 weeks, remission was significantly higher for the group that received text messages compared to the control group (intervention group = 51.2%; control group = 36.1%, p = .05). The study authors speculate that three mechanisms may account for this better outcome: (1) increased compliance with self-monitoring, (2) a decrease in symptoms due to tailored feedback showing continuous support as well as reminders of CBT skills, and (3) that ongoing text messages encouraged participants to seek additional support when needed.

While there are certainly some additional challenges including ethical considerations inherent when recommending or intervening with technology-based interventions, there are also a number of benefits. While it is doubtful that e-mail and texting will ever completely replace face-to-face treatment interaction, it is clear that the field is moving toward a more expansive view of what can be considered effective treatment modalities. With future generations becoming increasingly technologically integrated, developing and researching its benefits is a necessary step for the future of ED treatment.

CONCLUSION

EDs have complex etiologies and require clinical flexibility in developing sophisticated and personalized treatment. The term *effective treatment* should be used cautiously. Well-trained psychotherapists are likely to effectively use eclectic and integrative methods, and rely on their hard won clinical intuition to make astute choices. Psychotherapists would strengthen their capacity to treat clients with EDs by developing further expertise in already practiced methods or one or more methods addressed in this chapter. Multidisciplinary team members who are not psychotherapists would benefit from acquiring the Certified Eating Disorder Professional credential, which provides some training in counseling those with EDs, and would benefit by learning about the methods used by the treating psychotherapist. Self-help recommendations will likely become increasingly popular adjunctive or primary referral sources as technology sharpens efficacy and engagement. By working to understand the complex and diverse approaches to working with EDs, providers can help to treat this population with the greatest possible efficacy and compassion.

APPENDIX 4.1: Integrative Thought Record

Situation

Describe the situation in a few words.   Feeling uncomfortable with my weight at a party.

Rate Emotion

Read emotions lists found on the Internet to expand your emotion vocabulary. Rate the emotions, not relative to each other, but individually, from 0 to 10, 0 = no intensity and 10 = high intensity.	

Humiliated	9
Sad	8
Angry (at myself)	10

Body Experience

This integrates somatic and mindfulness therapies.   Pain in stomach, tense back, holding breath.

Negative Thought (NT) about Self

From Michael Balint's (1968) psychoanalytic concept of the basic fault, attempt to find a fundamental negative message captures the essence of almost all of one's negative thoughts. The most common ones are listed, and an extensive list of negative cognitions may be found in the EMDR literature. It is helpful to work primarily on the basic fault; the working-through process will generalize to other negative thoughts.

There is something wrong with me.
Other common basic faults are:
  I am alone.
  I am not good enough.
  I am bad.
  I am too much.
  I am unwanted.
  I am not enough.

Evidence for the NT

The problem may be addressed at the level of the situation or at the level of the basic fault. Generally, it is more helpful to work at the level of the basic fault. Often these messages have been repeated internally so often that they seem consistent with a sense of self.

List two.

I felt bad, so that is evidence there is something wrong with me.

I do not have a perfect body and I could if I didn't make mistakes in the way I eat.

Evidence against the NT

This may be more challenging than evidence against and may initially require therapist assistance.

List two.

I realize that my body looks at least normal to other people.

Something being wrong with me is an old thought that comes out of nowhere for no good reason.

(Continued)

APPENDIX 4.1 (*Continued*): Integrative Thought Record

Good Parent Message(s)

From Integrative Body Psychotherapy *(Rosenberg and Rand 1985), a somatic, psychodynamic, and object relations approach, these are the messages that every child should have received energetically. The parent can no longer repair the absence of these, and the client must learn to give these messages to self, from the wise, compassionate self, to the wounded self.*

Choose 1–3 messages to give from the competent wise self to the vulnerable self.

I love you, and I give you permission to be different from me. I see you and I hear you.

I love you. I want you. You are special to me. I see you and I hear you. It is not what you do, but who you are that I love.

I love you, and I give you permission to be different from me. I'll take care of you. I'll be there for you; I will be there for you even when you die. You don't have to be alone anymore. You can trust me. You can trust your inner voice. Sometimes I will tell you "no," and that's because I love you. You don't have to be afraid anymore. My love will make you well. I welcome and cherish your love. I can set limits, and I am willing to enforce them. If you fall down I will pick you up.

I am proud of you. I have confidence in you, I am sure you will succeed. I give you permission to be the same as I, to be more or less. You are beautiful/handsome. I give you permission to love and enjoy your erotic sexuality with a partner of your choice and not lose me (Rosenberg and Rand 1985).

My self-encouraging, rational, self-supportive, productive, wise, relational voice states a more helpful way to think which will move me toward my goal of being kinder toward self, happier, having better relationships, being more hopeful, and wiser.

EMDR and DBT literatures have excellent lists of positive coping thoughts.

I can focus on something other than my body so that I can enjoy being with friends. I can focus on the music and on conversation.

Re-rate Emotion	Hopeful	7
(3)	Courageous	7
	Peaceful	8

Body Experience?   Breathing; shoulders are relaxed, feeling more present.

This sample thought record is based on CBT theory unless otherwise noted as integrating somatic, mindfulness, and psychodynamic theory (Fries, 2012).

REFERENCES

Aardoom, JJ, Dingemans AE, Spinhoven P, and Van Furth EF. Treating eating disorders over the Internet: A systematic review and future research directions. *International Journal of Eating Disorders* 46, no. 6 (2013): 539–552.

American Psychiatric Association. *Diagnostic and Statistical Manual of Mental Disorders* (5th ed.). Washington, DC: Author, 2013.

American Psychological Association, Division 12. "Training in and Dissemination of Empirically-Validated Psychological Treatments: Report and Recommendations and Future Research Directions." Society of Clinical Psychology. APA Division 12 Task Force on Promotion and Dissemination of Psychological Procedures. 1995. http://www .div12.org/PsychologicalTreatments/index.html (accessed August 2013, 2013).

American Psychological Association Presidential Task Force on Evidence-Based Practice. Evidence-based practice in psychology. *American Psychologist* 61, no. 4 (2006): 271–285.

Arcelus, J, Whight D, Langham C, Baggott J, McGrain L, Meadows L, and Meyer C. A case series evaluation of a modified version of interpersonal psychotherapy for the treatment of bulimic eating disorders: A pilot study. *European Eating Disorders Review* 17, no. 4 (2009): 260–268.

Balint, M. *The Basic Fault: Therapeutic Aspects of Regression*. New York, NY: Brunner/ Mazel, 1968.

Bauer, S, and Moessner M. Harnessing the power of technology for the treatment and prevention of eating disorders. *International Journal of Eating Disorders* 46, no. 5 (2013): 508–515.

Bauer, S, Okon E, Meermann R, and Kordy H. Technology-enhanced maintenance of treatment gains in eating disorders: Efficacy of an intervention delivered via text messaging. *Journal of Consulting and Clinical Psychology* 80, no. 4 (2012): 700–706.

Bauer, S, Percevic R, Okon E, Meerman R, and Kordy H. Use of text messaging in the aftercare of patients with bulimia nervosa. *European Eating Disorders Review* 11, no. 3 (2003): 279–290.

Bell, L. The spectrum of psychological problems in people with eating disorders, an analysis of 30 eating disordered patients treated with cognitive analytic therapy. *Clinical Psychology and Psychotherapy* 6, no. 1 (1999): 29–38.

Beutler, L. Identifying empirically supported treatments: What if we didn't? *Journal of Consulting and Clinical Psychology* 66, no. 1 (1998): 113–120.

Birchall, H. Interpersonal psychotherapy in the treatment of eating disorders. *European Eating Disorders Review* 7, no. 5 (1999): 315–320.

Blagys, M, and Hilsenroth M. Distinctive features of short-term psychodynamic-interpersonal psychotherapy: A review of the comparative psychotherapy process literature. *Clinical Psychology: Science and Practice* 7, no. 2 (2000): 167–188.

Boh, B, Lemmens LH, Jansen A, Nederkoorn C, Kerkhofs V, Spanakis G, Weiss G, and Roefs A. An ecological momentary intervention for weight loss and healthy eating via smartphone and internet: Study protocol for a randomised controlled trial. *Trials* 17, no. 154 (2016): 1–12.

Boudette, R. Question and answer: Yoga in the treatment of disordered eating and body image disturbance: How can the practice of yoga be helpful in recovery from an eating disorder? *Eating Disorders* 14, no. 2 (2006): 167–170.

Bulik, CM, Berkman ND, Brownley KA, Sedway JA, and Lohr KN. Anorexia nervosa treatment: A systematic review of randomized controlled trials. *International Journal of Eating Disorders* 40, no. 4 (2007): 310–320.

Chambless, DL, Baker MJ, Baucom DH, Beutler LE, Calhoun KS, Crits-Christoph P, Daiuto A, DeRubeis R, Detweiler J, Haaga DAF, Bennett Johnson S, McCurry S, Mueser KT, Pope KS, Sanderson WC, Shoham V, Stickle T, Williams DA, and Woody SR. Update on empirically validated therapies, II. *Clinical Psychologist* 51, no. 1 (1998): 3–16.

Chambless, D, and Hollon S. Defining empirically supported therapies. *Journal of Consulting and Clinical Psychology* 66, no. 1 (1998): 7–18.

Cooper, Z, and Fairburn CG. The evolution of "enhanced" cognitive behavior therapy for eating disorders: Learning from treatment nonresponse. *Cognitive and Behavioral Practice* 18, no. 3 (2011): 394–402.

Costin, C, interview by J Fries. *Monte Nido Founder and Chief Clinical Officer*. Los Angeles, CA. 12 October 2012.

Couturier, J, Kimber M, and Szatmari P. Efficacy of family-based treatment for adolescents with eating disorders: A systematic review and meta-analysis. *International Journal of Eating Disorders* 46, no. 1 (2013): 3–11.

Dare, C. The family therapy of anorexia nervosa. *Journal of Psychiatric Research* 19, no. 2–3 (1985): 435–443.

Dare, C, Eisler I, Russell G, Treasure J, and Dodge L. Psychological therapies for adults with anorexia nervosa: Randomised controlled trial of out-patient treatments. *British Journal of Psychiatry* 178, (2001): 216–221.

Daubenmier, J. The relationship of yoga, body awareness and body responsiveness to self-objectification and disordered eating. *Psychology of Women Quarterly* 29, no. 2 (2005): 207–219.

Dölemeyer, R, Tietjen A, Kersting A, and Wagner B. Internet-based interventions for eating disorders in adults: A systematic review. *BMC Psychiatry* 13, (2013): 207.

Douglass, L. Thinking through the body: The conceptualization of yoga as therapy for individuals with eating disorders. *Eating Disorders* 19, no. 1 (2011): 83–96.

Douglass, L. Yoga as an intervention for eating disorders: Does it help? *Eating Disorders* 17, no. 2 (2009): 126–139.

Enright, A, Butterfield P, and Berkowitz B. Self-help and support groups in the management of eating disorders. In *Handbook of Psychotherapy for Anorexia Nervosa and Bulimia*, edited by DM Garner, and PE Garfinkel, pp. 491–512. New York, NY: Guilford Press, 1985.

Fairburn, C. A cognitive behavioural approach to the management of bulimia. *Psychological Medicine* 11, no. 4 (1981): 707–711.

Fairburn, C. Cognitive-behavioral treatment for bulimia. In *Handbook of Psychotherapy for Anorexia Nervosa and Bulimia*, edited by D Garner, and P Garfinkel, pp. 160–192. New York, NY: Guilford Press, 1985.

Fairburn, C. Eating disorders: The transdiagnostic view and the cognitive behavioral theory. In *Cognitive Behavior Therapy and Eating Disorders*, edited by C Fairburn, pp. 7–22. New York, NY: Guilford Press, 2008.

Fairburn, CG, Bailey-Straebler S, Basden S, Doll HA, Jones R, Murphy R, O'Connor ME, and Cooper Z. A transdiagnostic comparison of enhanced cognitive behaviour therapy (CBT-E) and interpersonal psychotherapy in the treatment of eating disorders. *Behavior Research and Therapy* 70 (2015): 64–71.

Fairburn, CG, Cooper Z, Doll HA, O'Connor ME, Bohn K, Hawker DM, Wales JA, and Palmer RL. Transdiagnostic cognitive-behavioral therapy for patients with eating disorders: A two-site trial with 60-week follow-up. *American Journal of Psychiatry* 166, no. 3 (2009): 311–319.

Fairburn, C, Cooper Z, and Shafran R. Cognitive behavior therapy for eating disorders: A "transdiagnostic" theory and treatment. *Behaviour Research and Therapy* 41, no. 5 (2003): 509–528.

Fairburn, C, Marcus M, and Wilson GT. Cognitive-behavioral therapy for binge eating and bulimia nervosa: A comprehensive treatment manual. In *Binge Eating: Nature, Assessment and Treatment*, edited by C Fairburn, and GT Wilson, pp. 361–404. New York, NY: Guilford Press, 1993.

Fettes, P, and Peters JM. A meta-analysis of group treatments for bulimia nervosa. *International Journal of Eating Disorders* 11, no. 2 (1992): 97–110.

Fichter, MM, Quadflieg N, Nisslmüller K, Lindner S, Osen B, Huber T, and Wünsch-Leiteritz W. Does Internet-based prevention reduce the risk of relapse for anorexia nervosa? *Behaviour Research and Therapy* 50, no. 3 (2012): 180–190.

Fischer, S, Meyer AH, Dremmel D, Schlup B, and Munsch S. Short-term cognitive-behavioral therapy for binge eating disorder: Long-term efficacy and predictors of long-term treatment success. *Behavior Research and Therapy* 58, (2014): 36–42.

Fonagy, P, Roth A, and Higgitt A. The outcome of psychodynamic psychotherapy for psychological disorders. *Clinical Neuroscience Research* 4, no. 5–6 (2005): 367–377.

Gale, C, Gilbert P, Read N, and Goss K. An evaluation of the impact of introducing compassion focused therapy to a standard treatment programme for people with eating disorders. *Clinical Psychology & Psychotherapy* 21, no. 1 (2014): 1–12.

Galsworthy-Francis, L, and Allan S. Cognitive behavioural therapy for anorexia nervosa: A systematic review. *Clinical Psychology Review* 34, no. 1 (2014): 54–72.

Garner, D, and Bemis K. A cognitive-behavioral approach to anorexia nervosa. *Cognitive Therapy and Research* 6, no. 2 (1982): 123–150.

Garner, D, and Bemis K. Cognitive therapy for anorexia. In *Handbook of Psychotherapy for Anorexia Nervosa and Bulimia*, edited by D Garner, and P Garfinkel, pp. 107–146. New York, NY: Guilford Press, 1985.

Garner, D, Vitousek K, and Pike K. Cognitive-behavioral therapy for anorexia nervosa. In *Handbook of Treatment for Eating Disorders*, edited by D Garner, and P Garfinkel, pp. 94–144. New York, NY: Guildford Press, 1997.

Goldenberg, H, and Goldenberg I. *Family Therapy: An Overview* (8th ed.). Belmont, CA: Brooks/Cole, 2013.

Halvgaard, K. Single case study: Does EMDR psychotherapy work on emotional eating? *Journal of EMDR Practice and Research* 9, no. 4 (2015): 188–197.

Heenan, C. A feminist psychotherapeutic approach to working with women who eat compulsively. *Counseling and Psychotherapy Research* 5, no. 3 (2005): 238–245.

Hepworth, N. A mindful eating group as an adjunct to individual treatment for eating disorders: A pilot study. *Eating Disorders* 19, no. 1 (2011): 6–16.

Hurst, K, Read S, and Wallis A. Anorexia nervosa in adolescence and Maudsley family-based treatment. *Journal of Counseling and Development* 90, no. 3 (2012): 339–345.

Inbody, DR, and Ellis JJ. Group therapy with anorexic and bulimic patients: Implications for therapeutic intervention. *American Journal of Psychotherapy* 39, no. 3 (1983): 411–420.

Kazdin, AE. Evidence-based treatment and practice: New opportunities to bridge clinical research and practice, enhance the knowledge base, and improve patient care. *American Psychologist* 63, no. 3 (2008): 146–159.

Katterman, SN, Kleinman BM, Hood MM, Nackers LM, and Corsica JA. Mindfulness meditation as an intervention for binge eating, emotional eating, and weight loss: A systematic review. *Eating Behaviors* 15, no. 2 (2014): 197–204.

Kelly, AC, Carter JC, and Borairi S. Are improvements in shame and self-compassion early in eating disorders treatment associated with better patient outcomes? *International Journal of Eating Disorders* 47, no. 1 (2014): 54–64.

Le Grange, D, Lock J, Agras WS, Bryson SW, and Jo B. Randomized clinical trial of family-based treatment and cognitive-behavioral therapy for adolescent bulimia nervosa. *Journal of the American Academy of Child and Adolescent Psychiatry* 54, no. 11 (2015): 886–894.

Lenz, AS, Taylor R, Fleming M, and Serman N. Effectiveness of dialectical behavior therapy for eating disorders. *Journal of Counseling and Development* 92, no. 1 (2014): 26–35.

Lock, J. Evaluation of family treatment models for eating disorders. *Current Opinion in Psychiatry* 24, no. 4 (2011): 274–279.

Lock, J, Le Grange D, Agras WS, and Dare C. *Treatment Manual for Anorexia Nervosa: A Family-Based Approach*. New York, NY: Guildford Press, 2001.

Loeb, K. Eating Disorders and Obesity. Society of Clinical Psychology, American Psychological Association, Division 12. 27 August 2016. Available at http://www.div12.org/psychological-treatments/disorders/eating-disorders-and-obesity/

Loucas, CE, Fairburn CG, Whittington C, Pennant ME, Stockton S, and Kendall T. E-therapy in the treatment and prevention of eating disorders: A systematic review and meta-analysis. *Behavior Research and Therapy* 63 (2014): 122–131.

Malenbaum, R, Herzog D, Eisenthal S, and Wyshak G. Overeaters anonymous: Impact on bulimia. *International Journal of Eating Disorders* 7, no. 1 (1988): 139–143.

Markowitz, J, and Weissman M. Interpersonal psychotherapy: Past, present and future. *Journal of Clinical Psychology and Psychotherapy* 19, no. 2 (2012): 99–105.

Masheb, RM, and Grilo CM. Binge eating disorder: A need for additional diagnostic criteria. *Comprehensive Psychiatry* 41, no. 3 (2000): 159–162.

McIver, S, O'Halloran P, and McGartland M. Yoga as treatment for binge eating disorder: A preliminary study. *Complementary Therapies in Medicine* 17, no. 4 (2009): 196–202.

Minuchin, S, Rosman B, and Baker L. *Psychosomatic Families: Anorexia Nervosa in Context.* Cambridge, MA: Harvard University Press, 1978.

Mitchell, KS, Mazzeo SE, Rausch SM, and Cooke KL. Innovative interventions for disordered eating: Evaluating dissonance-based and yoga intervention. *International Journal of Eating Disorders* 40, no. 2 (2007): 120–128.

Murphy, S, Russell L, and Waller G. Integrated psychodynamic therapy for bulimia nervosa and binge eating disorder: Theory, practice and preliminary findings. *European Eating Disorders Review* 13, no. 6 (2005): 383–391.

National Collaborating Centre for Mental Health. *Eating Disorders: Core Interventions in the Treatment and Management of Anorexia Nervosa, Bulimia Nervosa and Related Eating Disorders; Clinical Guideline 9.* London, UK: National Institute for Clinical Excellence. 2004. Available at http://guidance.nice.org.uk/CG9/QuickRefGuide/pdf/English.

Neacsiu, A, Ward-Ciesielski E, and Linehan M. Emerging approaches to counseling intervention: Dialectical behavior therapy. *Counseling Psychologist* 40, no. 7 (2012): 1003–1032.

Nevonen, L, and Broberg AG. A comparison of sequenced individual and group psychotherapy for patients with bulimia nervosa. *International Journal of Eating Disorders* 39, no. 2 (2006): 117–127.

Norcross, J. Collegially validated limitations of empirically validated treatments. *Clinical Psychology: Science and Practice* 6, no. 4 (1999): 472–476.

Orbach, S. Social dimensions in compulsive eating in women. *Psychotherapy: Theory, Research and Practice* 15, no. 2 (1978): 180–189.

Paxton, SJ, McLean SA, Gollings EK, Faulkner C, and Wertheim EH. Comparison of face-to-face and internet interventions for body image and eating problems in adult Women: An RCT. *International Journal of Eating Disorders* 40, no. 8 (2007): 692–704.

Piazza, E, Carni J, Kelly J, and Plante S. Group psychotherapy for anorexia nervosa. *Journal of the American Academy of Child Psychiatry* 22, no. 3 (1983): 276–278.

Piazza, E, and Stenier-Adair C. Recent trends in group therapy for anorexia nervosa and bulimia. In *Eating Disorders: Effective Care and Treatment*, edited by F Larocca, pp. 25–51. New York, NY: Wiley, 1986.

Polivy, J, and Federoff I. Group psychotherapy. In *Handbook of Treatment for Eating Disorders*, edited by D Garner and P Garfinkel, pp. 462–475. New York, NY: Guilford Press, 1997.

Poulsen, S, Lunn S, Daniel SI, Folke S, Mathiesen BB, Katznelson H, and Fairburn CG. A randomized controlled trial of psychoanalytic psychotherapy or cognitive-behavioral therapy for bulimia nervosa. *American Journal of Psychiatry* 171, no. 1 (2014): 109–116.

Ricca, V, Castellini G, Mannucci E, Lo Sauro C, Ravaldi C, Rotella CM, and Faravelli C. Comparison of individual and group cognitive behavioral therapy for binge eating disorder: A randomized, three-year follow-up study. *Appetite* 55, no. 3 (2010): 656–665.

Ronel, N, and Libman G. Eating disorders and recovery: Lessons from overeaters anonymous. *Clinical Social Work Journal* 31, no. 2 (2003): 155–171.

Rosenberg, J, and Rand M. *Body, Self, and Soul: Sustaining Integration.* Atlanta, GA: Humanics Limited, 1985.

Rust, J, and Beck M. The healing of Isabel. In International Association of Eating Disorder Professionals, October 2012.

Ryle, A, and Kerr I. Cognitive analytic therapy. *British Journal of Psychiatry* 183, no. 79 (2003): 75–81.

Schiff, M. Helping characteristics of self-help and support groups. *Small Group Research* 31, no. 3 (2000): 275–305.

Scime, M, and Cook-Cottone C. Primary prevention of eating disorders: A constructivist integration of mind and body strategies. *International Journal of Eating Disorders* 41, no. 2 (2008): 134–142.

Shapiro, R. *EMDR Solutions II: For Depression, Eating Disorders, Performance, and More.* New York, NY: W.W. Norton & Company, 2009.

Shedler, J. The efficacy of psychodynamic psychotherapy. *American Psychologist* 65, no. 2 (2010): 98–109.

Silver, AL, and White J. Dynamic psychiatry and the treatment of anorexia psychosis. *Journal of the American Academy of Psychoanalysis and Dynamic Psychiatry* 39, no. 1 (2011): 63–76.

Smith, D, and Robbins T. The neurobiological underpinnings of obesity and binge eating: A rationale for adopting the food addiction model. *Biological Psychiatry* 73, no. 9 (2013): 804–810.

Spring, B, Pagoto S, Kaufmann PG, Whitlock EP, Glasgow RE, Smith TW, Trudeau KJ, and Davidson KW. Invitation to a dialogue between researchers and clinicians about evidence-based behavioral medicine. *Annals of Behavioral Medicine* 30, no. 2 (2005): 125–137.

Stein, KF, Wing J, Lewis A, and Raghunathan T. An eating disorder randomized clinical trial and attrition: Profiles and determinants of dropout. *International Journal of Eating Disorders* 44, no. 4 (2011): 356–368.

Sugarman, A. Bulimia: A displacement from psychological self to body self. In *Psychodynamic Treatment of Anorexia Nervosa and Bulimia*, edited by C Johnson, pp. 3–33. New York, NY: Guilford Press, 1991.

Suler, J, and Bartholomew E. The ideology of overeaters anonymous. *Social Policy* 16, no. 4 (1986): 48–53.

Tanofsky-Kraff, M, Wilfley DE, Young JF, Mufson L, Yanovski SZ, Glasofer DR, Salaita CG, and Schvey NA. A pilot study of interpersonal psychotherapy for preventing excess weight gain in adolescent girls at-risk for obesity. *International Journal of eating Disorders* 43, no. 8 (2010): 701–706.

Tasca, G, and Bone M. Individual versus group psychotherapy for eating disorders. *International Journal of Group Psychotherapy* 57, no. 3 (2007): 399–403.

Telch, C, Agras WS, and Linehan M. Dialectical behavior therapy for binge eating disorder. *Journal of Consulting and Clinical Psychology* 69, no. 6 (2001): 1061–1065.

Thompson-Brenner, H, Boisseau C, and Satir D. Adolescent eating disorders: Treatment and response in a naturalistic setting. *Journal of Clinical Psychology* 66, no. 3 (2010): 277–301.

Thompson-Brenner, H, and Westen D. A naturalistic study of psychotherapy for bulimia nervosa, part 2: Therapeutic interventions in the community. *Journal of Nervous and Mental Disease* 193, no. 9 (2005): 585–595.

Tolin, DF, McKay D, Forman EM, Klonsky ED, and Thombs BD. Empirically supported treatment: Recommendations for a new model. *Clinical Psychology: Science and Practice* 22, no. 4 (2015): 317–338.

Treasure, J, Claudino AM, and Zucker N. Eating disorders. *Lancet* 375, no. 9714 (2010): 583–593.

Treasure, J, Smith G, and Crane A. *Skills-Based Learning for Caring for a Loved One with an Eating Disorder: The New Maudsley Method.* New York, NY: Routledge, 2007.

Vandereycken, W. Can eating disorders become 'contagious' in group therapy and specialized inpatient care? *European Eating Disorder Review* 19, no. 4 (2011): 289–295.

Wade, TD, Treasure J, and Schmidt U. A case series evaluation of the Maudsley model for treatment of adults with anorexia nervosa. *European Eating Disorders Review* 19, no. 5 (2011): 382–389.

Wampold, B. *The Great Psychotherapy Debate: Models, Methods, and Findings.* Mahwah, NJ: Lawrence Erlbaum Publishers, 2001.

Wasson, DH, and Jackson M. An analysis of the role of overeaters anonymous in women's recovery from bulimia nervosa. *Eating Disorders* 12, no. 4 (2004): 337–356.

Weltzin, T, Weisensel N, Cornella-Carlson T, and Bean P. Improvements in the severity of eating disorder symptoms and weight changes in a large population of males undergoing treatment for eating disorders. *Best Practices in Mental Health* 3, no. 1 (2007): 52–65.

Wilfley, DE, Agras WS, Telch CF, Rossiter EM, Schneider JA, Cole AG, Sifford LA, and Raeburn SD. Group cognitive-behavioral therapy and group interpersonal psychotherapy for the nonpurging bulimic individual: A controlled comparison. *Journal of Consulting and Clinical Psychology* 61, no. 2 (1993): 296–305.

Wilfley, D, Mackenzie R, Welch R, Ayers V, and Weissman M. *Interpersonal Psychotherapy for Group.* New York, NY: Basic Books, 2000.

Wilfley, DE, Welch RR, Stein RI, Spurrell EB, Cohen LR, Saelens BE, Dounchis JZ, Frank MA, Wiseman CV, and Matt GE. A randomized comparison of group cognitive-behavioral therapy and group interpersonal psychotherapy for the treatment of overweight individuals with binge-eating disorder. *Archives of General Psychiatry* 59, no. 8 (2002): 713–721.

Wilson, GT. The addiction model of eating disorders: A critical analysis. *Advances in Behavior Research and Therapy* 13, no. 1 (1991): 27–72.

Wilson, GT, Grilo C, and Vitousek K. Psychological treatment of eating disorders. *American Psychologist* 62, no. 3 (2007): 199–216.

Wood, LL, and Schneider, C. Setting the stage for self-attunement: Drama therapy as a guide for neural integration in the treatment of eating disorders. *Drama Therapy Review* 1, no. 1 (2015): 55–70.

Wyer, K. Mirror image: Yoga classes at the Monte Nido clinic are changing how women with eating disorders see themselves. *Yoga Journal* 158, (2001): 70–73.

Yager, J. Email therapy for anorexia nervosa: Prospects and limitations. *European Eating Disorders Review* 11, no. 3 (2003): 189–209.

Yalom, I. *The Theory and Practice of Group Psychotherapy* (4th ed.). New York, NY: Basic Books, 1995.

Yellowlees, P. Group psychotherapy in anorexia nervosa. *International Journal of Eating Disorders* 7, no. 5 (1988): 649–655.

Zipfel, S, Wild B, Groß G, Friederich HC, Teufel M, Schellberg D, Giel KE, de Zwaan M, Dinkel A, Herpertz S, Burgmer M, Löwe B, Tagay S, von Wietersheim J, Zeeck A, Schade-Brittinger C, Schauenburg H, and Herzog W. Focal psychodynamic therapy, cognitive behaviour therapy, and optimised treatment as usual in outpatients with anorexia nervosa (ANTOP study): Randomised controlled trial. *Lancet* 383, no. 9912 (2014): 127–137.

RECOMMENDED READINGS

BOOKS FOR THERAPISTS

Cash TF. *The Body Image Workbook: An Eight Step Program for Learning to Like Your Looks* (2nd ed), 2008. Oakland, CA: New Harbinger Publications.

Duncan BL, Miller SD, and Sparks JA. *The Heroic Client.* 2000. San Francisco, CA: Jossey-Bass.

Duncan BL, Miller SD, Wampold BE, and Hubble MA (eds). *The Heart and Soul of Change* (2nd ed). 2010. Washington, DC: The American Psychological Association.

Nelson T. *What's Eating You?: A Workbook for Teens with Anorexia, Bulimia, and other Eating Disorders.* 2008. Oakland, CA: New Harbinger Publications.

Norcross JC (ed). *Psychotherapy Relationships That Work* (2nd ed). 2012. New York, NY: Oxford University Press.

BOOKS FOR CLIENTS

Astrachan-Fletcher E and Maslar M. *The Dialectical Behavior Therapy Skills Workbook for Bulimia: Using DBT to Break the Cycle and Regain Control of Your Life.* 2009. Oakland, CA: New Harbinger Publications.

Brown H. *Brave Girl Eating: A Family's Struggle with Anorexia.* New York, NY: Harper-Collins Publishers.

Fairburn CG. *Overcoming Binge Eating* (2nd ed). 2013. New York, NY: The Guilford Press.

Gold SS. *Food: The Good Girls Drug: How to Stop Using Food to Control Your Feelings.* 2011. New York, NY: Penguin Books.

Liu A. *Gaining: The Truth about Life After Eating Disorders.* 2007. New York, NY: Warner Books.

McCabe RE, McFarlane TL, and Olmsted MP. *The Overcoming Bulimia Workbook: Your Comprehensive Step-by-Step Guide to Recovery.* 2003. Oakland, CA: New Harbinger Publications.

Schaefer J. Goodbye ED, *Hello Me: Recover from Your Eating Disorder and Fall in Love with Life.* 2010. (edit date: 2009) New York, NY: McGraw-Hill.

Schaefer J. *Life without ED: How One Woman Declared Independence from Her Eating Disorder and How You Can Too.* 2004. (edit date: 2003) New York, NY: McGraw-Hill.

5 Nutrition Therapy
Evolution, Collaboration, and Counseling Skills

Sondra Kronberg, MS, RD, CDN, CEDRD

CONTENTS

LEARNING OBJECTIVES

After reading this chapter, the reader should be able to do the following:

- Understand how the value and the role of the nutrition therapist has evolved and changed throughout the years
- Identify the criteria needed for a registered dietitian (RD) to become a nutrition therapist and understand the importance for patients and treatment providers to work with an RD who specializes in eating disorders and has obtained the Certified Eating Disorder Registered Dietitian (CEDRD) certification from the International Association of Eating Disorder Professionals (IAEDP)
- Understand the multidisciplinary approach and the importance of consistent, cohesive, and respectful collaboration among the treatment team members
- Better understand the role of nutrition therapists and their importance in the multidisciplinary team approach in the treatment of eating disorders
- Become aware of how potential coping mechanisms, including manipulation of food and weight, as symptoms of the eating disorder, are serving the client
- Recognize the overlap between nutrition therapy and psychotherapy and distinguish the differences in the scope of practice
- Provide an overview of the cognitive-behavioral thinking skills that nutrition therapists may employ with their clients and that may be helpful for other team members
- Be familiar with the stages of change and how they may be relevant to nutrition therapy when working with eating-disorder clients
- Become aware of how a variety of eating and meal support programs are developing and how these programs are being used to expose, challenge, and support clients with food and eating behaviors in their recovery process

INTRODUCTION

Current best practices for the treatment of eating disorders recommend a multidisciplinary team approach throughout the continuum of care with treatment lasting up to 10 years (Appendix A; Wolfe 2003; Wentz et al. 2009). All professionals treating

eating-disordered clients benefit from knowledge of the behavioral, psychological, nutritional, and physiological aspects of disordered eating, eating disorders, and their consequences, irrespective of their discipline, training, or roles in the treatment (Mittnacht and Bulik 2015). In order to provide a cohesive, consistent, and persistent message to the clients, all members of the team and family are best served by being aware of the roles, language, and approaches of their collaborators (Braham and Sampson 2013). This book is a resource for all professionals who wish to enhance their knowledge of eating disorders, their ability to collaborate, and their treatment efficacy. This chapter informs all members of the treatment team of the evolving role of the nutrition therapist within the multidisciplinary eating-disorder treatment team and the cognitive-behavioral counseling skills that facilitate the difficult process of food, eating, weight, exercise, and body image changes. With the overall mission of this book being to positively impact treatment and recovery outcomes, sharing this information will enhance the knowledge and ability of professionals treating eating-disorder clients while improving interactions between all treatment team members, including a trained nutrition therapist.

EVOLUTION OF COLLABORATIVE TREATMENT OF EATING DISORDERS

Eating-disorder treatment in general was in its infancy when the author of this chapter entered the field almost 30 years ago. There were few treatment centers, little research, and a void of validated treatment protocols. Most of the information came from the writings and first-hand accounts of psychotherapists or physicians who treated a handful of patients with extreme eating behaviors and a variety of severe medical consequences. Providers were using psychodynamic and psycho-analytic talk therapies and/or medical interventions, applying their trainings to uncover the underlying psychotherapeutic causes or correct the physiological con-sequences of the eating-disorder behaviors. There were few established protocols specific to eating disorders and little understanding of how to treat these compli-cated biopsychosocial disorders (Grilo and Mitchell 2010). Each modality worked within their scope of practice to manage their piece of the illness with little or no collaboration.

Early on, nutritionists often applied their didactic skills to set up a meal plan, explain physiological occurrences, balance energy consumptions with expen-ditures, and make nutrient recommendations to clients who sought them out look-ing for an alliance or for advice about their food, weight, and eating behaviors. In the effort to effect changes in behaviors and provide the desired service to the client, these nutritionists, with no official eating-disorders schooling, learned more about eating behavior with each new client that presented. Sometimes unknowingly, they colluded with the client's eating disorder to help them lose weight, introduce new dieting ideas, and foster their disordered thinking. Today, this still remains a potential risk when a client is working with or the team is collaborating with a nutritionist who has not been trained to treat eating disorders.

The psychotherapists, whose work focused on the client's emotional distress and the impact of their eating disorder on their emotional well-being, processed issues related to trauma, abuse, relationships, and self-esteem (Gehart 2016). These psychotherapists with minimal nutritional training often unknowingly ignored the nutritional and overall physical dangers of the eating disorder. Physicians, historically, focused on treating the medical complications that were consequences of the self-destructive eating-disorder behaviors and were hard-pressed to address the psychological and nutritional underpinnings. Physicians, therapists, and nutritionists often worked relatively independently using the skills they had been trained in to try to effect positive change. As psychiatrically diagnosable illnesses, treatment continued for years with a focus on addressing the underlying emotional issues and the repair of the psychological damage or deficits. The role of the nutritionist was marginalized as there was little history, written documentation, or perceived value in consulting a nutritionist for these psychologically based illnesses. The fact that a nutrition degree did not include eating-disorder education and nutritionists were unable to diagnose illness under their scope of practice may have further hampered the importance of the nutritionist's contribution. Treatment remained trying and difficult for all professionals, with outcomes poor.

Gradually, it became more evident and imperative that treating these complex disorders required a multidimensional approach, one where all modalities work together, share information, learn from each other, and collaborate around the needs of the clients to cohesively address the emotional, behavioral, physiological, and nutritional components of the disorder in order to provide a more interconnected and effective treatment.

As the awareness, incidence, and need for more effective, available, and collaborative treatment of eating disorders ensued, professional, research, educational, political, public action, and training organizations evolved locally and eventually nationally and internationally. The number of skilled treatment providers has increased, informed treatment protocols have developed, and treatment centers have grown rapidly to meet the needs of the clients. Over the past 10 years, the opening of residential treatment centers has exploded creating an abundance of intensive settings, which provide a more inclusive, progressive, and contained environment in which the eating-disorder behaviors can be extinguished and positive change can occur (Frisch et al. 2006). A continuum of care, which includes partial hospitalization (PHP), intensive outpatient (IOP), and creative meal support programs have been developed. These step-down levels of care, which offer continued but varied levels of supervision and support therapy for the emotional, behavioral, and nutritional progressions and regressions, were previously nonexistent in most areas. Today when clients move out of residential care and return to their lives, there are many outpatient treatment programs developing that provide ongoing coaching, support, and socialization around food, eating, and recovery. Several of these facilities are owned or directed by nutrition therapists.

As a result of this growth, best therapeutic treatment perspectives have shifted from focusing solely on psychotherapeutic treatment approaches and addressing the underlying psychodynamics to include a variety of cognitive and behavioral therapies (Mittnacht and Bulik 2015). Therapeutic strategies, which help clients recognize their thoughts and change their thinking patterns in order to change their actions and their identification with the eating disorder, have become critical to all treatment, giving new importance to the role and function of the nutritionist. Nutritionists learned quickly the value of developing relational and therapeutic counseling skills in order to effectively apply their nutritional knowledge when working with disordered eating sufferers (see Appendix B). In the field of eating disorders, a specialized group of nutritionists, nutrition therapists, evolved. Throughout the continuum of care, nutrition therapists have become an important component of treatment protocols and they continue to expand the role of the nutritionist in the treatment of eating disorders.

WHAT IS A NUTRITION THERAPIST?

There is limited research, outcome studies, and written manuscripts regarding this evolution of the nutrition therapist and the treatment developments that are still in progress. Much of what is written in this chapter comes from the author's 30 years of experience as a forerunner in the field of nutrition therapy, as a founder and director of a treatment center with innovative eating programs, and as a clinician who has trained and supervised many nutrition therapists and psychotherapists working in the field today.

Nutritional counseling for eating disorders is a specialized form of nutrition counseling in that there is a significant degree of psychological expertise and counseling skill required to effectively foster a trusting relationship and facilitate change in these often resistant clients suffering from complex biopsychosocial disorders (Grilo and Mitchell 2010). Many health professionals may offer nutritional advice and can call themselves nutritionists, without having a recognized license, certification, or degree. The Academy of Nutrition and Dietetics (formerly the American Dietetic Association) certifies the RD as the only nutrition professional qualified to provide medical nutrition therapy (MNT; American Dietetic Association 2011). RDs are trained experts in food science, physiology, nutrition science, and the impact of foods on body wellness and disease function. They provide MNT while functioning as an integral part of numerous healthcare teams. Medical nutrition therapists are key components of maintenance and restoration on metabolic support, diabetes care, oncology treatment, and gastrointestinal disease teams. They work with sports medicine, obstetrics, and pediatric units to provide well care. Registered dietitians are trained through education and field experience to understand the intricate relationship between food intake, nutrient and energy usage, metabolic functions, and physiological health. They have been trained to educate and impart information to clients as part of MNT. There is, however, little to no formal education about eating disorders or, furthermore, how to treat them. The increased awareness and incidence of eating disorders and the value of a nutritionist on the team have made it essential for RDs to seek additional training outside of the official nutrition science degree.

In the treatment of eating disorders, the term "nutrition therapist" has been adapted to distinguish those RDs who have gone through additional psychotherapeutic and advanced counseling training, continued education, experience, self-study, and supervision under professionals who are experts in this field (Wolfe 2003).

Nutrition therapists develop an expertise and many skills specific to the needs of the eating-disordered client. They become qualified to direct all treatment aspects related to nutrition, physiology, and behavior change. The trained nutrition therapist will provide the patient with a safe place to discuss food and any thoughts or actions that surround the food (King and Klawitter 2007). The role of the nutrition therapist varies slightly depending on the level of care.

Eating-disordered behaviors and poor nourishment impact physiological and psychological functioning (American Dietetic Association 2011). Nutrition therapists are also well versed and skilled in the information and communication related to physiology through the lifespan and process of health and disease. Cognitive therapies have long been instrumental nutrition counseling tools used in facilitating progressive changes in food, weight, exercise, and eating behaviors. Nutrition therapists effectively utilize their counseling skills, advanced cognitive strategies, and their knowledge base to elicit behavioral change, in a population where thought and behavior change is challenging.

In 1985, the IAEDP established the Certified Eating Disorder Specialist (CEDS) certification for psychotherapists and physicians, in recognition of the need for advanced training for eating disorders and the necessity for clients, families, and other treatment professionals to access professionals who are experts in treating these disorders. Qualified physicians and psychotherapists with advanced expertise in eating disorders would have the opportunity to distinguish themselves from noneating-disorder professionals with the CEDS credential (IAEDP 2003).

In 2004, with increased awareness of the crucial role of the nutritionist and need to identify nutrition therapists demonstrating an expertise in eating disorders, IAEDP developed an advanced certification program for nutritionists. Registered dietitians with advanced training and specific counseling skills specializing in eating disorders could acquire a CEDRD credential (IAEDP 2003). The CEDRD for RDs is the equivalent of the CEDS for physicians and psychologists, certifying the expert and advanced training of the respective professions. The CEDRD is an experienced nutrition therapist with advanced psychotherapeutic training who has met exceptional educational and skill requirements and has accumulated the number of hours of qualifying work experience under an experienced eating-disorder treatment supervisor (IAEDP 2003). In 2010, the author received IAEDP's CEDS award. It was the first time this annual award was given to a nutrition therapist. The author considered this a paradigm shift and long-awaited validation by the field of the importance of the role of the nutrition therapist in the treatment of eating disorders.

For the remainder of this chapter, the term "nutrition therapist" is used to describe RDs who also have advanced psychological training and are dedicated to ongoing learning through self-study hours, continuing education, and supervision from a master's level experienced eating disorder specialist, either a CEDS or CEDRD. They have either been certified as eating-disorder nutrition specialists, CEDRDs, or are working toward acquiring that certification under an approved supervisor (see Appendix C).

THE ROLE OF THE NUTRITION THERAPIST

Frequently, the most tangible and easily recognized symptoms and behaviors of an eating disorder have to do with changes in food, weight, exercise, and eating (Murphy et al. 2010). These symptoms are not always perceived by the client, or the family, as having psychological underpinnings and medical consequences. Therefore, clients often seek consultation with a nutritionist before considering a psychotherapist or physician. In addition, clients might opt to consult a nutritionist, perceiving that avenue as being more culturally accepted and/or less threatening, shameful, or confronting of the underlying issues (Costin and Schubert Grabb 2012). The nutrition therapist may often be the first person to see and assess the client (Murphy et al. 2010). These initial visits place the nutritionist in a unique position as the first professional to recognize, evaluate, or identify the disordered potential. If the client has come to the nutrition therapist for the first time without having sought treatment from any other eating-disorder professionals, it is the first responsibility of the nutrition therapist to educate the client about eating disorders and address the importance of a treatment team in eating-disorder recovery.

The nutrition therapist is in the crucial role of evaluating the patient's nutritional status, assessing eating-disorder risk factors, creating a therapeutic meal plan, educating the client and family, suggesting a course of treatment, making essential referrals for an effective treatment team, and assisting in the determination of the level of care needed. While a nutrition therapist is not able to make a diagnosis (outside of the nutritionist scope of practice), he or she does provide valuable information to the team physician and psychotherapist who will then diagnose the client (Graves and Reiter 2010).

The nutrition therapist conducts a thorough nutritional and physiological assessment according to Nutrition Care Process Standards, which includes lab results, menses history, food recall, body mass index, percentage of ideal body weight, exercise regimen, and an extensive eating-disorder history (American Dietetic Association 2011). By conducting a full intake, the nutrition therapist will become informed of the client's current and past dietary intake, weight and body perspectives, eating patterns, beliefs about food, and eating-disorder behaviors.

Beyond the initial assessment and throughout treatment, nutrition therapists play a major role in facilitating and monitoring goals regarding food, eating, eating-disorder symptoms, weight, and activity (Fairburn et al. 2003). Ongoing sessions will include inquiry and planning about methods and responsibility for food shopping, purchasing and preparing of foods, and food-related relationships and traditions in the home environment. Information on the values and relationships with food, eating, weight, exercise, and body image within the client's family and social circles is gathered. Additionally, it may be necessary to explore the family values in general and specifically regarding expectations, education, money, satisfaction, and success, as all of these have the potential to influence treatment compliance, length of treatment, and payment issues (Siegel et al. 1988). The client's motivation, goals, and supports are established and revisited periodically. The nutrition therapist assesses this clinical information with nonjudgmental curiosity. He or she maintains an awareness of the eating disorder's presence and the client's internal suffering. The nutrition therapist is hopeful that the safety of their connection will enable the client to share their often unspoken thoughts, beliefs, fantasies, goals, and fears associated with food, weight, and their body, as well as what drives those thoughts and motivates their behavior (Cardi et al. 2015).

The nutrition therapist will teach the client ways to change food, exercise, and weight-related behaviors. He or she will educate the client about normal and abnormal food intake, hunger patterns, and metabolic processes (King and Klawitter 2007). The nutrition therapist will also educate and assist clients in awareness of the physiological, biological, emotional, and somatic reactions to food, exercise, and substance misuse (Graves and Reiter 2010). He or she will aid clients in understanding the connection between emotions and eating-disordered behaviors. The nutrition therapist will guide the client by teaching them how to develop a healthy relationship with food while developing normal eating patterns and maintaining their weight within a healthy range (Graves and Reiter 2010). The nutrition therapist will work on behavioral change through cognitive awareness and changes in motivation, thinking, and action patterns, while the therapist will additionally work on a deeper level to bring awareness of genetics, familial, and sociocultural dynamics contributing to the development and maintenance of an eating disorder, and increase the client's ability and potential to make the necessary behavioral changes (Grilo and Mitchell 2010).

A nutrition therapist who is well trained in therapeutic counseling and eating disorders is in the unique position to elicit the thoughts that keep the eating-disorder behaviors in place. The skilled nutrition therapist can uncover, through the language of food, weight, and body often spoken by clients, where the client is entrenched. The nutrition therapist listens for the beliefs and thoughts that precipitate and perpetuate the eating disorder. Through the development of a trusting relationship, the nutrition therapist will work with the client on detaching from the thoughts, beliefs, and consequent actions that are keeping the eating disorder cemented. The nutrition therapist who specializes in eating disorders listens to the messages and deciphers the eating-disorder language codes to help the client and team understand how the eating-disorder functions in the client's life. For example, a client who is struggling at college and would feel like a failure and a disappointment to his or her parents if he or she decided to come home may be unable to communicate that with words. They may consciously or unconsciously become so medically compromised that his or her parents, psychotherapist, and nutrition therapist make the decision that it is no longer safe for them to stay in school. The eating-disorder consequences become the language that communicates what he or she may not be able to express with words.

The nutrition therapist apprises the multidisciplinary treatment team of the changes in the client's eating behaviors, weight, resistance, exercise, and progressive or regressive shifts in eating-disordered cognitions, and symptoms, at all levels of treatment. It is important for other team members to be familiar with the roles, skills, and dialogues of the nutrition therapist, and how to utilize the nutrition therapist's abilities to complement the overall treatment. In geographic areas where trained eating-disorder nutrition therapists are not available to a treatment team or where finances or other factors make consulting with the nutrition therapist not possible, the other team members may have to assume some of a nutrition therapist's role, integrate nutritional dialogues, and incorporate nutritional therapeutics into their treatment strategies.

The nutrition therapist imparts a wealth of psychoeducational information and a language that he or she uses to inform the clients, their family, and their support systems. It is most helpful if this information, while under the scope of practice of the nutrition therapist, is available to the entire team. The author has developed standard modules of nutrition "savvy" EDucation dialogues (Appendix D) to inform and counter the erroneous beliefs of clients. These are learning/teaching modules that nutrition therapists currently use in many treatment centers around the country to educate their clients and families. These same modules are shared with all collaborating treatment professionals. This enables families and other team members to learn what clients are learning in nutrition therapy and be able to reinforce the same dialogues in a common language. The more consistent and cohesive the message, the greater the likelihood that message will empower the client and prevent the eating-disordered voice from prevailing. These shared modules help clients and treatment members become informed and unified in battling the disordered messages, especially if they are going to discuss, participate, or supervise meals with the client.

COLLABORATION WITH THE TREATMENT TEAM

Collaboration among the treatment team and across the continuum of care increases the potential success of the treatment. This collaboration is enhanced when all members are unified in dialogues, display confidence, and trust in each other, and have a means of communicating that keeps them up to date. When treatment team members are knowledgeable of the other team members' practice techniques and strategies, clients experience treatment as more cohesive (Lyster-Mensh 2012).

Clients may enter treatment through a variety of avenues or consultations with the different disciplines. It is important for all modalities to be able to recognize the medical, psychological, and nutritional risks and have enough information, counseling skill, and resources to facilitate the client's movement into the appropriate treatment.

Shared perspectives and dialogues that help all members of the team and the family understand the eating disorder will foster a more cohesive net and environment for the client's recovery to take place. Eating-disorder behaviors, though ultimately destructive, often are initially creative adaptations for emotional survival. They are a perfect storm of genetics and environment organized to manage feelings of pain, shame, guilt, worthlessness, anxiety, anger, and fear resulting from past abuse, trauma, chaotic surroundings, sensitivity, excessive need for control, or perfectionism (Reiff and Reiff 1992). Eating disorders often serve as a vehicle for expressing or coping with uncomfortable circumstances and feelings. The eating disorder may be a veil that conceals the client's feelings of inadequacy, and low sense of self that often filters their perceptions of life and the world. It may be an outlet for feelings, needs, or hungers that the client is unaware of or unwilling to embrace. It is helpful to understand that the eating-disorder behavior and identity often give definition, value, control, and substance to clients struggling with an inner sense of worthlessness (Reiff and Reiff 1992). It may become a voice, a container for feelings, an escape, or a confidante. There is usually ambivalence if not resistance to relinquishing the behavior and recovering.

This collaborative team understanding and congruent messages aim to provide consistency and continuity throughout the client's treatment course. Effective communication and unified management are essential not only in the nutrition therapist's relationship with the client and family but also in the relationship with team members and any adjunct treatment facilities, which may become part of the client's care.

The nutrition therapist will collaborate with each of the members of the team or with adjunctive treatment facilities at different stages and with varying frequency based on a client's medical, psychological, and behavioral status (Vandereycken 2003). Collaborating with the physician is based on ongoing physical monitoring and will change with the criticalness of the medical and physical state of the client. There will also be collaboration with the family regarding their concerns or involvement with weight changes or food behaviors and how they may support or should handle circumstances. There will be collaboration with the providers at facilities that are adjunctive for periods of time when the client needs different levels of care and to provide smooth transitions in and out of higher levels of care. For example, if a client is suffering from gastroparesis, or slow stomach emptying, the nutrition therapist will collaborate with greater regularity with the physician, sharing each other's findings throughout treatment. If a client slips into a deep zone of depression, the frequency of collaboration may increase between the nutrition therapist, the psychotherapist, and the psychiatrist when there is a pharmacological team member.

COLLABORATION BETWEEN PSYCHOTHERAPIST AND NUTRITION THERAPIST

Throughout the continuum of care of treatment, the psychotherapist and the nutrition therapist are in the unique collaborative position regarding ongoing strategies and evaluation of client's progress. They are usually the most frequently and consistently consulted of the long-term providers on the multidisciplinary treatment team (Costin 2007). The nature of this long-term relationship places both the nutrition therapist and psychotherapist in a dynamic relationship with the client, the family, and each other. As such it is important that they distinguish and respect their unique roles as well as balance the overlaps to prevent impasses, disruptions, or disconnections with the client or each other.

The psychotherapist is responsible for all psychological aspects of treatment. The therapist explores the underlying emotional, behavioral, and psychological issues that precipitate or perpetuate the disorder (Siegel 1988). Psychotherapists help their clients understand how circumstances and people affect them, which includes the ability for the client to develop, communicate, and function in their environments at home, in school, and with friends. The treatment also involves processing the client's biopsychosocial history including family dynamics, previous relationships, and experiences including abuse, trauma, neglect, and the ways in which these experiences impact the client's sense of self, worth, and ego (Costin 2007). Psychotherapists assess and diagnose psychological well-being and illness and set forth treatment protocols that help the client become aware of and address underlying issues. They will also determine levels of participation of family and provide input on the appropriate level of care for the client.

Nutrition therapists are responsible for assessing and monitoring physiological and nutritional consequences related to food and eating. They continually determine macro- and micronutrient requirements, calculate caloric intake and expenditures, establish weight and exercise goals, and create meal plans and eating challenges. These tasks all fall into the scope of the nutrition therapist and distinguish the nutrition therapist's role from the psychotherapist's in these complex disorders which have psychological origins and physiological consequences.

However, there is a natural overlap which occurs in the collaboration of these two modalities in the effective collaborative treatment of eating disorders. Both treatment processes involve aiding clients in understanding the irrational thoughts and behaviors that surround food, understanding the importance of normalized eating, and paths to overcoming disordered thoughts and feelings to change their behaviors (Spahn et al. 2010). Both nutrition therapy and psychotherapy will help families understand the complexities of eating disorders and both collaborate with associated physicians. More recently, as psychotherapists are either trained or work in higher levels of care and meal support programs, they are more involved with meal therapy and are often eating with or coaching clients at meals. For best care of the client, the nutrition therapist and psychotherapist benefit by effective communication toward developing a working balance, which allows them to stay within their scope of practice and practice in a united manner. This minimizes the potential for splitting with patient or team members and enhances the usefulness of the collaboration (Siegel et al. 1988; Spahn et al. 2010).

Together, through the therapeutic relationships with the client and their relationship with each other, using respective therapeutic processes, the nutrition therapist and psychotherapist, as well as other members of the team will enable the client to

- Become aware of their behaviors, thoughts, feelings, and/or needs
- Understand the purpose the eating disorder serves
- Find alternative ways to express those feelings or meet those needs
- Take action to change the behavior
- Develop the courage to cope with the consequences of the change
- Challenge old patterns relating to eating food, weight and body
- Develop healthy patterns of self-care and eventually a healthy self (see Appendix E)

Another function of the collaborative team will be to help the client establish supports that allow them to move from isolation, deprivation, and perfectionism into connectedness. Eating-disordered clients have learned to isolate, to count only on themselves, and not to depend on others, which the author has labeled self-adamancy. Learning to trust and allow the nutrition therapist, psychotherapist, and others such as family and friends into their lives to support them in their struggle is an important part of recovery. The team helps clients develop significant supports and healthy relationships that will cushion ups and downs and contribute to building self-worth. All supports must be tailored to the needs and ability of the client at the time. The purpose of support, whether a person, a strategy, or a group, is to help the client move through a difficult emotion, circumstance, or anxiety-producing experience without using their eating-disordered symptoms to cope. The communication and collaboration of the team once again are essential for effective support of the client.

The ultimate goal of treatment collaboration is to create a cohesive net that fosters effective communication, authentic feeling states, and an environment of trust. Creating hope and awareness among the treatment team provides a nurturing space in which the client can develop a new sense of self and leave behind the self that was dependent on the eating disorder for identity, structure, and purpose (Grilo and Mitchell 2010; Olmsted et al. 2012).

NUTRITION THERAPY COUNSELING SKILLS AND THERAPEUTIC PROCESSES

Successful nutritional treatment of eating disorders requires specialized counseling skills and the incorporation of processes that address the psychological components of eating. The emotional and behavioral entanglements that revolve around food, weight, and body image dissatisfaction require that the nutrition therapist develop a long-term relationship with the client to facilitate positive changes. In order to evoke this positive change, the nutrition therapist must be well versed with the means to do so.

This section discusses advanced therapeutic and counseling skills that are employed in a nutrition therapist's session. With these learned and practiced skills, the nutrition therapist can strengthen the relationship with the eating-disordered client, and provide the treatment team with a deeper understanding of how the client's eating disorder is manifesting physiologically, emotionally, and behaviorally. In addition to nutrition therapists, the other members of the treatment team may benefit and be more effective in their roles by incorporating and reinforcing the cognitive tools and nutritional modules that the nutrition therapist employs.

Individuals with eating disorders often have not experienced healthy relationships (Grilo and Mitchell 2010). The therapeutic process provides an opportunity to experience such relationships. An environment of acceptance, trust, and safety nourishes communication, a critical medium for the development of any relationship. It is the vehicle through which connection, change, and worth become established. The collaboration between psychotherapist and nutritionist, nutritionist and physician, nutritionist and family, and team and client can benefit the client by modeling effective communication. The ability to disagree, compromise, discuss, conclude, support, inform, be honest, and maintain boundaries enables the client to experience how healthy relationships function and fosters the client's trust in the team. The therapeutic process enables the nutrition therapist to safely explore the client's needs, hungers, violations, and past disappointments to help them identify what they currently need. Understanding one's needs is empowering; lack of awareness or denial often leads to an increase in eating-disorder behavior (Reiff and Reiff 1992). In the therapeutic relationship, clients learn to manage relationships, food, and self by learning to speak up, assert a boundary, ask for help, negotiate for their needs, voice a desire, and satisfy their hungers (Costin 2007). The nutrition therapist uses food and eating exercises to develop these abilities (Graves and Reiter 2010). Learning these cognitive and communication skills helps clients to better navigate relationships, make choices, and learn to trust themselves around people and experience. Ultimately, therapeutic work leads the client to a deeper connection with his or her own inner experience. Over time, as they eventually learn to listen and trust their internal cues, they are able to disconnect from distorted thoughts and external cues that have immobilized their being.

The therapeutic process guides clients through periods of engagement, exploration, grieving, integration, acceptance, maintenance, and termination (Braham and Sampson 2013). This process of change and recovery occurs over an extended period of time (Wentz et al. 2009; Wolfe 2003). Paralleling the flow of the overall treatment, the flow of each session includes combinations of change, trust building, awareness development, active listening, exploration, reflection, feedback, direction, goal setting, agreements, minimizing sabotage and fear of success, support, progress, maintenance of change, relapse prevention, and closure or termination. Discussion of food, eating patterns, and weight actually and metaphorically demonstrates how one is able to make choices that are nurturing and enhancing and not restrictive, depriving, chaotic, or impulsive.

CHANGE

Change may be difficult for a majority of people but is especially difficult for those recovering from an eating disorder (Vitousek et al. 1998). According to Prochaska, permanent change occurs as a process in predictable stages or steps that usually take place over an extended period in a supportive environment (Prochaska et al. 1995). The transtheoretical model (TTM) is an integrative, biopsychosocial model used to conceptualize the process of intentional behavior change (Prochaska et al. 1995; see Appendix F).

The stages of change

1. Precontemplation
2. Contemplation
3. Preparation
4. Action
5. Maintenance
6. Relapse

In eating-disorder treatment, change occurs through awareness, self-observation, contemplation of alternatives, production of an environment that encourages new behaviors, support from others, and maintenance of those behaviors (Costin and Schubert Grabb 2012). While progress takes place in all the stages, changes in awareness, self-observation, self-image, emotions, and thinking occur before the new behaviors are visible (see Box 5.1). Visible, tangible change takes place after the risk of action has taken place.

The therapeutic process and communication are essential instruments for producing change (Fruggeri 1992). The psychotherapist, nutrition therapist, and client work to become aware of the function of the eating-disorder behavior. When the

BOX 5.1   PROGRESS VERSUS RELAPSE

PROGRESS

- Takes place in all stages
- Moving from stage to stage is also progress
- Invisible changes take place in the first three stages (e.g., change in awareness, emotions, self-image, and thinking)
- Visible changes take place in the last three stages

RECYCLE/RELAPSE

- Progress is not linear
- Relapse is the rule, not the exception
- It is not uncommon to "spiral" through several progressions and regressions before exiting
- Complications should be expected
- Distress and social pressure often precipitate relapse
- Guilt and self-blame exacerbate the relapse

Source: Prochaska, JO et al., *Changing for Good*, Avon Books, New York, 1995.

needs behind the eating disorder are uncovered, alternative ways to meet those needs can be developed (Costin and Schubert Grabb 2012). Change requires patience, creativity, support, and competence to enable a client to give up a survival mechanism or system that has contributed to their identity.

Trust Building

Successful communication and change depend on the nutrition therapist's ability to create a safe place and to develop trust. The client's success depends upon their willingness to explore, to learn how to trust and express their feelings, and to take some risks within the safety of the relationship and eventually in the world. The nutrition therapist's office may be more frightening than any other professional's offices. In nutrition therapy, clients often fear the confrontation about their food and are anxious about the attempts that will be made to alter their food choices or weight (King and Klawitter 2007). There is usually increased anxiety over need for them to take action as opposed to other components of treatment where they are asked to freely talk about how the eating behaviors make them feel or discuss the consequences of the behaviors (King and Klawitter 2007).

The nutrition therapist must understand that, to the client, the eating disorder has functioned almost like a life preserver (Costin and Schubert Grabb 2012). Threatening to take away the eating disorder or giving the client the idea that this will happen may scare them away. Despite any pain and suffering it inflicts in the present, it is also a source of comfort, protection, accomplishment, intimacy, and salvation (Reiff and Reiff 1992). It is critical to allow the client these attachments and to recognize how valuable the eating disorder has been. The goal is to strengthen the part of the client's self that does want to get better by teaching the client the tools they need to do so.

The eating-disorder client may also carry a myriad of noncommunicated thoughts and feelings, including any combination of the following (but not limited to):

- Not feeling worthy of the nutrition therapist's time
- Feeling ashamed of the presenting behavior
- Fearing abandonment, abuse, or rejection
- Not thinking there is a problem (denial)

A variety of distorted thinking modes support these thoughts and feelings. There are often strongly developed feelings of worthlessness and a repertoire of self-loathing thoughts and behaviors (Costin 2007). The eating-disordered client is typically self-judgmental and overly sensitive to the surrounding environment (Reiff and Reiff 1992).

The client's perception of the nutrition therapist and the subsequent barrier building will begin long before the actual session. The therapist's voice, how she or he answers the phone, and where the office is located will all be evaluated. Once the client is at the office, they will judge the furniture and the nutrition therapist's hair, clothing, body language, and weight. He or she will probably experience transference, likening the nutrition therapist to someone else in their life (Abbate-Daga et al. 2013; Mittnacht and Bulik 2015). Each of these thoughts or feelings will be a potential reason for not trusting the nutrition therapist in a therapeutic relationship. What the client is really thinking is, "Can I trust this person? Will I be understood? Can I let anyone get close to me?" The nutrition therapist needs to be aware of how the client's conscious and unconscious feelings will affect the sessions and the relationship.

From the initial moment of connection, the nutrition therapist will have an impact on the client and vice versa. Early sessions can be an opportunity for the client to find fault. They are also the nutrition therapist's opportunity for acceptance, to foster trust, and to provide hope. The client may push or provoke to prove that the nutrition therapist is not to be trusted or that they themselves are again unworthy. Food and eating negotiations are the medium through which this takes place. This testing period is emotionally stressful, creating uncomfortable feelings for both participants. Practice and professional supervision will develop skills that enable the nutrition therapist to manage personal feelings in a manner that supports a constructive therapeutic relationship and the client's progress. The nutrition therapists also will have to learn to be aware of their own food weight and body beliefs, feelings, strengths, and deficits so they can explore and empathize with their client's feelings in an accepting and nonjudgmental manner.

In the therapeutic moments, the eating-disordered client requires unconditional acceptance of their behavior, as well as of their potential for growth.

Many of these clients have been in relationships in which they have been overly controlled, neglected, abandoned, or abused (emotionally, sexually, or physically; Zucker et al. 2012). They may fear relationships, lean toward isolation, or have an obsessive relationship with food or its absence. The prospect of relating to people presents the potential for hurt and the fear of reliving past patterns of abuse.

The client needs to know that the nutrition therapist is aware of their fear. It is helpful to acknowledge the client for the courage required in making the initial call and showing up for the appointment and give them a sense that they will be respected and listened to in your office. The nutrition therapist's focus, silence, words, and demeanor are important. The nutrition therapist fosters trust by listening carefully to everything that is said without judgment or ridicule, while also listening for things that may not be said. Actions of the nutrition therapist that promote the development of trust include

- Beginning and ending appointments on time
- Making as few changes as possible in the appointment schedule
- Informing clients far in advance of any vacations or off-time
- Setting firm limits and boundaries for both the client and oneself
- Adhering to these limits and boundaries
- Keeping one's word
- Telling the truth
- Modeling integrity
- Being consistent
- Admitting mistakes or uncertainties
- Respecting the client's self-knowledge
- Maintaining confidentiality
- Listening
- Following through with agreements
- Exhibiting patience

These behaviors not only earn trust but also teach the client to be trustworthy. Eventually, the client will learn to trust self. This process may be long and fragile (Wentz et al. 2009; Wolfe 2003). It will continue throughout treatment. It will be constantly tested. It may ebb and flow according to other traumas and betrayals perceived or encountered during treatment. If a client was referred by a psychotherapist, physician, or someone else who earned their trust, the nutrition therapist can ride on that trust for a while, but he or she must work quickly to earn his or her own. Clients who present for treatment under less cooperative circumstances will be more reluctant to trust their treatment team, particularly the nutrition therapist who by the nature of the perceived role is the member of the team who will "require change" (King and Klawitter 2007). In psychotherapy patients are asked to show up and talk about how they feel; in nutrition therapy patients are asked to show up and change, often making showing up for nutrition therapy a more difficult task (Costin 2007).

AWARENESS DEVELOPMENT

The nutrition therapist must clearly identify that the first stage of treatment is about awareness—the first step in all permanent change (Prochaska et al. 1995). Developing the client's awareness allows the nutrition therapist and client to observe how foods, circumstances, and other people affect the client and are managed through the eating disorder (King and Klawitter 2007). The client is best served when the nutrition therapist is able to meet the client where they are and move them forward at a pace that does not exacerbate the need for the eating-disorder behaviors. For example, the nutrition therapist can make the client a partner in treatment by saying, "You are the expert on *you*, I am the expert on food, eating, and the eating disorder; and your psychotherapist is the expert on feelings, emotions, and the eating disorder. We will all work together on this as a team." This engages the client by making him or her a member of the team by creating allegiance and partnership, not giving the client a sense that they are being dictated to or forced to change. Creating the opportunity for choice, by encouraging them to show up, be real, tell the truth, and not be attached to the outcome (Costin and Schubert Grabb 2012).

Identifying awareness of the client's values is another major goal of treatment rather than imposing therapist-centered goals on the client such as "fixing" or controlling the client. Nutrition therapists who work within a medical model often use this method of counseling (Academy for Eating Disorders 2012). Clients come to them with nutritional and medical issues and they are asked to provide nutritional solutions: what to eat, how to exercise, what vitamins to take, and so on. This is part of traditional training for the unspecialized nutritionist and the medical culture. In the treatment of eating disorders, the team, including the client, works toward mutually agreed-upon goals with a focus on what the client values. "Fixing" would not teach the client to take responsibility for self nor would it foster the development of choice, critical to recovering and growth. Treatment sessions would become a battleground for control thwarting progress. Engaging and directing the client by asking how they feel about things or what things mean to them not only deepens the client's self-awareness but also serves to deepen the therapist–client connection. Nutrition therapists help the client become aware of what they value, what they want, what the outcome will be, where their actions take them, or what the long-term result of behaviors are, essentially, what they are choosing by not choosing to get better or what the potential is when choosing new, different, or opposite actions.

The therapeutic process uses open-ended questions as opposed to close-ended questions (Mittnacht and Bulik 2015). Nutrition therapists, through their Motivational Interviewing (MI) studies, learn how to communicate using this dialogue (Wentz et al. 2009; Wolfe 2003). For example, rather than asking "Did you like that?" and leaving the client to reply with "Yes" or "No," the nutrition therapist would ask "What was that like?" The difference in wording is slight, but the possible responses are dramatically different. The open-ended question calls for thought, words, and sentences. Open-ended questions engage the client and encourage him or her to go deeper. Finding out where the client is and how he or she feels about being there will help the nutrition therapist gauge how to continue. Examples include

- What made you want to see a nutrition therapist?
- What were you hoping I would tell you?
- What did eating/not eating do for you?
- What events in the past influence your behavior today?
- How did you feel when you got here today?
- How do you feel after not eating/overeating/purging?

Exploring where the client is and reassessing is imperative, not just at the first session but throughout the recovery process. Asking the client to gauge what they are feeling or what they are hungry for models a skill they will hopefully later be able to use themselves. Eventually, the client's feelings and hungers will provide information on how to proceed through certain situations, and not represent something to suppress, avoid, or fear. Our feelings and hungers actually and metaphorically are our antennae for navigating life and determining our preferences: what we like, what makes us feel good, who we want to be with, and what we need to leave behind. Hungers and feelings help us learn who we are. We teach our clients how to embrace them and listen to them. Demonstrating a neutral comfort when talking and asking about symptoms and behaviors will help clients feel less shameful, guilty, and be more willing to talk about their feelings, symptoms, and behaviors.

Acceptance of the client and their actions will allow further exploration of what their thoughts or actions mean through the use of open-ended questions:

- What does it mean when you lose or gain weight?
- How does it feel when you eat two extra graham crackers?
- What does it mean when someone tells you that you look healthier?

It is recommended that the nutrition therapist allow the client to express the thoughts behind their behavior and share their concerns. It is important that the nutrition therapist be mindful not to place either good or bad value on the information shared. He or she will have to address the client's concerns and not minimize their feelings: being interested in what the client has to say and flexible enough to focus on their agenda increases the possibility of the client feeling listened to.

The nutrition therapist will continue to search for disordered thoughts by asking questions that promote exploration and awareness:

- What messages were you giving yourself?
- What did that feeling make you want to act on?
- What happens when you eat 12 slices of pizza?
- How does it affect you when you skip lunch and dinner? Physically, emotionally, socially?

Again, open-ended questions, coupled with active listening in a safe environment, may help the client to look inward and become aware of the feelings the eating disorder has been covering (King and Klawitter 2007).

The nutrition therapist's own values and feelings (e.g., sadness, frustration, anger, or discouragement) will naturally be challenged by topics discussed in the session

(Costin 2007). This phenomenon is called *countertransference* (Spahn et al. 2010). The nutrition therapist would benefit by learning to recognize these feelings and using them as a gauge. Feelings that arise in session provide useful information. For the client, their feelings will be processed in their psychotherapy session; for the nutrition therapist, they can be discussed in supervision. Nutrition therapists must also learn to accept and express their own food weight and body beliefs. It is understood that everyone has their own unique beliefs and it is expected that in a supervisory setting, any practitioner can express their feelings on these issues, receive feedback, and get help reconciling their own beliefs with what they are working on with their clients.

ACTIVE LISTENING

Of equal importance to the way we ask the questions is our willingness and ability to listen to the responses. Active listening is a skill, which is important in all stages of the therapeutic counseling process, particularly in engagement and exploration. The client needs to know that his or her words were heard and their meaning understood. The nutrition therapist shows concern and interest, not judgment, disappointment, or disapproval (Martin et al. 2000). He or she listens actively. Nonjudgmental listening is neither positive nor negative. It merely acknowledges that information has been heard, without judging the information as shocking, mundane, or exciting. Clients will watch closely for signs of approval or disapproval because they may be used to being judged or judging themselves. We want to demonstrate that their emotions and actions are not good or bad, right or wrong, and healthy or unhealthy. Remaining neutral will help the nutrition therapist gain understanding of what the client is thinking and the thoughts that are catalyzing their actions. Knowing that the nutrition therapist (and, ideally, each treatment professional) is an accepting and nonthreatening audience is helpful in enabling the client to be able to voice his or her inner thoughts. The greater the nutrition therapist's awareness and the more neutral his or her listening and acceptance of eating-disordered thinking and behaviors, the more comfortable clients will feel disclosing inner thoughts, feelings, and behaviors in the session. In their lives, clients will often feel misunderstood or not listened to. They may feel shamed by their behaviors or believe they are the only one who behaves in this manner. Knowing that nothing they could share will shock the nutrition therapist and that the nutrition therapist has an understanding of them, something the client may not have experienced before, is significant. It is important that the clients know they count and that what they say and who they are has value. The nutrition therapist will use his or her voice, eyes, and body language to communicate that he or she has heard the client and accepts what the client has communicated or experienced without judgment.

Allowing the client to lead the session with his or her concerns and agenda can also demonstrate interest and flexibility on the part of the nutrition therapist, a concept encouraged in recovery. Often clients struggling with eating disorders have experienced years of feeling devalued (Reiff and Reiff 1992). Care may need to be taken so as not to recreate these feelings in the session by placing another agenda ahead of the client's, or by suggesting that anyone else's feelings

or thoughts are more important or valuable than the client's. The nutrition therapists will find it useful to provide data, articles, examples, and handouts with new
and accurate information, while taking care not to disregard the client's beliefs
or perspective.

EXPLORATION

Exploration is about introspection and discovery. It is the process by which the client
discovers the purpose of the eating disorder through such questions as

- How does it help you function?
- When do you need it?
- How do you use it to protect yourself?
- What are the benefits? Consequences?
- How does that support your goal?

During exploration, the nutrition therapist helps the client uncover their feelings,
expose their needs, and unveil past hurts (King and Klawitter 2007). This is often
more effective when done gently, entering only when, where, and at the speed the
client is willing to go. All discoveries can be shared with the psychotherapist.

Exploration techniques provide the opportunity to connect the eating-disordered
behavior to life circumstances and feelings. It may connect purging to shame,
restricting to feelings of worthlessness, overeating to a fear of intimacy, and bingeing to sense of deprivation (Engel 2006). The quest to identify situations and feelings
that require the coping mechanism of the eating disorder will include questions like
these:

- How did you feel when your sister did that?
- What were you telling yourself when you got the job interview?
- Can you remember what you were feeling when no one asked you to go?

The first line of questioning provides the opportunity to explore the circumstance.
The next step is to connect the circumstance or feeling to the eating-disordered
behavior:

- So how did your friend's comment affect your restricting?
- How do you think weighing yourself more often this week was connected
  to your new relationship?
- How was your eating affected by what happened?
- How was your feeling connected to your need to purge?

In early stages, clients will likely have difficulty acknowledging emotions and
expressing feelings (Fairburn 2008). Words are often scary and threatening. The
nutrition therapist needs to be creative when exploring the connection between

eating-disordered behaviors and the client's emotions. It is important to develop a repertoire of ways to interpret the metaphors and repave the path of expression.

Exploration techniques vary, and range from provocation to empathy. A mix of humor, confrontation, sarcasm, modeling, and silence can be effectively integrated to facilitate exploration and discovery (Fairburn 2008). Creative exercises that incorporate various modes of expression promote this process. Examples include food play, guided imagery, journal writing, dance and movement exercises, music, role-playing, writing assignments, and art projects. Each offers an opportunity to express hidden messages that have eluded verbal expression. Through these activities, connections between behaviors and feelings are encouraged. Eventually, the treatment team guides the client toward more direct expression through verbal communication.

REFLECTION

An important goal of treatment is to teach clients to effectively communicate their thoughts and feelings in order to have their needs met (Costin 2007). The nutrition therapist's reflection of messages that are heard, seen, or experienced in the exploration process helps communication in the session and models for the client ways to communicate in the world. It clears up miscommunications and lessens the damage incurred by noncommunicated assumptions. It also provides a soft summary of what has been heard and connects feelings to actions. For example, the nutrition therapist might say

- I am hearing that you were able to say no to your son and not feel guilty and need to eat over it.
- It sounds as if you were very angry when your father did not call you and you started to restrict instead of tell him how you felt.
- What I am hearing is that you were confused about what we had talked about last week and because you were confused you were disappointed in me so you binged and purged to feel better.

Eating-disordered clients often presuppose that others view them negatively (Reiff and Reiff 1992). Reflection provides a means of testing that assumption. It ensures that the client has been heard correctly and encourages them to clarify if not heard correctly. It allows the client to express feelings that make them uncomfortable, such as loneliness and anger, as well as allowing the nutrition therapist to note the absence of appropriate feelings, often replaced by food or weight thoughts or behaviors. It allows the nutrition therapist to clarify the client's often negative perspective and responses. The nutrition therapist may also reframe the behavior and the client's self-judgment in a more positive way (see Box 5.2). The ability to appropriately communicate difficult emotions such as anger will be evidence of the client's increasing ability to express how he or she is feeling. Through reflection, the nutrition therapist helps the client begin to be more curious and less judgmental of his or her thoughts, feelings, and behaviors (Golden and Meyer 2004).

BOX 5.2   CASE STUDY: CONNECTING EMOTIONS TO EATING-DISORDER BEHAVIORS

In one session Allison related how a friend had called to cancel plans right before an evening they had planned long ago. She said that when the friend gave her the news, she responded, "No problem. We can do it another day." Allison ended up staying home and bingeing. In the session, she reported this incident without signs of anger, frustration, sadness, or disappointment. In fact, she told the story with a smile on her face. I am aware from collaboration with her psychotherapist that a focus of treatment to this point had been that Allison's inability to handle anger and her continual suppression of her feelings repeatedly led her to eating and bingeing.

At this point, reflection was used to heighten awareness of the conflict between what Allison had heard and how she had responded.

NUTRITION THERAPIST: How did that feel when your friend cancelled so late?
ALLISON: Okay.
NUTRITION THERAPIST: Okay, huh? I'm hearing that you ended up bingeing and noticing that you are telling me this story with a smile on your face. Can you tell me more about this? I get the sense that you are not so okay with this. Let's go back there. Was it really okay? I'm thinking about the last time you felt she disregarded your feelings. Can you remember that? What were you feeling? Would it be okay for you to be angry, sad, or disappointed with her? And how might you experience those feelings if you allowed yourself, if you were not bingeing?

The nutrition therapist is helping Allison connect bingeing with her inability to acknowledge or express her feelings. The nutrition therapist also pointed out the inconsistency between what Allison felt and how she was describing it. In addition, the nutrition therapist validated those appropriate feelings of sadness, anger, and disappointment and offered the possibility that expressing those feelings would be a healthy, positive response that may decrease the need to binge.

FEEDBACK AND DIRECTION

Up to this point, the focus has been on recognizing circumstances, the resulting painful thoughts and feelings, and the disordered eating behaviors that develop out of those thoughts and feelings. Once this has been accomplished, the focus changes to altering some of these behaviors. The goals of recovery are to separate thoughts and feelings from food, weight, and body image behaviors and to find healthier ways of expressing and coping with feelings. Healing occurs when connections to people, places, and life itself replace the dysfunctional relationship with food and effort or need to control their body and weight. Helping a client give up a thought and the consequent actions that have brought security, control, structure, and comfort must be done in a gentle and caring way over time. Though respectful of the way in which the eating disorder gives structure, identity, and power to the client, the nutrition therapist must help the client develop the thinking skills that move the client's actions toward wholeness and recovery.

NUTRITION THERAPY TREATMENT APPROACHES

The successful approach of the nutrition therapist depends less on imparting nutritional information and more on forming a trusting relationship for conveying this information and providing the necessary support. It is the treatment team's ability to guide the client toward the development of a more positive sense of self, one willing to listen to and meet their nutritional and biological needs, that will ultimately heal them (Costin 2007). The client becomes an essential and highly valued element in the treatment, rather than an object to be treated. As mentioned in the beginning of this chapter, psychotherapeutic techniques are not traditionally taught to nutrition students. The traditional role of the RD in the medical model is to provide information to the client to devise and implement a plan that fixes the problem in a relatively short-term time structure. Solely conveying information on the biochemistry of foods, the physiology of the illness, and constructing a treatment plan will not change the eating-disorder behavior. However, creating nutritional, behavioral, and physiological awareness in a therapeutic environment supported by a positive framework and a sense of hope, over a longer period of time, can be very effective (Cardi et al. 2015).

EXPOSURE AND RESPONSE THERAPY

Currently at all levels of care, nutrition therapists practice cognitive-behavioral therapy (CBT) coupled with exposure and response therapy (ERT) to first observe, then discover and challenge their client's food, weight, body, thoughts, and actions (Steinglass et al. 2011). Experiential sessions that build on cognitive and behavioral progressions which expand the client's comfort zone with food, weight, and their bodies are an essential part of the recovery process (Yager et al. 2006). The development of ERT in nutrition treatment is in a quantum growth phase in which the nutrition therapists and client experience exposure to food and eating through a variety of venues and food-related activities. Eating and meal support activities challenge the client's fears and beliefs both in and out of the treatment facility. This work enables the nutrition therapist to be present with clients in authentic life situations and with real food, in actual restaurants or grocery stores. The nutrition therapist supervises the client through the agreed-upon challenges and helps them to modulate their responses using tools they have acquired in treatment.

Planned experiential meals, spontaneous exposure exercises, and eating events that foster a healthy, flexible, and balanced relationship with one's food and body include (but are not limited to)

- Creating recipes and meals
- Developing grocery lists and grocery shopping for foods
- Preparing both simple and elaborate recipes
- Portioning and serving themselves and others
- Planning foods for celebrations
- Social and multicultural foods and eating events
- Dining out at unique, fearful, or unfamiliar places
- Experimenting with new food
- Group meals and group challenges

These experiential and exposure exercises afford the nutrition therapist an entirely new perspective on how the eating disorder operates in the outside world. Eating events provide the nutrition therapist and team with a wealth of information often not available in talk therapy, while providing the client with a variety of supportive experiences.

Clients often return to past eating-disorder behaviors as a means of coping when external circumstances, transitions, or conflicts prove too stressful (Bailey et al. 2015). By actually being present at experiential eating events or food challenges and through meal supervision, coaching, and support therapy, nutrition therapists can observe first-hand the obstacles of anxiety, obsession, fear, and anger. For the client experiencing stressful emotions, challenging circumstances, and triggering environments, this in vivo approach offers previously unavailable levels of supervision and support.

Nutrition therapists are not the only professionals who eat with clients. Especially in treatment centers, psychotherapists, recovery coaches, family members, and additional trained staff may eat with clients (Center for Substance Abuse Treatment 2006). It is important for any professional eating with a client to be knowledgeable of the client's meal plan, their eating-disorder behaviors or rituals before, during, or after a meal, and how to address these behaviors (Costin 2007). Many psychotherapists who have been trained in treatment centers where they have eaten with patients often choose to continue this practice in their outpatient offices to be able to garner the wealth of information that comes with the exposure to and direct contact with the behaviors.

Eating Coaches

Because nutrition therapists in outpatient work can only eat with a limited number of patients each day, a new category of professional help has emerged—eating coaches—who are supervised by nutrition therapists and trained specifically to support or supervise meals with an eating-disordered client as an adjunct to the nutrition therapist's eating work.

The nutrition therapist, psychotherapist, or eating coach will need to model all of the concepts that the treatment has introduced and fostered with clients during their recovery process:

- Joy in eating
- Nonjudgmental thoughts, feelings, or actions about food
- Full range of food choices
- Self-acceptance
- Body love and acceptance
- Mindfulness
- Connectedness
- Flexibility
- Balance
- Freedom
- Choice
- Assertiveness

Eating with a nutrition therapist, psychotherapist, or coach allows the client to be guided through the challenge and have time to process thoughts and feelings about the meal or challenge in a supportive environment. Clients pay attention to the professional's communications, balance, decision-making, and assertiveness throughout the process. It is helpful that clients observe the professional's joy, satisfaction, and intuitiveness around eating as well as an overall comfort with their natural body size and shape. This exposure often offers the client more confidence in the therapeutic and recovery messages they are learning in treatment. Often these experiences make the client even more vulnerable and connected to his or her nutrition therapist or psychotherapist. The level of visibility and trust that occurs may be unique for the client and professional as they are often entering areas that have not even been experienced or witnessed in the therapeutic setting. These eating events and exposure interactions allow the nutrition therapist or psychotherapist into places that once remained secret or shameful. The new level of trust and visibility can be pivotal to the client's progress and continued recovery. Stepping outside the therapeutic box also leaves the nutrition therapist more personally exposed; it has inherent pitfalls and changes the traditional therapeutic boundaries, further reinforcing the need for the nutrition therapist to develop the therapeutic counseling expertise that makes it safe for both the client and the nutrition therapist to go into these uncharted waters.

COGNITIVE-BEHAVIORAL THERAPY

One of the most successful techniques for helping clients move their thoughts is CBT (Fairburn et al. 2003; Graves and Reiter 2010; Spahn et al. 2010). CBT increases awareness of thoughts, behaviors, and functions of the eating disorder. The process of CBT involves discovering what the client is thinking, and becoming aware of how those thoughts move the client into action and are connected to their eating-disorder behaviors. Thoughts about certain foods or their body can move the clients to eat or not eat, purge or not purge, and binge or not binge. The job of the nutrition therapist is to help the client to develop healthier thoughts and actions, which are more congruous with movement toward their recovery goals. Nutrition therapists incorporate CBT as one of their primary techniques to facilitate behavior change (Grilo and Mitchell 2010). CBT effectively applied to eating disorders is an advanced counseling skill that distinguishes a nutrition therapist from a nutritionist (Mittnacht and Bulik 2015). All professionals and family members, however, will have the opportunity in their dialogues with clients to identify eating-disordered thinking, and support the client in incorporating healthier thoughts.

In eating-disordered clients, negative thoughts prompt negative feelings, which foster negative behaviors, which eventually reinforce a negative belief system and ultimately support a negative identity (see Box 5.3). Recognizing the earliest disordered thoughts and changing them to positive, more constructive thoughts will ultimately change the ensuing behavior. Examples of tools that support this treatment technique include positive self-talk exercises, positive affirmations, handouts that expose the client to positive, motivating thoughts about life and people, and books that reinforce self-empowerment. These tools feed positive thinking and feeling. Handouts and books serve as reinforcements of positive thoughts between appointments. These objects represent the nutrition therapist's presence and support on a daily basis helping to create a more constructive culture and positive environment in the client's life.

In session, the nutrition therapist models positive thinking by emphasizing the client's success and de-emphasizing perceived failures. Thoughts that precipitated the eating-disordered behavior are replaced with more constructive thoughts. CBT concepts help the client to create new thoughts, which increase his or her ability to

---

BOX 5.3   THE CONSEQUENCES OF NEGATIVE THOUGHTS

Negative Words
"A magazine suggests that I am fat."
↓
Negative Thoughts
"I must be fat."
↓
Negative Behavior
"I act as if I am fat."
↓
Negative Belief System
"I am a failure because I am fat."
↓
Negative Identity
"I am a fat failure who can't succeed at anything."

create new behaviors. Sessions provide the environment for these new thoughts to develop. For example, the nutrition therapist might ask

- What was it you were telling yourself?
- Can you focus on the thoughts or feelings you had before you began purging?
- What were you telling yourself about the graham cracker?
- What were the rules or messages you were hearing before you decided not to eat?

The client may need help identifying specific negative thoughts. The nutrition therapist might prompt, "Let us go through the day together." Self-monitoring tools, such as journal writing and lists of rules, messages, and thoughts identified outside the session, can help to make the client's thoughts more accessible during the session:

- I was wondering if you would be willing to write down your thoughts the next time you were to purge?
- Would you be willing to keep an ongoing list of the rules that your eating disorder requires you to follow as you hear them this week?

Once the thought or feeling that triggers the behavior has been identified, the team works to create a new thought and a new response, and encourages a new, more productive behavior. It is at this stage that negative thought patterns, attitudes, and errors in thinking are challenged. Trust and willingness to change allow for the active challenge of distorted thoughts through CBT. Recovery requires continued practice in identifying errors in thinking and using a positive frame for constructing new thoughts (see Box 5.4).

BOX 5.4   ERRORS IN THINKING AND ATTITUDES THAT PERPETUATE EATING DISORDERS

ALL-OR-NONE REASONING

There are no intermediate states. Frequently used words include "control" and "chaos," "binge" and "starve," "thin" and "fat," and "everything" and "nothing." "I messed up and ate one cookie, so I might as well just eat the whole box now."

PERSONALIZATION

Self-worth depends on what others think. Everything that happens in the world reflects one's personal failures and others' disapproval. "I did not get invited to the party. I know it is because I am a fat, disgusting, ugly, loser."

(Continued)

**BOX 5.4   ERRORS IN THINKING AND ATTITUDES THAT
PERPETUATE EATING DISORDERS (*CONTINUED*)**

OVERGENERALIZATION

If something turns out badly once, it will always turn out badly. "I can't ever go to the movies again. Every time I go, I eat the entire box of popcorn and a whole bag of candy."

MAGICAL OR SUPERSTITIOUS THINKING

When some thing or state is acquired, everything will be perfect. "When I am the thinnest in class, everyone will want to be my friend and I will get a boyfriend."

CATASTROPHIZING/MAGNIFICATION

The outcome or potential outcome is thought of as the worst of all possible consequences to validate negative feelings. "If I eat carbs, I will get fat and my parents will hate me."

ABSTRACTION

The individual focuses on a single aspect of a situation, even though the whole picture may be quite different. "My therapist misunderstood what I was saying today, therefore I do not think he ever understands me, nor does anyone else, for that matter."

PERFECTIONISTIC THINKING

Rigid thinking prevents deviation from a task or behavior because of (often unfounded) fear of negative consequences. "I have to follow my exchange meal plan and I cannot have any less or any more than what my nutritionist says. If I mess up it will prove I am a failure."

SOLUTION-FOCUSED BEHAVIORAL THERAPY

An approach that is usually coupled with CBT is solution-focused behavioral therapy (SBT). This form of advanced counseling therapy is another effective tool for nutrition therapists treating eating disorders. SBT does not investigate the reasons for feelings behind actions, but rather explores solutions. The goal is to help the client to find different solutions and ways to diminish the need for the behavior.

This technique encourages the client to create an ideal solution: a magical or ideal day, situation, or behavior. From there, they are asked to gauge where they are in relation to the ideal, on a scale from 1 to 10. The client is encouraged to create solutions that help them to get closer to that ideal or improve the outcome. Typical questions include

- What would the ideal dinner with your husband/wife be like?
- On a scale from 1 to 10, where would last night's dinner be?
- What would have to happen for you to get closer to the ideal dinner, closer to a 10?

The nutrition therapist asks questions that generate client introspection or proposes possible solutions in a neutral context, opening the door to alternatives:

- What would you like to happen?
- What would happen if you did not go to the candy store?
- What would have to happen for you to get through the day without exercising?
- What would you be willing to do to prevent, delay, or minimize your bingeing after lunch?

The idea is to create solutions and help the client to incorporate them. Questions are aimed at getting the client to provide the solutions. If the client cannot create the solutions, the nutrition therapist can make suggestions through questions:

- Would it be more relaxing if you played soft music while you were eating with your husband/wife tonight?
- I am wondering what would happen if you wrote in your journal instead of going to the refrigerator?
- Would you be willing to eat more of your food earlier in the day so that you would not be so hungry at night?
- Do you think if you were able to make a phone call at that time, you might be able to take better care of yourself? How does that sound to you?

The nutrition therapist should not instruct the client but rather provide them with as much information as necessary to back up the suggestions. For example, information on blood sugar, metabolism, and the binge/purge cycle would all support the suggestion that eating earlier would decrease the tendency to overeat at night: leveraging your partnership to create value and goals that motivate the client to take different actions.

ACCEPTANCE AND COMMITMENT THERAPY

Acceptance and commitment therapy (ACT) strategies may be used in this process. ACT is an empirically based psychological intervention that uses acceptance and mindfulness strategies, together with commitment and behavior change strategies (Cardi et al. 2015). The idea is to help the client accept their reactions or feelings to a situation while remaining present and choose a reaction or action that will take them in a valued direction. Sessions are used to help determine what the client values or wants to achieve and what the risk/challenge will be, as well as when, how, and with whom the risks will be taken.

NUTRITION THERAPY: MOTIVATION, GOAL SETTING, AND RECOVERY

Motivational interviewing (MI) is a method that works on facilitating and engaging intrinsic motivation within the client in order to change behavior. Using MI, the practitioner can better help the client move forward in their desire to make changes. MI is a goal-oriented, client-centered counseling style for eliciting behavior change by helping clients to explore and resolve ambivalence (Golan 2013; Wilson and Schlam 2004). The nutrition therapist must proceed with a strong sense of purpose, clear strategies, and skills for pursuing that purpose. They can point out discrepancies between the client's values and goals, and their current behavior, in a nonargumentative or accusatory manner (Wilson and Schlam 2004; Golan 2013). The goal for the nutrition therapist is to assist the client in finding the motivation to make these changes. If the client is not intrinsically motivated, it will be more difficult for them to put in the effort to make the necessary behavior changes.

No matter the selected treatment approach, the overarching goal is for the client to develop a life that brings them closer to their true self and their values. By taking action that supports their goals, the patient gradually moves from destructive-disordered behavior to a healthy relationship with food, weight, body, self, and others. Interim goals are tiny steps along the way. All steps are progress because they reflect the brain's ability to change. These include changing the quantity, quality, and variety of food the client eats and the freedom and choice involved. Fostering the process of making, supporting, and maintaining these changes requires a wealth of information, alternatives, and tools, including alternative behaviors, shared eating activities, calming techniques, buffering skills, cognitive-behavioral dialogues, guided imageries, self-care techniques, support groups, and constant reinforcement of the physiological, metabolic, and food facts that have been distorted by the eating disorder (Costin 2007; Costin and Schubert Grabb 2012).

It is important to impress upon the client that their growth and progress will be unique to the individual. Not all tools will work for them, and they will need to practice all the tools to determine which are most effective and best develop their skills. With time, they will become better at assessing which tools to use in which situations. The more frequently a healthier behavior is practiced, the more skilled the client will become. The goal is to learn to be persistent, patient, and self-compassionate.

During treatment, nutrition therapists must develop and model the qualities they are guiding the clients toward, continually affirming that there is hope and that they will not give up on the client or the client's recovery. Actions and demeanor, as well as words, will communicate this. Healing takes place out of self-compassion and not out of self-loathing. Clients are often prone to all-or-none thinking, and frequently give up if they slip or fall because of the fear of failure or the unwillingness to risk success. The nutrition therapist's commitment, compassion, and understanding, as well as their strength and determination, provide a model to follow.

Moving into action is a crucial part of recovery. Like a fork in the road, it requires active decisions and effort. The client will need guidance onto a new, different, hard, and scary path and toward a more productive way of handling old situations. A strong therapeutic relationship with demonstrated caring will help move them forward, if they are ready. However, all the caring in the world will not facilitate progress if the client is not ready. It is not the nutrition therapist's responsibility to make the client change. The client has to be willing to work hard on changing himself or herself to move from the fork in the road. Standing in place or retreating down the old path cannot be prevented if the client chooses to do so. Some clients may never be ready, no matter how hard the nutrition therapist works, or they may be ready with the next nutrition therapist. Recognizing this and setting professional limits are necessary for the nutrition therapist's self-care.

In negotiating changes with the client, it is mutually beneficial for the nutrition therapist to work out agreements with the client about what they are willing to strive for between sessions. The nutrition therapist may ask the client for suggestions and solutions:

- What do you think you would like to see happen this week?
- What are you willing to do this week?
- How do you think we might accomplish that?
- Whose support do you need to get that to happen?

The goals should be achievable and match what the client is willing or ready to agree to doing. The nutrition therapist should not set the client up for failure or let them set themselves up for failure by setting unachievable goals, which may reconfirm to them that he or she is worthless. The nutrition therapist should avoid tendencies to have an agenda and planned solutions, to get the job done quickly, or to do the work for the client (King and Klawitter 2007).

The nutrition therapist should be leery of the words "I will try." These usually signal that the goal that has been set up is too risky or that the client is not prepared for it. The two answers that follow the nutrition therapist's question in this scenario show the difference:

NT: It sounds as if you recognize how important it has been for you to monitor your
         feelings. Are you willing to resume writing in your journal this week?
Client response 1: Yes, I can do that.
Client response 2: I will try.

If the first response is clear and accompanied by a confident manner, it suggests that both the nutrition therapist and the client are comfortable with the goal. The second response suggests that further questioning is needed:

- It sounds as if you are uncertain whether you will be able to resume your writing. What is in the way of that happening?
- What are your concerns or what is your unwillingness about?
- What do you think is a better goal for you this week?

The client might respond, "Well, I really do not like the book I have and I do not have money to buy a new one." The goal could then be adjusted to remove some of these barriers or to discover what the real resistance is. If the stated barriers are not cleared or true barriers are not uncovered, the client will not write. "I will try" is often a way for many clients to say "no" without confrontation.

Every client needs to have their individualized treatment plan. Agreements should be simple, clear, and few. Each goal should be broken into small steps that lead to its completion. Techniques should be chosen that will help this particular client comply. Agreements can be made to simply observe something or to take action. The client will need help to think through what has to happen to achieve the goal. What thoughts, behaviors, and actions need to be considered? The nutrition therapist should attempt to uncover thoughts that might get in the way of the goal. CBT will promote changing a thought or creating a new image to help the client change their behavior (Fairburn et al. 2003; Fairburn 2008). The nutrition therapist and team will frequently remind the client of what they value and what they want to accomplish, and continually connect the change in thoughts and actions to achieving those values.

Through treatment, the client will become willing to take small risks, to do things differently, to fall, and to learn from the fall instead of feel defeated. They become willing to experiment with behaviors that have been difficult for them. It is important to take small and realistic risks. The nutrition therapist directs the client toward changes in food choices (Academy for Eating Disorders 2012). The psychotherapist works with similar goals in other aspects of the client's life (Costin 2007). For example, when the psychotherapist is working with a client who cannot ask for what they need from their husband/wife, the nutrition therapist can work with the client on asking for some special food or preparation in a restaurant. Taking a risk to ask for what they need in either circumstance fosters growth in both areas. In addition, helping clients accept that the important step of asking does not mean they have the power to control the answer, only how they respond to the answer.

RECOVERY

Recovery is the ongoing process of creating value in one's life (Olmsted et al. 2012). Throughout treatment, the nutrition therapist will work with the client to change her thinking processes and replace eating-disordered behaviors and thoughts with healthy behaviors and thoughts (Graves and Reiter 2010). The nutrition therapist needs to help the client to establish value in life beyond the eating disorder, shift the value from their eating disorder to themself, and constructively deal with the uncomfortable feelings that the eating disorder was masking. This can be difficult and painful.

Through the process of mirroring and discovery, the treatment team works to help the client see themself through different eyes. The nutrition therapist reflects a nurturing, accepting view of the client, and teaches skills the client will eventually master. Eventually, the client becomes increasingly willing to take risks and to experiment with experiences that are difficult, and is no longer willing or able to hide from themselves or their feelings. The nutrition therapist continues to direct the client toward making changes in their foods, as well as finding other ways to cope with their feelings (Graves and Reiter 2010).

The clients actively work at breaking the eating-disordered rules and patterns they previously considered untouchable. They expand their circle of foods, their relationships in the world, and their life. All actions are learning experiences and deserve applause. Uncompleted goals are never failures. Every action provides information. Inability to complete a task suggests that the need for the original behavior requires reexamination (Spahn et al. 2010). More achievable solutions can then be created, strengthening the overall concept of nonjudgment and acceptance. Helping the client accept who they are and where they are is essential to moving forward.

MINIMIZING SABOTAGE/FEAR OF SUCCESS

Roadblocks often develop situations, thoughts, and behaviors that keep clients immobilized or set them back. The nutrition therapist should anticipate roadblocks and sabotage. He or she should help clients think through the week ahead, plan for challenges, and learn how to better take care of themselves. Clients must look at the upcoming hour, day, and week to identify places, people, thoughts, behaviors, or circumstances that might be barriers to completing goals, and the nutrition therapist should discuss solutions with them, encouraging safe risks. The nutrition therapist might ask, "So what is happening this week that will get in the way of you taking care of yourself or following your plan?" It is important to be specific, to get into details, and help create healthier and more realistic solutions.

Clients will have difficulties with certain occasions. They are often impacted by certain vacations and holidays, particularly the gift-giving and food-consuming holidays (De LA Rie et al. 2006). Anniversaries of deaths and past traumas will trigger uncomfortable feelings, and it is helpful for the nutrition therapist to be aware and discuss these events with the client in advance (Treasure and Kanakam 2012). It is important that together the nutrition therapist and client process other special occasions or events, particularly weddings and proms, sports competitions, or try-outs, where there are a conglomerate of emotional elements, including wearing special clothes, exposing more of the body, being bombarded by an abundance of food, or dealing with feelings about acceptance, rejection, visibility, exclusion, and comparison. Helping the client learn how to anticipate, think through, solve problems, cope with feelings, and get needs met without the use of eating-disordered behaviors is part of the nutrition therapist's role.

The nutrition therapist will also need to watch for ambivalence about success on the part of the client (Wilson and Schlam 2004). Fear of success produces many side effects that the client must deal with to move forward. It may be one thing to desire to change and struggle to do so, but the actual achievement of progress may be scary. Succeeding will mean surrendering their eating-disorder identity or at least parts of it. Clients may fear this because they do not know what to expect. "Who am I? Will there be anything there? What will I become?" "Will you or others still care about me?" The known, the eating disorder, although painful, is consciously or unconsciously perceived as more desirable than the unknown of success and even more frightening may be the fear of never succeeding.

Success is also difficult because many clients feel they are not entitled to anything good. They are unable to give to themselves and are uncomfortable with the unfamiliarity of positive feelings. Finally, succeeding is arduous. As eating-disordered behaviors are discontinued, the painful or submerged feelings the eating-disorder behaviors have served to cover up begin to surface. Clients often choose the comfort of the eating disorder over the discomfort of painful feelings or the unknown territory of success (see Box 5.5).

BOX 5.5   CASE STUDY: CONNECTING EMOTIONS TO BEHAVIORS FOSTERS GROWTH AND SUCCESS

Alexis was a client who continued to binge and gain weight despite her ongoing desire to lose weight and follow a mindful eating plan. She had an underlying fear that if she lost weight, she would be obligated to be in an intimate romantic relationship. The bingeing and weight gain served as protection from having to deal with this fear.

Psychotherapy helped her to identify that unconsciously she defeated her work with the nutrition therapist because she was fearful that any progress or success would make her vulnerable. She became aware of the uncomfortable feelings and the need to avoid being hurt that would arise in any close relationship.

Alexis's psychotherapy focused on resolving her fear of intimacy, and involved examining her relationships, while experiencing, expressing, and challenging feelings without using food. The nutrition therapy explored the connection between foods, bingeing patterns, and these feelings through supervised exposure to new thoughts, foods, and eating experiences. Alexis was asked to take daily notes of even small challenges she succeeded at and record those marks of progress in her journal. This process allowed her to feel more successful and enabled her to continue to take more risks.

Gradually, they all worked together on slow steps, small risks and successes with her food, eating-disorder behaviors, and relationships. Throughout the process, in both her therapeutic and real-life relationships, these steps were acknowledged as growth. The treatment allowed for Alexis to connect her fear of intimacy and success with her eating-disorder behaviors. She began to experience relationships and food with less fear and viewed them as an opportunity to learn more about herself.

Over time, Alexis was successful at having an intimate romantic relationship and stopped bingeing as she learned to express herself, have increased tolerance and respect for her feelings, and perceive all experience with the potential of growth and success.

Monitoring Progress

The nutrition therapist must promote all work as progress and an opportunity to learn more, not simply a matter of whether the task was completed or not (Costin 2007). He or she will continually teach the client to create new thoughts and behaviors to replace the eating-disordered distortions and to manage the actions that result. Though initial work will focus on the client's relationship with food, that relationship is actually a metaphor for how he or she deals with life. Clients are learning to negotiate life and its difficulties. This process is ultimately about learning good self-care. Self-care skills need ongoing development and continued support (Olmsted et al. 2012). Practice is what allows the skills to be effective.

It is important that the nutrition therapist continually impress upon the client that change does not take place overnight. Old behavior has been reinforced over many years, and creating new thoughts and behaviors takes time, compassion, patience, practice, and repetition. It is a long process with many ups and downs. Many feelings will be aroused in both the client and the nutrition therapist, including frustrations, disappointment, hopelessness, incompetence, empowerment, fear, success, failure, dependency, inadequacy, and anger (Costin 2007). These are intense feelings, and may have led to the abandonment of relationships and therapy in the past.

Helping the client learn to tolerate these feelings is part of the process. Feelings have a beginning, middle, and an end. Learning to ride out an intense feeling is an important skill that therapy facilitates. With time, the client will learn to embrace their feelings and understand that they are their guides to self-awareness. Incorporating new thoughts and behaviors will promote change; reinforcing and supporting this change will help the client to leave the old behavior behind. Ultimately being able to label and express feelings will become an invaluable skill that diminishes the need for the eating-disordered behaviors.

Maintenance of Change

Equally important to making changes is maintaining them. As treatment continues and progress is made, a big part of the work will be to help the client adjust to the consequences of the changed behaviors. This is a difficult but crucial part of recovery. The client may have difficulty tolerating changes that occur as emotional and physical needs begin to be met. Even positive feelings will be part of this process.

Clients often express discomfort with positive feelings. They are uncomfortable feeling happy or fulfilled and often frightened about success. Up to this point, they may have been devalued or devalued themselves and are often incapable of letting in positive feelings. They will hopefully learn to use positive and negative feelings as guides. They will learn to understand to embrace their feelings, needs, and hungers and work through the consequences. It is an ongoing process that requires constant work in which curious and self-compassionate self-examination is productive.

- What am I frightened about?
- What can I do to change the situation?

- Who can I talk to about it?
- What can I do to feel better?
- How can I take care of myself?
- What am I hungry for?
- Do I want something hot or cold?
- Do I want to eat by myself?
- When do I want to eat?
- Where will I find what I want?
- How will I know if I am satisfied?

The nutrition therapist's function is to help the client learn to allow positive thoughts to flourish and to help the client tolerate a full range of feelings through the language of food and self-care (Costin 2007; Olmsted et al. 2012). He or she will foster movement away from perfectionist, all-or-none, black-and-white thinking and encourage adventuring into the gray or middle (Olmsted et al. 2012). Messages of acceptance, balance, and flexibility will replace perfectionistic and rigid thinking (Kaye et al. 2012). Each day is a new day, and each meal is a new meal. Though the sun does not shine every day, there is something positive to be found in each day. Teaching the client to accept where he or she is and to learn from whatever that day brings is a crucial part of recovery.

RELAPSE PREVENTION

Relapse, or recycling, is typically part of the process (Kaye et al. 2012). Along the path to recovery, relapses identify areas that the client may have trouble with, areas that need to be explored. The client is reminding themselves and the nutrition therapist that progress is not a straight line and success and growth may be frightening. Each setback communicates something not yet identified, which may still be painful, anxiety producing, or terrifying.

When a client's symptoms resurface or they are unable to achieve their goals, this is a message that some event, feeling, or circumstance needs to be addressed. The nutrition therapist might ask

- What do you think was happening?
- What were you feeling?
- What happened that day?

When something causes the client pain, anxiety, or fear, the resulting bingeing or restricting enables the client and nutrition therapist to pinpoint the cause without judgment and work on ways to handle it (Vitousek et al. 1998).

Sometimes, a client's unwillingness or inability to look at their feelings keeps them immersed in their eating-disordered behaviors (Braham and Sampson 2013). They may strongly resist doing any work on food or food-related behaviors because they feel they desperately need them to survive (Vitousek et al. 1998). It is important for the nutrition therapist to recognize this, keep the psychotherapist informed and, if necessary, allow the client to take a break from challenging issues. This may mean that the nutrition therapist will see the client less often for a time, or that sessions will be suspended until the treatment team (the client included) determines that it is appropriate to resume them. The client must view any break as part of the process, rather than failure or rejection by the nutrition therapist. It is an opportunity to let things settle and perhaps concentrate on emotional issues before returning to address food issues.

Clients can still be seen during this period, with a focus on communication and support, and the work may shift to the psychotherapist. Clients usually welcome the support, even though they are not "producing results." Maintaining the connection may shorten the "downtime" and reduce the likelihood of the client's perceiving herself as a failure. If a client is uncomfortable with sessions in which he or she is unable to work directly on food behaviors, it may be helpful to make an appointment for a specified time 4–6 weeks in the future. This keeps the client and nutrition therapist connected. From there, appointments can be scheduled every 4–6 weeks until the client expresses, or the treatment team observes, that they are ready to resume work.

Closure/Termination

Clients are loaned to therapists. Treatment is a mutual process. Every client learns from their nutrition therapist, but does his or her own teaching as well. As clients change, so too do the nutrition therapists change. The goal of treatment is to teach clients self-care and to connect with their inner strength. To help them recognize their hungers and to feed themselves physically, emotionally, and spiritually. Both the client and the nutrition therapist are rewarded by this transformation.

The client begins treatment dependent on their nutrition therapist. During treatment, they learn how to be independent (Golan 2013); then they move on to function in and be part of a larger world. The process is similar to raising a child, then watching the child develop and go out into the world. Both the child and the parent have ambivalent feelings. There is a sense of both joy and loss.

Clients experience varying degrees of anxiety about the loss of their therapeutic relationship. Some even choose to hold on to some aspect of their eating disorder as a way of remaining in need of help and staying in treatment. There is often fear of getting better for fear that the relationship will be lost (Erskine 2011).

This fear should be discussed several times during treatment. It is important at the time of closure to assure the client that this is not the end of the relationship, but the beginning of a new phase. When it is time for the client to end treatment, the nutrition therapist will discuss with the client the possibility of seeing them less and less frequently. This helps decrease the client's sense of dependence, lessens their sense of loss, and assures them of their capabilities and stability.

One technique for closure is to set up a series of two or three closing sessions once a mutual decision has been reached that it is time for the client to leave treatment and fly on their own. In the sessions, the nutrition therapist and client will review progress made, strengths, weaknesses, tools, and current life circumstances. They will acknowledge growth that has occurred, potential challenges, and confidence that the client will succeed. The nutrition therapist will assure the client that they can schedule an appointment when necessary, but remind them that they now have the tools they need for problem-solving. The client will need to also be reminded that there will be ups and downs, and that they know how to work through both.

Closure and termination will be less complete for clients who are frustrated with themselves or with the nutrition therapist, frightened that they are getting better, or discouraged that they are not getting better. Some may just not show up or cancel appointments and not reschedule them. It is important for the nutrition therapist to call and encourage them to come in and talk about what is happening face to face. A client may be angry at the nutrition therapist for her lack of success or avoid the therapist because they do not want to succeed. In either case, they should be encouraged to come in. In that session, the nutrition therapist will help the client to identify their need to leave and share any negative emotions he or she was unwilling to verbalize or found easier to cope with through not coming to appointments. There are several approaches the nutrition therapist could take:

- Perhaps something you want/need is not happening here.
- I am wondering if I disappointed you.
- I am wondering how long you have wanted to leave and why you did not say anything?
- What has given you the courage to leave now?
- Where else do you leave when you feel disappointed, angry, frustrated, and so on?
- Is there any other way you could handle that feeling?
- Would you like me to help you to stay or help you to leave?

Even in the process of leaving, the goal is to explore, reflect, and then plan the action (Cardi et al. 2015). If the client still wants to leave, the nutrition therapist should close as with any other client, outlining the progress thus far and the potential seen. He or she should ask if the client would like to be referred to someone else, and leave the door open to return if they ever choose to do so.

If the client will not come to a closure session, phone sessions or letters are other options. Completion models responsibility in relationships and the importance of communicating what is happening (Bodell and Keel 2010). It is an important part of the therapeutic process because it teaches clients to face uncomfortable emotions, instead of simply running away.

CONCLUSION

Nutrition therapists treating eating disorders must develop their own strong psychotherapeutic skills, network, and therapeutic alliances. The nutrition therapist, through practice, professional supervision, and self-examination, can learn how to engage clients, sharpen his or her own communication skills, and deepen inquiry into clients' issues. A nutrition therapist, who already holds the RD credential, can become certified by IAEDP, the accrediting body, as a CEDS (CEDRD). Multidisciplinary treatment is currently considered best practice for eating disorders and the nutrition therapist has an important role on the multidisciplinary team throughout the continuum of care. Trust building and counseling skills are essential to be effective with both the clients and the collaborative team. Nutrition therapists often integrate a number of treatment modalities to help clients change behaviors related to food, weight, activity, and body dissatisfaction. The nutrition therapist guides the client through the process of change from awareness to alternative actions and finally to the elimination of the eating-disordered behaviors. Changes include taking risks to replace distorted beliefs and behaviors with healthier ones. The nutrition therapist should not do the work for the client, but rather guide him or her through the work. Changes in behavior result when the client recognizes the purpose of the eating disorder and is able to find new ways to satisfy their needs. Change takes place in stages over a period of time. Nutrition therapists and some therapists may work with clients at meals, in restaurants, grocery stores, and in eating groups through planned exposure to expand the comfort around foods and social eating circumstances. It is important for a nutrition therapist to engage in eating events with the client in order for the client to be able to fully share his or her personal eating experiences. The client can share the thoughts and feelings as they arise and the nutrition therapist can then help them work through these feelings. It is important for the client to gain exposure to these uncomfortable eating events when in the company of a safe, therapeutic treatment team member, in hopes of making it easier for the client to face the different eating events that may arise in day-to-day life with friends and family in various settings such as restaurants, take out, buffets, and so on. Since the nutrition therapist has the responsibility to discuss the food with the client, he or she may also be in the position to uncover and address the feelings that surround the food, and the choices that the individual is making. This information, when shared with the entire treatment team, can enhance the work of the other team members, strengthening the treatment path for that client. The nutrition therapist will adapt advanced therapeutic counseling skills and merge them with nutrition language. This unique combination of physiological knowledge and understanding of underlying psychological issues is what makes the nutrition therapist's role so crucial in treatment. The learning process takes a great amount of skill, continued practice, and supervision with seasoned nutrition therapists, psychotherapists, physicians, and psychiatrists who specialize in the treatment of eating disorders.

It is the focus of this chapter to create a better understanding of the role of nutrition therapists in the treatment of eating disorders so that clients, families, and the collaborative team are able to utilize a nutrition therapist to enhance treatment. It is beyond the scope of this chapter to detail specific protocols or give nutritional recommendations for clients and for nutrition conditions that coexist with eating disorders. Additional research and documentation are necessary to support the evolving role of the nutrition therapist.

APPENDIX A: THE TREATMENT TEAM

A *multidisciplinary approach* is imperative for the treatment of eating disorders

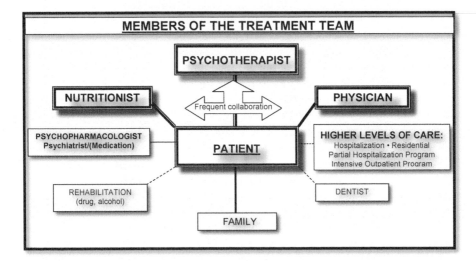

MEMBERS OF THE TREATMENT TEAM

Successful collaborative treatment must simultaneously address these aspects of the eating disorder.

1. **Physiological:** *the physician* - medical aspects of treatment, hospitalization.
2. **Nutritional:** *the nutritionist* - all aspects of food, weight and eating behaviors.
3. **Pharmacological:** *the psychiatrist* - psychotropic medication and brain chemistry.
4. **Psychological:** *the therapist* - emotional and underlying issues.

APPENDIX B: THERAPEUTIC COUNSELING SKILLS –
BASIC, ADVANCED AND EXPERIENTIAL

Be aware of the uniqueness and the differences in each client in every session.

- Backgrounds
- Expectations
- Processing skills
- Supports
- Resources
- Present stage of recovery

And meet the client where they are at, ALWAYS!

Successful counseling skills equal successful communication skills. Improved skills result in increased: compliance, commitment, motivation and success.

Use your feelings and the client's feelings as your compass in negotiating the treatment path. Learning to use and communicate your feelings effectively will deepen the therapeutic relationship and model productive forms of communication for your client. Practice. Be patient, persistent and compassionate.

A healing relationship fosters:
Validation, Mutuality, Self-Empathy and Empowerment

BASIC SKILLS

Ambiance
Is your office friendly, professional, comfortable?
Will it foster communication?
Will you be interrupted?
Is it private?

Expectations/Goal Setting
Discuss and agree. Don't mandate.
Take baby steps.
Make goals attainable.
Monitor expectations.

Engagement
Make the client feel welcome and at ease. Build a rapport, communicate your willingness to be related, connected.

Exploratory Questioning
Use open-ended questions.
Probe into the meaning of vague adjectives or descriptions.

Listening
Listen without interrupting.
Don't make assumptions.

Reflection/Clarification
Summarize what you hear.
Ask what the client heard you say.

Non-Judgmental Responsiveness
Take yourself and your beliefs out of the picture. Respond from your client's perspective.

Building Trust/Showing Respect
Set limits and boundaries. Keep them!
Keep your word/commitments.
Keep your time frame.
Respect their confidentiality.

Silence
Use the silence. Sit with it. Do not try to fill the space or take away uncomfortable moments or feelings.

Feedback
Give your feedback without an agenda or position. Be able to receive feedback and remain neutral.

ADVANCED SKILLS

Dealing with Emotions in the Session
Develop your ability to tolerate a wide range: anger, sadness, fear, hopelessness and rage.
Learn to use emotions as warning signs.
Direct emotions in a productive direction.

Fostering Connectedness
Become comfortable with connecting and building intimate relationships.
Balance the responsibility and power of being so important to the well being of another.

Self-Disclosure
Remain cognizant of effects of revealing personal data and your feelings.
Maintain a check on whose needs you are meeting when you disclose.

Developing Patience and Tolerance
Ability to withstand the pace, intensity and destructive behaviors which manifest.

Transference
Identifying the role which you have taken on in your client's eyes or subconscious. (good mother, teacher, authority figure).

Countertransference
Notice the issues the client brings out in you.
Deal with your own food, weight, relationship and sexuality issues in supervision.

Acknowledge Errors
Learn to acknowledge and discuss errors, breaches of contract or poor judgement that you have made as well as the patient. Deal with feelings that arise for both of you.

Psychiatric Diagnosis
Learn more about psychiatric diagnosis and personality disorders.
Develop your ability to work with severely depressed, borderline and dissociative patients.
Familiarize yourself with indications for and side affects of psychopharmacological medications.

Resources and Referrals
Establish a network of professionals and treatment facilities that you can refer to.
Become aware of ongoing support groups, conferences and other resources available in your community.

EXPERIENTIAL SKILLS

Offers a variety of means for expression and self-awareness. Ultimately develops self-love and self-empathy.

Role Playing – Acting out fearful or difficult situations.

Guided Imagery – Uses the power of imagination to create and visualize the future or reconstruction of past trauma.

Biofeedback – Teaches attunement to stressful body responses and offers relaxation techniques for handling emotional and body stress.

Eating Awareness – Actual planned eating events for increasing focus on thoughts, feelings and behaviors which exist during the eating process.

Art Therapy/Music Therapy – Alternative mechanisms of expression of feelings. Use of cut or drawn pictures, played or taped music to create visual or auditory images of self, pain, pleasure, past and future.

Spiritual Development – Development of spiritual connection and nourishment. Including but not limited to: authentic self, higher power, universal energy, nature.

Body Awareness – Movement work to help client get in touch with their bodies and ultimately release the pain and enjoy the pleasure. Including but not limited to: dance, yoga, massage, walking.

Meditation – Calming and reflective tool. May be used as a stress intervention or as a self-care tool to increase awareness, focus and purpose in one's life.

Journaling – Writing brings focus and awareness to the page. A cost effective, reflective tool for depositing feelings in private forum.

Food Play – Hands on sculpting, drawing and storytelling with food becomes a medium for feelings to arise. Also may be used to desensitize clients with food phobias.

APPENDIX C: THE PATH FROM RD TO CEDRD

Registered Dietitian (RD):

- Completion of a 4-year Baccalaureate Degree accredited by the Accreditation Council for Education in Nutrition and Dietetics (ACEND) and the Commission on Dietetic Registration (CDR). Coursework includes food and nutrition sciences, organic chemistry, nutrition biochemistry, genetics, microbiology, psychology, sociology, anatomy and physiology, foodservice systems management, community nutrition, lifespan nutrition, communications, business, and computer science
- Supervised practice through a Didactic Program in Dietetics and Dietetic Internship or a Coordinated Program in Dietetics accredited by ACEND.
- Completion with a passing score on the national Registration Examination for Registered Dietitians administered by CDR. This RD credential is maintained with yearly CDR-approved continuing education.

Nutrition Therapist/Counselor:

- Responsibilities can vary depending on the division of responsibilities within the treatment team.
- The nutrition therapist practices under the scope of practice within his or her state, as well as the code of ethics for nutrition counselors established by the Academy of Nutrition and Dietetics/Commission on Dietetic Registration.
- Advanced level of study of the eating disorder population is achieved through self-study, continued education, and supervision under eating disorder specialists/professionals.

Certified Eating Disorders Registered Dietitian (CEDRD):

- Education and Registration Status: RD status (requirements stated above)
- Supervised Patient Requirements: 2,500 supervised patient care hours directly in the field of eating disorders by an IAEDP Approved Supervisor
- Continuing Education Requirements
- Core Course Examination Requirements
- Case Study Requirements
- Recommendation Letter Requirements

Be Proactive – National Organizations to Become Involved With:

- AED (Academy for Eating Disorder Professionals)
- BEDA (Binge Eating Disorder Association)
- IAEDP (International Academy of Eating Disorder Professionals)
- IFEDD (International Federation of Eating Disorder Dietitians)
- NEDA (National Eating Disorders Association)
- SCAN (Sports, Cardiovascular, and Wellness Nutrition)

Source: "The CEDRD in Eating Disorder Care", IAEDP 2015
American Dietetic Association "Journal of American Dietetic Association"

APPENDIX D: NUTRITION SAVVY THERAPY AND FAMILY EDUCATION MODULES

Treatment is most successful when professionals (medical, psychological, nutrition), client and family members learn and teach cohesive messages. Having a common language and the skills to discuss these topics is key for client's continued progression and recovery.

Being unified and knowledgeable allows clients to be more confident and trusting of the team.
Nutrition "savvy" ED dialogs will help all to understand the clients eating disordered behavior and even more importantly help the client to feel understood.

- Weight
  - Energy expenditure and replenishment
  - Re-feeding realities
  - Fluid fluctuations
  - Normal factors that influence weight changes
  - Weighing (#, <,>)

- Nutrient requirements and Functions
  - Protein
  - Carbohydrates
  - Fat

- Food and Mood Connection
  - Brain and blood chemistry

- Food (Triggers and Solutions)
  - Choosing
  - Shopping
  - Preparing

- Mind Traps
  - Perfectionism
  - Comparison (comparativism)
  - Self-adamancy

- Non-diet Approach
  - No good or bad foods
  - Restrict-Binge cycle
  - Relaxed/Mindful eating

- Body Perspectives and Beliefs/ Social Circumstance
  - Clothing shopping
  - Vulnerable events (for body exposure or focus)
    - Prom
    - Summer
    - Sexual experiences
    - Real or virtual

- Normal Body Development
  - Growth patterns
  - Hormonal changes
  - Menstrual regularity

- Healthful Exercise
  - Muscle vs. weight vs. fat
  - Exercise obsession
  - Movement and activity

- Cultural Over Exposure
  - Embedded messages
  - Accepted dialogs
  - Current fads/clean eating

- Progress: Means and Modes
  - Relapse circle
  - Staircase up and down
  - Realistic length of time

APPENDIX E: COLLABORATION BETWEEN THE NUTRITIONIST AND THERAPIST FOR THE TREATMENT OF EATING DISORDERS

Therapist's Role	Nutritionist's Role
1. Responsible for the psychological aspects of treatment.	1. Teaches eating disordered client ways to change food, exercise and weight related behaviors.
2. Determines when individual, family or group therapy is appropriate for the eating disordered patient.	2. Educates the client about normal and abnormal food intake patterns, hunger patterns, metabolic rate and somatic sensations or symptoms of each.
3. Needs to keep other team members apprised of progress in therapy.	3. Educates and helps patient become aware of the physiological, biological and emotional body reactions to food, exercise, and substance misuse.
4. Explains to team members the issues that a person has that might affect the client's relationship with them.	4. Assists client in understanding connection between emotions and behaviors.
5. Helps client make the connection between the underlying issues and eating disordered behavior.	5. Guides and teaches client how to develop a healthy relationship with food. Developing normal eating patterns and eventually maintaining their weight within a healthy range.
6. Educates, discusses and prepares the client for working collaboratively as part of a treatment team.	6. Keeps other members of the team apprised of changes in eating, weight and food behaviors.
7. Helps client and family understand the purpose the eating disorder serves and explores client's willingness to get better.	

Shared Roles of the Therapist and Nutritionist

1. Continuously reinforce the purpose of team treatment and the roles of each member. Model for client your connection in regard to their issues.

2. Continuously reveal to client how food, weight and body image behaviors mirror their relationship behaviors and often act as a means of expression or protection.

3. Work with clients to repair damaged self and body images. Develop exercises to improve positive self-talk and recreate a positive self-image.

4. Help client develop a sense of trust, relationship and connectedness to other people and self, not their eating disorder behavior.

5. Help client learn what their needs are and how to meet those needs in appropriate ways.

6. Help client develop other tools for dealing and coping with issues and emotions in their lives.

7. Support and encourage risk and change of eating disordered behaviors that will catalyze and foster developmental and emotional growth.

APPENDIX F: SUCCESSFUL CHANGE

Successful change is scientific, predictable and controllable.

Failure often occurs when people try to change by themselves and get burnt out trying to reinvent the wheel. The struggle often leaves them exhausted and self-defeated.

The path of successful change requires that you:

- Be open and willing to learn.
- Make change a top priority.
- Increase your understanding of how the problem works for and against you.
- Develop new coping skills.
  - **(These ingredients create the best possible chance of success when you are ready for action).**

If you **believe** that you **can change** you are more likely to be **successful.** Beliefs stem from words, thoughts and images.
THEREFORE WE CAN USE OUR MIND POWER TO CREATE CHANGE.

Stages of Change

There are predictable, well-defined stages to change. Each stage requires a period of time and entails a series of tasks that need to be completed before moving on to the next stage.

1. Precontemplation- You are not aware of or able to acknowledge the problem. Not able to admit or acknowledge that it bothers you.

2. Contemplation- You acknowledge that you have a problem and begin to struggle to understand and wonder about solutions. Focus is more on the problem than the solution. You think more about the past than the future.

3. Preparation- You plan to take action. Make public your intent. You have not necessarily resolved your ambivalence.
   Short cutting the preparation stage decreases your chance of success.

4. Action- You make overt modifications of behavior or surroundings. Action is predicated on a commitment of time and energy. Action elicits increased recognition from others.
5. Maintenance- You struggle to prevent lapses and relapses. (Lasts from six months to a lifetime).
   Easy/quick change fails in maintenance.

6. Termination- You eliminate the problem or need for the behavior. No fear or threat that the behavior will return. Confident that you can cope without fear of relapse.

Progress

- Progress takes place in all stages.
- **Moving from stage to stage is progress.**
- **Invisible changes** will take place in the first three stages. Changes in awareness, emotions, self-image and thinking.
- **Visible changes** take place in the last three stages, **(action, termination and maintenance).**

Recycle/(Relapse)

- Progress is **not linear**.
- Relapse is the rule not the exception.
- Often you spiral through the stages 3 or 4 times or more before you exit.
- Be prepared for complications.
- Distress and social pressure precipitate relapse.
- Guilt and self-blame exacerbate the relapse.

THE KEY TO SUCCESSFUL CHANGE IS TO KNOW WHAT STAGE YOU ARE IN!

Source: Changing for Good.© 1994, James Prochaska, Phd., John Norcross, Phd., and Carlo DiClemente, Phd

REFERENCES

Abbate-Daga, G, Amianto F, Delsedime N, De-Bacco C, and Fassino S. Resistance to treatment and change in anorexia nervosa: A clinical overview. *BMC Psychiatry* 13, (2013): 294.

Academy for Eating Disorders. *Eating Disorders: Critical Points for Early Recognition and Medical Risk Management in the Care of Individuals with Eating Disorders* (2nd ed.). Deerfield, IL: Academy for Eating Disorders, 2012.

American Dietetic Association. Position of the American Dietetic Association: Nutrition intervention in the treatment of eating disorders. *Journal of the American Dietetic Association* 111, (2011): 1236–1241.

Bailey, AP, Parker AG, Colautti LA, Hart LM, Liu P, and Hetrick SE. Mapping the evidence for the prevention and treatment of eating disorders in young people. *Journal of Eating Disorders* 2, (2015): 1–12.

Bodell, LP, and Keel, P. Current treatment for anorexia nervosa: Efficacy, safety, and adherence. *Journal of Psychology Research and Behavior Management* 3 (2010): 91–108.

Braham, S, and Sampson K. A cohesive multidisciplinary team approach to the management of patients with eating disorders. *Journal of Eating Disorders* 1, no. S1 (2013): O15.

Cardi, V, Ambwani S, Crosby R, Macdonald P, Todd G, Park J, Moss S, Schmidt U, and Treasure J. Self-help and recovery guide for eating disorders (SHARED): Study protocol for a randomized controlled trial. *Trials* 16, no. 165 (2015): 1–11.

Center for Substance Abuse Treatment. *Substance Abuse: Clinical Issues in Intensive Outpatient Treatment. Treatment Improvement Protocol (TIP) Series 47. DHHS Publication No. (SMA) 06-4182.* Rockville, MD: Substance Abuse and Mental Health Services Administration, 2006.

Costin, C. *The Eating Disorder Sourcebook* (3rd ed.). New York, NY: McGraw-Hill, 2007.

Costin, C, and Schubert Grabb G. *8 Keys to Recovery from an Eating Disorder: Effective Strategies from Therapeutic Practice and Personal Experience.* New York, NY: W.W. Norton & Company, 2012.

De LA Rie, SM, Van Furth EF, De Koning A, Noordenbos G, and Donker MCH. The quality of life of family caregivers of eating disorder patients. *Eating Disorders: Journal of Treatment and Prevention* 13 (2006): 345–351.

Engel, B. *Healing Your Emotional Self: A Powerful Program to Help You Raise Your Self-Esteem, Quiet Your Inner Critic, and Overcome Your Shame.* Hoboken, NJ: John Wiley & Sons, 2006.

Erskine, RG. Attachment, relational-needs, and psychotherapeutic presence. *Institute for Integrative Psychotherapy Articles* 2, no. 1 (2011): 12–14.

Fairburn, CG. *Cognitive Behavioral Therapy and Eating Disorders.* New York, NY: Guilford Press, 2008.

Fairburn, CG, Cooper Z, and Shafran R. Cognitive behavioral therapy for eating disorders: A "transdiagnostic" theory and treatment. *Behaviour Research and Therapy* 41, no. 5 (2003): 509–528.

Frisch, MJ, Herzog DB, and Franko DL. Residential treatment for eating disorders. *International Journal of Eating Disorders* 39, no. 5 (2006): 434–442.

Fruggeri, L. Therapeutic process as the social construction of change. In *Therapy as Social Construction,* edited by S McNamee and KJL Gerden. Thousand Oaks, CA: Sage Publications, 1992.

Gehart, D. *Theory and Treatment Planning in Counseling and Psychotherapy* (2nd ed.). Boston, MA: Cengage Learning, 2016.

Golan, M. The journey from opposition to recovery from eating disorders: Multidisciplinary model integrating narrative counseling and motivational interviewing in traditional approaches. *Journal of Eating Disorders* 1 (2013), 19.

Golden, NH, and Meyer W. Nutritional rehabilitation of anorexia nervosa. Goals and dangers. *International Journal of Adolescent Medicine and Health* 16, no. 2 (2004): 131–144.

Graves, CS, and Reiter L. Nutrition therapy for eating disorders. *Nutrition in Clinical Practice* 25, no. 2 (2010): 122–136.

Grilo, CM, and Mitchell JE. *The Treatment of Eating Disorders: A Clinical Handbook.* New York, NY: Guilford Press, 2010.

International Association of Eating Disorder Professionals (IAEDP). The CEDRD in eating disorder care, American Dietetic Association. *Journal of American Dietetic Association* (2015): 4–9.

International Association of Eating Disorder Professionals. *CEDS Certification Manual.* Pekin, IL: IAEDP, 2003.

Kaye, WH, Bailer UF, and Klabunde, M. Neurobiology explanations for puzzling behaviours. In *A Collaborative Approach to Eating Disorders*, edited by J Alexander and J Treasure. New York, NY: Routledge, 2012.

King, K, and Klawitter B. *Nutrition Therapy: Advanced Counseling Skills* (3rd ed.). Baltimore, MD: Lippincott Williams & Wilkins, 2007.

Kronberg, S. *Eating Disorder Learning/Teaching Handout Manual.* New York, NY: Wellness Publishing, 2003.

Lyster-Mensh, L. Introduction: Part 2. In *A Collaborative Approach to Eating Disorders*, edited by J Alexander and J Treasure. New York, NY: Routledge, 2012.

Martin, DJ, Garske JP, and Davis MK. Relation of the therapeutic alliance with outcome and other variables: A meta-analytic review. *Journal of Consulting and Clinical Psychology* 68, no. 3 (2000): 438–450.

Mittnacht, AM, and Bulik CM. Best nutrition counseling practices for the treatment of anorexia nervosa: A Delphi study. *International Journal of Eating Disorders* 48, no. 1 (2015): 111–122.

Murphy, M, Straebler S, Cooper Z, and Fairburn CG. Cognitive behavioral therapy for eating disorders. *Psychiatric Clinics of North America* 33, no. 3 (2010): 611–627.

Olmsted, MP, Carter, JC, and Pike, KM. Relapse prevention. In *A Collaborative Approach to Eating Disorders*, edited by J Alexander and J Treasure. New York, NY: Routledge, 2012.

Prochaska, JO, Norcross, J, and DiClemente, C. *Changing for Good.* New York, NY: Avon Books, 1995.

Reiff, DW, and Reiff KK. *Eating Disorders: Nutrition Therapy in the Recovery Process.* Gaithersburg, MD: Aspen Publishers, 1992.

Siegel, M, Brisman J, and Weinshel M. *Surviving an Eating Disorder: Strategies for Family and Friends.* New York, NY: Harper and Row Publishers, 1988.

Spahn, JM, Reeves RS, Keim KS, Laquatra I, Kellogg M, Jortberg B, and Clark NA. State of the evidence regarding behavior change theories and strategies in nutrition counseling to facilitate health and food behavior change. *Journal of the American Dietetic Association* 110, no. 6 (2010): 879–891.

Steinglass, JE, Sysko R, Glasofer D, Albano AM, Simpson HB, and Walsh BT. Rationale for the application of exposure and response prevention to the treatment of anorexia nervosa. *International Journal of Eating Disorders* 44, no. 2 (2011): 134–141.

Treasure, J, and Kanakam N. The link between genes and the environment in the shaping of a personality. In *A Collaborative Approach to Eating Disorders*, edited by J Alexander and J Treasure. New York, NY: Routledge, 2012.

Vandereycken, W. The place of inpatient care in the treatment of anorexia nervosa: Questions to be answered. *International Journal of Eating Disorders* 34, no. 4 (2003): 409–422.

Vitousek, K, Watson S, and Wilson GT. Enhancing motivation for change in treatment-resistant eating disorders. *Clinical Psychology Review* 18, no. 4 (1998): 391–420.

Wentz, E, Gillberg IC, Anckarsäter H, Gillberg C, and Råstam M. Adolescent-onset anorexia nervosa: 18-year outcome. *British Journal of Psychiatry* 194, no. 2 (2009): 168–174.

Wilson, TG, and Schlam TR. The transtheoretical model and motivational interviewing in the treatment of eating and weight disorders. *Clinical Psychology Review* 24 (2004): 361–378.

Wolfe, KB. Treatment transitions: Improving patient recovery through effective collaboration. *Eating Disorders Review* (Gurze Books) 14, no. 5 (2003).

Yager J, Devlin MJ, Halmi KA, Herzog DB, Mitchell JE, Powers P, and Zerbe KJ. Practice guideline for the treatment of patients with eating disorders, 3rd edition. *American Journal of Psychiatry* 163, no. S7 (2006): 4–54.

Zucker, N, Moskovich A, Vinson M, and Watson K. Emotions and empathetic understanding: Capitalizing our relationships in those with eating disorders. In *A Collaborative Approach to Eating Disorders*, edited by J Alexander and J Treasure. New York, NY:

Section II

Special Populations

6 Eating Disorders in College Students

Mandy Golman, PhD, MS, MCHES, Marilyn Massey-Stokes, EdD, CHES, CWHC, FASHA, and Susan Karpiel, MS, RDN, LD

CONTENTS

LEARNING OBJECTIVES

After completing this chapter, you should be able to do the following:

- Identify prevalence rates of eating disorders in college students
- Describe the most commonly used measures in assessment and evaluation of eating disorders
- Identify the risk factors specific to college students that contribute to the development of eating disorders
- Address the physiological consequences of eating disorders in college students
- Address the psychosocial consequences of eating disorders in college students
- Describe the most common treatment approaches for college students with eating disorders

Dear Mom and Dad,

Well, I have just completed my first month at college. I'm not really sure what to say. I have made some nice new friends, but feel pretty homesick. I haven't slept too well in my new bed-it is really hard. My classes are tough and I feel overwhelmed by the work.

I think I flunked my first test! I can't find anything to eat in the cafeteria-everything is gross. I don't want to gain the Freshman 15. I'm not sure I'm ready for college at all!

This note, sent home from a first-year college student, summarizes many of the stressors college students can experience during this significant life transition. New environments, sometimes far from home, coupled with pressures to excel academically, make new friends, and manage new responsibilities, can create a very challenging situation for any student. For those struggling with negative body image, disordered eating (DE), or clinical eating disorders, the college campus can be even more daunting and become a perilous environment. Even though research shows that freshman gain between 2.5 and 3.5 lb. and that this is only 1/2 lb. greater than peers their same age who do not attend college, the dreaded Freshman 15 causes much concern for many college women (Zagorsky and Smith 2011). This concern can lead to obsessive thoughts of dieting, dietary restraint, and negative body image, even when no weight gain exists (Delinsky and Wilson 2008; Graham and Jones 2002). Substantial evidence has been found to support that pressure to be thin is predictive of dieting behaviors and onset of bulimic pathology (Cattarin and Thompson 1994; Stice 1998). The pressure to adhere to the thin ideal, the lack of support services, and the freedom of unmonitored behaviors makes the transition to college a period of high risk for the development of an eating disorder (Delinsky and Wilson 2008; National Eating Disorders Association [NEDA] 2013; Striegel-Moore et al. 1986).

PREVALENCE

It is estimated that 30 million people in the United States have an eating disorder at some point in their life (NEDA 2015). The Healthcare Cost and Utilization Project reported that between 1999 and 2006, hospitalizations involving eating disorders increased by 19% for patients aged 19–30 (Zhao and Encinosa 2009; American College Health Association 2015). In addition, eating disorders in the college population are on the rise and show no signs of slowing down. Three percent of females and 0.4% of males reported receiving a diagnosis of anorexia; 2% of females and 0.2% of males reported a previous diagnosis of bulimia; and 4% of females and 1% of males reported vomiting or taking laxatives to lose weight in the previous 30 days in the American College Health Association's National College Health Assessment (Hudson et al. 2007; American College Health Association 2015). In a recent random screening in a large midwestern university, prevalence rates appeared to be 9%–13% among females and 3%–4% among males significantly higher, than noncollege attending peers (Eisenberg et al. 2011). Mintz et al. (1997) found that while only 4% of college women in their sample had eating disorders, 19% of them had an identifiable risk factor for the development of an eating disorder. Although a small percentage of college students have a diagnosable eating disorder, some estimates predict that as many as 30% may be at risk for developing an eating disorder (Franko et al. 2005). Some studies report 64% of college women have reported dysfunctional eating behaviors (Mintz and Betz 1988). A survey conducted by Global Market Insite, Inc. for NEDA found similar startling results. Over 20% of those surveyed reported suffering from an eating disorder at some point in their life, and of that 20% who reported suffering, almost 75% did not seek treatment (NEDA 2015). In terms of mortality rates, eating disorders have the highest rate among mental illnesses with eating disorder not otherwise specified (EDNOS) having a higher mortality rate than anorexia nervosa or bulimia nervosa (Crow et al. 2009). Comorbidities are commonly seen with eating disorders and include depression, anxiety, and substance abuse (Jones et al. 2012). It is also found that these comorbidities can lead to eating disorders, especially in college students with body image concerns. The risk of developing an eating disorder increases from 4% to 60% when students have one or more comorbidities (Jones et al. 2012).

SPECIAL CONCERNS

THE FEMALE ATHLETE TRIAD

Disordered eating can be characterized by a range of unhealthy dietary and weight management attitudes and behaviors that don't warrant a clinical diagnosis of an eating disorder, yet still negatively impact health, wellness, and quality of life and potentially lead to actual eating disorders. Disordered eating includes, but is not limited to, excessive concerns about body weight, shape, and size; poor nutrition and/ or restrictive dieting; very rigid and unhealthy eating and exercise habits; feelings of guilt or shame when unable to meet self-imposed eating and exercise standards; binge eating; use of diuretics and diet pills; purging through laxatives, vomiting, or excessive exercise; and self-obsession with body weight and size, food, and exercise to the extent of causing distress and lowering quality of life (Anderson 2015). College athletes can be susceptible to DE due to the physiologic demands of sports (Granger et al. 2008) and the emphasis that some sports place on body weight and shape (e.g., gymnastics, dance, swimming, diving, cross-country, etc.). Furthermore, DE can lead to a condition referred to as the female athlete triad (Triad), which consists of three interrelated conditions—menstrual dysfunction, low energy availability (with or without an eating disorder), and decreased bone mineral density (Nazem and Ackerman 2012; Nattiv et al. 2007). Low energy availability (with or without an eating disorder) can negatively impact health, both physically and psychologically. Furthermore, the conditions associated with the Triad can lead to serious health issues, such as clinical diagnoses of eating disorders; functional hypothalamic amenorrhea; osteoporosis; bone stress injuries and decreased athletic performance; and complications in endocrine, gastrointestinal, renal, and neuropsychiatric functioning (Nattiv et al. 2007; De Souza et al. 2014).

Studies have indicated that female college athletes are at increased risk for experiencing problems related to DE and the Triad (Greenleaf et al. 2009; Mitchell and Robert-McComb 2014; Reinking and Alexander 2005). In a study of female college athletes from 17 sports at three universities, approximately 26% of the athletes exhibited subclinical symptoms of an eating disorder (Greenleaf et al. 2009). In another study, athletes in "lean" sports (e.g., dance, diving, distance running, gymnastics, and swimming) exhibited more DE than athletes in "nonlean" sports and nonathletes (Reinking and Alexander 2005). According to the National Athletic Trainers' Association (2008), prevalence estimates of eating-related problems have been as high as 62% among female athletes and 33% among male athletes (Granger et al. 2008). However, the extent to which college female athletes engage in pathogenic eating and weight management behaviors and experience clinical eating disorders is not clear (Mitchell and Robert-McComb 2014; Reinking and Alexander 2005; Smolak et al. 2000). Part of the uncertainty can be attributed to methodological differences that can affect findings. It also appears that college-level sports participation can increase risk for eating problems and yet be protective in some cases (Smolak et al. 2000). In addition, a systematic review revealed that the prevalence of the Triad conditions (subclinical and clinical) occurring simultaneously, in combination, and individually is not clear (Gibbs et al. 2013). It was contended that further prevalence research on the Triad is needed to better understand the scope of the problem and develop effective screening, prevention, and treatment strategies for the Triad conditions (alone or in combination).

A NEDA survey of 163 colleges and universities from across the nation revealed that there is a paucity of programs designed to prevent, screen for, and refer student athletes with eating problems, especially in high-risk sports such as gymnastics, wrestling, and swimming (NEDA 2013). Only 22% of the respondents indicated that their school's athletic department offers screening and counseling referrals for athletes in high-risk sports. Furthermore, only 2.5% of the colleges and universities surveyed have ongoing prevention education programs for athletes in high-risk sports. Of those who offer screening and referrals through the athletic department, 100% believe these services are very/extremely or somewhat important. Of all surveyed respondents, 91% stated that such programs are very/extremely or somewhat important. Overall, survey findings revealed that "there is a large unmet need for screenings and counseling services for athletes" (NEDA 2013).

There is general agreement that the most efficacious approach to addressing DE and the Triad conditions (alone or in combination) is early detection and prevention (Gibbs et al. 2013; Granger et al. 2008; Mountjoy et al. 2014; Nattiv et al. 2007; Nazem and Ackerman 2012). Possible warning signs of the Triad include performance regression, mood changes, noticeable weight loss, and frequent injury, particularly fractures. Therefore, maintaining keen awareness and creating an atmosphere that facilitates open communication can help with early detection and successful intervention (Nazem and Ackerman 2012). Moreover, published guidelines and tools are available to facilitate the prevention, detection, and management of DE in college athletes (Granger et al. 2008; Mitchell and Robert-McComb 2014; Nattiv et al. 2007; Rodriguez et al. 2009).

COLLEGE SORORITIES

College sororities are an important social system to target for eating disorder prevention interventions (Becker et al. 2008). Studies have suggested that sorority members highly value physical appearance and may be at increased risk for internalization of the thin ideal, body dissatisfaction, and eating disorders (Basow et al. 2007; Becker et al. 2005). Furthermore, it appears that social influence and modeling may play important roles in promoting DE, especially when sorority members live together (Basow et al. 2007; Crandall 1988; Hoerr et al. 2002). Social influence, particularly from family and peers, is thought to play a key role in the development of body dissatisfaction and internalization of the thin ideal, subthreshold eating problems, as well as clinical eating disorders such as bulimia (Basow et al. 2007; Crandall 1988; Luce et al. 2008; Stice 1998). In addition, social influence and modeling such as binge eating can be problematic within a social system like a sorority (Crandall 1988). In turn, these same social influences may function for compensatory weight control methods (Luce et al. 2008).

A study showed that college females at risk for developing negative body image and DE are attracted to sororities; findings showed that those who intended to join sororities were similar in body objectification to the women who were already members (Basow et al. 2007). In addition, women planning to join sororities rated perceived more social pressure to be attractive and social than nonsorority members and women who didn't plan to rush. Furthermore, the study revealed that women living together in a sorority house appear to be at increased risk for engaging in DE, thereby creating a potentially harmful reciprocal relationship. In contrast, Allison and Park (2004) examined DE prospectively among sorority and nonsorority women and found that DE did not differ between the groups before women joined sororities; however, sorority women maintained a drive for thinness throughout their college years.

Perfectionism is another possible factor that may increase sorority members' risk for experiencing body dissatisfaction and engaging in DE. Perfectionism has been associated with DE behaviors and has been identified as a specific risk factor for the development of eating disorders such as anorexia nervosa and bulimia nervosa (Burke et al. 2010; Macedo et al. 2007). Due to high personal standards (particularly those associated with physical appearance) that appear to be at play within sororities (Basow et al. 2007), perfectionism may play a role in increasing DE behaviors among members. In a study that compared undergraduate sorority women with sorority (Macedo et al. 2007) alumnae (Landa and Bybee 2007), eating problems were correlated with perfectionism and greater divergence between the real (current) and the ideal (desired) self-image. However, the discrepancies in both perfectionism and self-image were substantially lower among the alumnae, indicating important age-related changes in personality development. It is clear that more research is needed to examine the relationships that may be at play regarding sorority membership, body dissatisfaction, DE, and eating disorders. Nevertheless, existing research suggests that college sororities are a salient group to reach with interventions aimed at improving body image, reducing the drive for thinness, and preventing DE and eating disorders (Basow et al. 2007; Becker et al. 2005; Luce et al. 2008).

DRUNKOREXIA

Alcohol use and binge drinking are common among college-aged young adults (aged 18–25; Center for Behavioral Health Statistics and Quality 2015). According to the National Council on Alcoholism and Drug Dependence, Inc. (NCADD; 2015), approximately four out of five college students consume alcohol, and about half of those who drink engage in binge drinking. The negative consequences of alcohol use include, but are not limited to, increased risk for alcohol use disorder, alcohol poisoning, unsafe sex, impaired driving, physical assault, sexual assault, property damage, injury, involvement with the police, academic problems, health problems, and suicide attempts (National Council on Alcoholism and Drug Dependence, Inc. 2015; National Institute on Alcohol Abuse and Alcoholism 2015). First-year college students are considered a particularly high-risk group as they attempt to cope with various academic and social stressors during this key transitional period. Numerous first-year college students engage in episodic heavy drinking that often leads to negative outcomes during college and into young adulthood (Burke et al. 2010; Del Boca et al. 2004). Studies have also shown that members of sororities and fraternities tend to consume heavier amounts of alcohol than students who are not within the Greek system, and alcohol use of first-year students within the Greek system is particularly pronounced during initiation (Borsari et al. 2007).

Although "drunkorexia" is not a medically recognized term and is not listed in the American Psychiatric Association's *Diagnostic and Statistical Manual of Mental Disorders* (DSM-5; American Psychiatric Association 2013), it is increasingly recognized as a term to describe the phenomenon of purposefully restricting calories prior to alcohol consumption (Addiction Center 2016). Caloric restriction can manifest in different ways, such as skipping meals to account for increased caloric intake from alcoholic drinks, exercising excessively to compensate for the extra calories from alcohol consumption, and/or drinking alcohol excessively to become sick and purge food that was eaten earlier (Barry and Piazza-Gardner 2012). Restricting food intake prior to consuming alcohol increases the potential for becoming intoxicated, which, in turn, increases the risk for making poor decisions and experiencing negative consequences associated with alcohol intoxication (Giles et al. 2009).

Lupi et al. (2015) explained the phenomenon of drunkorexia as follows: "Social pressure to always be perfectly fit, combined with the culture of 'high,' may influence young people to resort to extreme measures in order to feel accepted by society." Multiple studies have demonstrated that drunkorexic behavior among college students is a problem that needs to be confronted. For example, Burke et al. (2010) found that 14% of first-year college students restricted calories on days they planned to drink alcohol and those who restricted calories were more likely to binge drink. However, there were no significant differences between males and females. In another study of a random sample of students attending a large university, Eisenberg et al. (2011) found that males who screened positive for eating disorders were less likely to binge drink than other males; however, they found the opposite to be true for females.

In a random sample of 4271 undergraduate students attending 10 universities, 67% reported drinking in the past 30 days. Of that group, 39% reported restricting food, fat, or calories prior to drinking alcohol. In addition, half of Greek pledges and 46% of Greek members reported restricting on days when they planned to consume alcohol. Of those students who reported restricting on drinking days, 47% of females and 32% of males reported that they restricted to control their weight (Giles et al. 2009). In another study conducted with undergraduate students enrolled in a private, urban university, participants reported that they engaged in drunkorexic behavior prior to 29.2% of all drinking events. Also, women were significantly more likely than men to restrict calories prior to consuming alcohol. Furthermore, women who were the heavier drinkers were the ones for whom the desire to control weight strongly predicted their drunkorexic behavior (Eisenberg and Fitz 2014). Research has shown that females who restrict calories and purge food to control body weight experience more severe consequences of alcohol use (Anderson et al. 2005; Burke et al. 2010).

Another line of investigation involves examining the relationship between physical activity and drunkorexia. In a study that was conducted with a nationally representative sample of college students, researchers determined that those students who engaged in vigorous exercise, strength training, and DE had greater odds of being binge drinkers. These findings validated other research findings in which highly physically active college students were more likely to binge drink than their nonactive peers and "highlight the potential of a drunkorexia perspective in explaining the counterintuitive alcohol–activity association among college students" (Barry and Piazza-Gardner 2012). In summary, given the disturbing frequency of drunkorexia and the likelihood of developing more serious health conditions later in life (Addiction Center 2016; Burke et al. 2010; Eisenberg and Fitz 2014; Giles et al. 2009), it is imperative that college campuses tackle the problem in a focused manner through increasing awareness and knowledge (e.g., via social marketing campaigns), improving screening mechanisms, and implementing effective health promotion interventions.

SCREENING AND ASSESSMENT

The demand for mental health care on college campuses is growing, as indicated by a reported increase in the student use of these services (NEDA 2013). In terms of eating disorders, students are often identified as having DE and clinical eating disorders because they took the initiative to seek help. However, there are countless at-risk students who do not seek help; therefore, it is important for health-care providers to be alert to possible risk factors and initiate a conversation with students. Nevertheless, a recent study found that only 6% of students with DE were questioned by their medical provider (White et al. 2011). In addition, although 87% of the universities surveyed agreed that screening is important, only 22.4% of those colleges surveyed offer year-round screening opportunities, which represents a substantial unmet need. Perhaps, mandatory screening of incoming students utilizing an online screening tool should be recommended for colleges (Jones et al. 2012).

No one screening or assessment tool is utilized in isolation for college students. As with other age groups, assessments most commonly used include Eating Disorder Inventory-3 (EDI-3), Sociocultural Attitudes Toward Appearance Questionnaire (SATAQ; Heinberg et al. 1995), Eating Disorder Examination Questionnaire (EDE-Q; Fairburn and Cooper 1993), and the Eating Attitudes Test (EAT-26; Garner et al. 1982).

The SCOFF questionnaire has been utilized frequently as an excellent screening tool for the college population (Morgan et al. 2000). Given the tremendous amounts of DE behaviors unreported, utilization of widespread screening tools is recommended. Early identification and intervention increase the chances for recovery (NEDA 2013).

The SCOFF Questions

- Do you make yourself **S**ick because you feel uncomfortably full?
- Do you worry that you have lost **C**ontrol over how much you eat?
- Have you recently lost more than **O**ne stone (14 lb.) in a 3-month period?
- Do you believe yourself to be **F**at when others say you are too thin?
- Would you say that **F**ood dominates your life? (Morgan et al. 1999)

When students present to the counseling center with an eating disorder, they are referred to college health services for a formal assessment. A campus physician examines the student and makes decisions for a treatment protocol. College officials are often in a difficult position as it relates to managing students with eating disorders. The majority of campuses are only able to provide limited psychological care for the illness, which often requires intense psychotherapy in combination with a physician and a nutritionist. Many student health centers lack personnel with specialized eating disorder training (Jones et al. 2012). Despite the challenges, many colleges and universities are taking a proactive approach to the assessment and treatment of eating disorders with the use of an eating disorder protocol. This protocol often involves a progression of events and evaluations that may result in a contract with the student whereby continued university enrollment is contingent upon treatment compliance. The universities that provide an eating disorder team approach to treatment are better able to manage the care of students with eating disorders. An eating disorder care team can quickly identify and refer students, as well as prevent students from having relapses after treatment (Choate 2010; Jones et al. 2012). However, it is not uncommon for a university to have to make the difficult decision to remove a student until he or she is deemed stable enough to return to the campus. This procedure is usually at no academic penalty to the student. Given that eating disorders are associated with mental illness, suicide, self-injury, binge drinking, cigarette smoking, and drug use, quick identification and treatment are of critical importance on college campuses (Jones et al. 2012).

TREATMENT RESOURCES

Although research is clear that early identification and intervention are the key to the recovery of an eating disorder; the treatment opportunities on college campuses are limited. These limitations vary from student's self-perceptions about their disorder, to schools having the resources to provide necessary services. Therefore, it is important for health-care providers and health educators to be vigilant to warning signs and assess college-aged individuals for possible eating disorders even when they don't present for specific calls for help. Eisenberg et al. (2011) found that many in their study that screened positive for eating disorder symptomology did not seek treatment.

It is important to examine the reasons that college students do not seek treatment. Many students with an eating disorder deny the seriousness of the disorder and are unlikely to seek help. They may feel ashamed or stigmatized by their mental health problem and refuse to confront their illness (Eisenberg et al. 2011; Jones et al. 2012). Often students believe they will grow out of DE (NEDA 2013). Additionally, there are some common personality traits among students with eating disorders that prevent them from seeking help, such as perfectionism and a desire for approval. Finally, lack of financial resources or insurance to pay for treatment is another major factor that limits treatment opportunities (Jones et al. 2012).

According to the NEDA Collegiate Survey Project, a comprehensive survey including 150 colleges and college service provider representatives, more students are requesting mental health services than in the past (NEDA 2013). In fact, the survey showed 23% of liberal arts students and 13% of students from universities nationwide use mental health services. However, the increased demand exceeds available services. In general, higher-education campuses lack the necessary resources to educate, screen, and treat students with eating disorders (NEDA 2013). Although most agree that services and education about eating disorders are important and needed on campus, this belief is most often unbalanced by a lack of services offered in the screening and treatment of this mental health problem. This gap is a serious problem given that eating disorders among college students are rising and early intervention is a key to recovery.

Another limitation is the large gap between how important respondents believe psychotherapy is for students with DE and the availability of counseling. Even though almost all respondents believe counseling is important, less than 80% offer this service. Additionally, only 43.2% of campuses offer group therapy for students dealing with body image or eating disorder issues, yet 80% of those who offer the service believe it is extremely important (NEDA 2013). Furthermore, many campus employees are positioned to identify and refer students at risk for an eating disorder. For example, coaches, athletic trainers, fitness trainers, health and fitness instructors, and dietitians work closely with students and make observations about exercise and eating patterns. As discussed earlier, research shows a high risk for eating disorders among high-level athletes and those participating in certain sports with an emphasis on body weight and size. Yet, there is a lack of training for those positioned to identify and screen athletes. Only 22% of respondent campuses provide training for these employees (NEDA 2013).

In summary, both national universities and liberal arts colleges are limited in the services they provide the students with eating disorders. The most significant challenges campuses have in providing the education and services needed is a lack of resources, such as insufficient funding, a lack of time, insufficient staffing, and the stigma attached to using eating disorder services (NEDA 2013).

PREVENTION

Eating disorder prevention efforts take many forms and prevention on the college campus is no different. Outreach programs and education events presented on college campuses have been demonstrated to be an effective way to increase awareness about eating disorders and encourage those students with DE to seek help (Napierski-Prancl 2011; NEDA 2013). Students who attend these programs have higher levels of knowledge of campus resources for body image and eating-disordered behaviors than those who have not attended campus programming, which has the potential to translate to increasing access to treatment and/or help-seeking behaviors (Tillman et al. 2012, 2015). Over the years, eating disorder prevention programs have gone through a transformation from primarily psychoeducational in content to a more targeted approach toward specific risk factors (NEDA 2013; Stice et al. 2003, 2013a; Tillman et al. 2012, 2015; Yager and O'Dea 2008). Widespread efforts might include informational resources with the goal of raising awareness about the symptoms and dangers of eating disorders, for example, brochures distributed at the health center, websites on campus servers, eating disorder awareness week programming, or programs in the residence halls, sororities, or classrooms. Other more targeted efforts might include more substantial programs or workshops with the goals of reducing risk factors such as body dissatisfaction, unhealthy dieting behaviors, and negative media influences; some efforts utilize a peer education model (Napierski-Prancl 2011; Yager and O'Dea 2008).

A frequent debate among prevention program directors is whether to implement a widespread universal prevention program for an entire campus or a more targeted prevention approach for those identified as high risk, such as athletes. While studies do demonstrate that a more selective approach increases effect sizes, sometimes it might be more feasible at a university to have a greater impact by doing a large-scale program, even if the effect size is smaller (Stice et al. 2013a). In an evaluation of the National Eating Disorders Awareness Week, studies support that these one-time programs are beneficial to students. For example, Dove™ has a widely disseminated positive body image program that is utilized frequently; however, only marginally positive results have been observed (Richardson et al. 2009). Several similar programs exist. Two programs that have been utilized both as targeted as well as universal are *The Body Project* and *A Healthy Weight. The Body Project* by Stice et al. (2013b) is a cognitive dissonance model utilizing peer educators. Researchers found that a treatment package consisting of dissonance-based eating disorder prevention along with psychoeducational and behavioral exposure components was effective in reducing thin-ideal internalization, body dissatisfaction, dieting behaviors, negative affect, and bulimic symptoms among at-risk college females (Stice et al. 2003; Roehrig et al. 2006). In addition, *A Body Project* is one of the few programs that have been demonstrated to be effectively utilized with both universal and targeted approaches (Stice et al. 2013a). *A Healthy Weight* focuses on dietary intake and physical activity and has demonstrated statistically significant reductions in eating pathology onset (Stice et al. 2008). These two projects are among the few that have been demonstrated to be effective with randomized trials. Although peer education programs are widely utilized in eating disorder prevention, evaluation studies supporting the effectiveness of these types of efforts are lacking; therefore more research is needed in this area (Yager and O'Dea 2008; Stice et al. 2013a).

Regardless of the approach, the need for prevention services on college campuses is overwhelming. In the NEDA Collegiate Survey Project, the majority of survey respondents stated that it is important to have peer advisors on campus to work with students, although only 35% of respondent campuses had an advisor (NEDA 2013). The majority also agreed that it is important to train resident advisors on how to identify and refer students with eating disorders, yet only 57% offered resident training. In addition, respondents identified education campaigns as the most successful service provided for eating disorders yet fewer than 20% of their campuses offer monthly or weekly events. These data underscore the importance of providing ongoing education programs on college campuses. Increasing education about the symptoms of DE for all campus health workers and resident assistants provides an excellent opportunity to assure an early diagnosis and intervention of the college student (Choate 2010; Jones et al. 2012; NEDA 2013).

CONCLUSION

Eating disorders are considered chronic, devastating, and potentially life-threatening health conditions; early diagnosis and intervention are critical to recovery. Due to the high prevalence of college-aged females struggling with eating disorders, university student health and counseling services staff should be trained to assess and work with eating disorders as well as potentially coexisting mental health issues (Prouty et al. 2002). Integrated teams of professionals need to be able to connect and interact with these young women and men in ways that are relevant to the student's lives.

CASE STUDY 6.1

Cassie

Cassie is a college freshman who was a heavily recruited soccer player at a large state high school. She had 13 college soccer scholarship offers in high school and was the #1 recruit of her team. She also excelled academically and graduated with a 4.0 grade point average. After accepting a full-ride soccer scholarship at a Division I university, Cassie and her mom met with her future college coaches. During the meeting, Cassie's mother disclosed that Cassie had "struggled off and on with some eating problems," but they were under control and she was fine. She assured the coaches that it was "nothing too serious to worry about." The coaches took Cassie's mom at her word and looked forward to gaining a great player.

As Cassie begins college, she is at a healthy weight. Her workouts on the team are rigorous, and she is a bit stunned at how hard they are compared to her high school practices. In addition, she quickly learns that she will need to earn respect from her upperclassmen teammates—very different from the "rockstar" status she maintained in high school. As school begins, she is exhausted from the workouts and finds that keeping up with her studies is quite challenging. She has always been able to stay on top of things and has never been one to ask for help, so she assumes she will "figure it out" and adjust soon. She makes some friends on the soccer team, but finds meeting other friends difficult. She misses her close knit group of friends from home.

(Continued)

CASE STUDY 6.1 *(CONTINUED)*

About 6 weeks into the semester, the coaches notice that Cassie looks tired and appears to have lost some weight. Despite her tired appearance, she is working out harder than the others. She is the first one to practice and the last to leave. The coaches talk to her after practice and she assures them she is just fine, just tired. One week later, Cassie appears wobbly on the field and almost passes out. The coaches take her out of the game. One of her teammates confides that she has noticed that Cassie doesn't eat much at the daily team meals. The coaches have another discussion with Cassie and call home to share their concerns with her mother. Cassie's mother gets very frustrated with Cassie and tells her to "not blow this" and "just get it together." Both Cassie and her mom assure the coaches that she will be fine. The next week Cassie seems to be more energetic, and the coaches put their concerns on the back burner.

Another 3 weeks go by and the girls are in the dressing room. One of the girls on the team notices Cassie's shockingly thin appearance and reports her concerns to the coach. The coaches meet with Cassie again to voice concern. She breaks down and begs them not to call her mom; she tearfully tells them that she will take care of it on her own.

QUESTIONS

1. What are the coaches' obligations in this situation?
2. What are some recommended steps the coaches can take?
3. What can the university do to help Cassie?

Crossover education and training, such as education about healthy body image and eating in campus-based health education activities (Prouty et al. 2002), may also be useful. Finally, considerably more effort into a coordinated approach of screening as well as implementation and evaluation of evidence-based widely disseminated prevention programs is likely to drastically reduce the incidence of eating disorders on college campuses (Jones et al. 2012; NEDA 2013).

REFERENCES

Addiction Center. Drunkorexia. 2016. Available at https://www.addictioncenter.com/alcohol/drunkorexia/ (accessed 30 May 2016).

Allison, KC, and Park CL. A prospective study of disordered eating among sorority and nonsorority women. *International Journal of Eating Disorders* 35, no. 3 (2004): 354–358.

American College Health Association. *American College Health Association-National College Health Assessment II: Reference Group Executive Summary Spring 2015.* Hanover, MD: Author, 2015.

American Psychiatric Association. *Diagnostic and Statistical Manual of Mental Disorders* (5th ed.). Washington, DC: Author, 2013.

Anderson, M. What Is Disordered Eating? eatright.org, Academy of Nutrition and Dietetics. 25 February 2015. Available at http://www.eatright.org/resource/health/diseases-and-conditions/eating-disorders/what-is-disordered-eating

Anderson, DA, Martens MP, and Cimini MD. Do female college students who purge report greater alcohol use and negative alcohol-related consequences? *International Journal of Eating Disorders* 37, no. 1 (2005): 65–68.

Barry, AE, and Piazza-Gardner AK. Drunkorexia: Understanding the co-occurrence of alcohol consumption and eating/exercise weight management behavior. *Journal of American College Health* 60, no. 3 (2012): 236–243.

Basow, SA, Foran KA, and Bookwala J. Body objectification, social pressure, and disordered eating behavior in college women: The role of sorority membership. *Psychology of Women Quarterly* 31, no. 4 (2007): 394–400.

Becker, CB, Ciao AC, and Smith LM. Moving from efficacy to effectiveness in eating disorders prevention: The sorority body image program. *Cognitive and Behavioral Practice* 15, no. 1 (2008): 18–27.

Becker, C, Smith LM, and Ciao AC. Reducing eating disorder risk factors in sorority members: A randomized trial. *Behavior Therapy* 36, no. 3 (2005): 245–253.

Borsari, B, Murphy JG, and Barnett NP. Predictors of alcohol use during the first year of college: Implications for prevention. *Addictive Behaviors* 32, no. 10 (2007): 2062–2086.

Burke, SC, Cremeens J, Vail-Smith K, and Woolsey CL. Drunkorexia: Calorie restriction prior to alcohol consumption among college freshman. *Journal of Alcohol and Drug Education* 54, no. 2 (2010): 17–35.

Cattarin, JA, and Thompson, JK. A three-year longitudinal study of body image, eating disturbance, and general psychological functioning in adolescent females. *Eating Disorders: Journal of Treatment and Prevention* 2, no. 2 (1994): 114–125.

Center for Behavioral Health Statistics and Quality. Behavioral Health Trends in the United States: Results from the 2014 National Survey on Drug Use and Health (HHS Publication No. SMA 15-4927, NSDUH Series H-50). S*ubstance Abuse and Mental Health Services Administration*. 2015. Available at http://www.samhsa.gov/data/

Choate, LH. Counseling college women experiencing eating disorder not otherwise specified: A cognitive behavior therapy model. *Journal of College Counseling* 13, no. 1 (2010): 73–86.

Crandall, CS. Social contagion of binge eating. *Journal of Personality and Social Psychology* 55, no. 4 (1988): 588–598.

Crow, SJ, Peterson CB, Swanson SA, Raymond NC, Specker S, Eckert ED, and Mitchell JE. Increased mortality in bulimia nervosa and other eating disorders. *American Journal of Psychiatry* 166, no. 12 (2009): 1342–1346.

De Souza, MJ, Nattiv A, Joy E, Misra M, Williams NI, Mallinson RJ, Gibbs JC, Olmsted M, Goolsby M, and Matheson G. 2014 Female Athlete Triad Coalition Consensus Statement on Treatment and Return to Play of the Female Athlete Triad: 1st International Conference held in San Francisco, California, May 2012 and 2nd International Conference held in Indianapolis, Indiana, May 2013. *British Journal of Sports Medicine* 48 (2014): 289.

Del Boca, FK, Darkes J, Greenbaum PE, and Goldman MS. Up close and personal: Temporal variability in the drinking of individual college students during their first year. *Journal of Consulting and Clinical Psychology* 72, no. 2 (2004): 155–164.

Delinsky, SS, and Wilson GT. Weight gain, dietary restraint, and disordered eating in the freshman year of college. *Eating Behaviors* 9, no. 1 (2008): 82–90.

Eisenberg, MH, and Fitz CC. "Drunkorexia": Exploring the who and why of a disturbing trend in college students' eating and drinking behavior. *Journal of American College Health* 62, no. 8 (2014): 570–577.

Eisenberg, D, Nicklett EJ, Roeder K, and Kirz NE. Eating disorder symptoms among college students: Prevalence, persistence, correlates, and treatment-seeking. *Journal of American College Health* 59, no. 8 (2011): 700–707.

Fairburn, CG, and Cooper Z. The eating disorder examination. In *Binge Eating: Nature, Assessment and Treatment* (12th ed.), edited by CG Fairburn and GT Wilson, pp. 317–360. New York, NY: Guilford Press, 1993.

Franko, DL, Mintz LB, Villapiano M, Green TC, Mainelli D, Folensbee L, Butler SF, Davidson MM, Hamilton E, Little D, Kearns M, and Budman SH. Food, mood, and attitude: Reducing risk for eating disorders in college women. *Health Psychology* 24, no. 6 (2005): 567–578.

Garner, DM, Olmsted MP, Bohr Y, and Garfinkel PE. The eating attitudes test: Psychometric features and clinical correlates. *Psychological Medicine* 12, no. 4 (1982): 871–878.

Gibbs, JC, Williams NI, and De Souza MJ. Prevalence of individual and combined components of the female athlete triad. *Medicine and Science in Sports and Exercise* 45, no. 5 (2013): 985–996.

Giles, SM, Champion H, Sutfin EL, McCoy TP, and Wagoner K. Calorie restriction on drinking days: An examination of drinking consequences among college students. *Journal of American College Health* 57, no. 6 (2009): 603–609.

Graham, M, and Jones A. Freshman 15: Valid theory or harmful myth? *Journal of American College Health* 46, no. 4 (2002): 189–191.

Granger, LR, Johnson CL, Malina RM, Milne LW, Ryan RR, and Vanderbunt EM. National Athletic Trainers' Association position statement: Preventing, detecting, and managing disordered eating in athletes. *Journal of Athletic Training* 43, no. 1 (2008): 80–108.

Greenleaf, C, Petrie TA, Carter J, and Reel JJ. Female collegiate athletes: Prevalence of eating disorders and disordered eating behaviors. *Journal of American College Health* 57, no. 5 (2009): 489–496.

Heinberg, LJ, Thompson JK, and Stormer S. Development and validation of the sociocultural attitudes towards appearance questionnaire. *International Journal of Eating Disorders* 17, no. 1 (1995): 81–89.

Hoerr, SL, Bokram R, Lugo B, Bivins T, and Keast DR. Risk for disordered eating relates to both gender and ethnicity for college student. *Journal of the American College of Nutrition* 21, (2002): 307–314.

Hudson, JI, Hiripi E, Pope HG Jr, and Kessler RC. The prevalence and correlates of eating disorders in the National Comorbidity Survey Replication. *Biological Psychiatry* 61, no. 3 (2007): 348–358.

Jones, M, Darcy A, Colborn D, Stewart MC, and Fitzpatrick K. Eating disorders on college campuses: Implications for prevention and treatment. *Harvard Health Policy Review* 13, no. 2 (2012): 28–32.

Landa, CE, and Bybee JA. Adaptive elements of aging: Self-image discrepancy, perfectionism, and eating problem. *Developmental Psychology* 43, no. 1 (2007): 83–93.

Luce, KH, Crowther JH, and Pole M. Eating Disorder Examination Questionnaire (EDE-Q): Norms for undergraduate women. *International Journal of Eating Disorders* 41, no. 3 (2008): 273–276.

Lupi, M, Acciavatti T, Santacroce R, Cinosi E, Martinotti G, and Di Giannantonio M. "Drunkorexia": A pilot study in an italian sample. *Research and Advances in Psychiatry* 2, no. 1 (2015): 28–32.

Macedo, A, João Soares M, Azevedo MH, Gomes A, Pereira AT, Maia B, and Pato M. Perfectionism and eating attitudes in Portuguese university students. *European Eating Disorders Review* 15, no. 4 (2007): 296–304.

Mintz, LB, and Betz NE. Prevalence and correlates of eating disordered behaviors among undergraduate women. *Journal of Counseling Psychology* 35, no. 4 (1988): 463–471.

Mintz LB, O'Halloran SM, Mulholland AM, and Schneider PA. Questionnaire for eating disorder diagnoses: Reliability and validity of operationalizing DSM-IV criteria into a self-report format. *Journal of Counseling Psychology* 44, no. 1 (1997): 63–79.

Mitchell, JJ and Robert-McComb JJ. Creening for disordered eating and eating disorders in female athletes. In *The Active Female: Health Issues throughout the Lifespan*, edited by JJ Robert-McComb, RL Norman, and M Zumwalt, pp. 191–206. New York, NY: Springer, 2014.

Morgan, JF, Reid F, and Lacey JH. The SCOFF questionnaire: A new screening tool for eating disorders. *Western Journal of Medicine* 172, no. 3 (2000): 164–165.

Mountjoy, M, Sundgot-Borgen J, Burke L, Carter S, Constantini N, Lebrun C, Meyer N, Sherman R, Steffen K, Budgett R, and Ljungqvis A. The IOC consensus statement: Beyond the Female Athlete Triad—Relative Energy Deficiency in Sport (RED-S). *British Journal of Sports Medicine* 48 (2014): 491–497.

Napierski-Prancl, M. Raising awareness: Incorporating a student-run campus awareness week in course objectives. *Teaching Sociology* 39, no. 1 (2011): 88–102.

National Council on Alcoholism and Drug Dependence, Inc. Underage and College Drinking. 2015. Available at https://www.ncadd.org/about-addiction/underage-issues/underage-and-college-drinking

National Eating Disorders Association (NEDA). Eating Disorders on the College Campus: A National Survey of Programs and Services. 2013. Available at http://www.nationaleatingdisorders.org/CollegiateSurveyProject

National Eating Disorders Association (NEDA). *Get the Facts on Eating Disorders*, 2015. Available at http://www.nationaleatingdisorders.org/get-the-facts-eating-disorders

National Institute on Alcohol Abuse and Alcoholism. College Drinking Fact Sheet. 2015. Available at http://pubs.niaaa.nih.gov/publications/CollegeFactSheet/CollegeFactSheet.pdf

Nattiv, A, Loucks AB, Manore MM, Sanborn CF, Sundgot-Borgen J, and Warren MP. American College of Sports Medicine position stand: The female athlete triad. *Medicine & Science in Sports & Exercise* 39, no. 10 (2007): 1867–1882.

Nazem, TG, and Ackerman KE. The female athlete triad. *Sports Health* 4, no. 4 (2012): 302–311.

Prouty, A, Protinsky H, and Canady D. College women: Eating behaviors and help seeking preferences. *Adolescence* 37, no. 146 (2002): 353–363.

Reinking, MF, and Alexander LE. Prevalence of disordered-eating behaviors in undergraduate female collegiate athletes and nonathlete. *Journal of Athletic Training* 40, no. 1 (2005): 47–51.

Richardson, SM, Paxton SJ, and Thomson JS. Is BodyThink an efficacious body image and self-esteem program? A controlled evaluation with adolescents. *Body Image* 6, no. 2 (2009): 75–82.

Rodriguez, NR, DiMarco NM, and Langley S. Position of the American Dietetic Association, Dietitians of Canada, and the American College of Sports Medicine: Nutrition and athletic performance. *Journal of the American Dietetic Association* 109, no. 3 (2009): 509–527.

Roehrig, M, Thompson JK, Brannick M, and van den Berg P. Dissonance induction treatment of body image disturbance: A dismantling investigation. *International Journal of Eating Disorders* 39, (2006): 1–10.

Smolak L, Murnen SK, and Ruble AE. Female athletes and eating problems: A meta-analysis. *International Journal of Eating Disorders* 27, no. 4 (2000): 371–380.

Stice, E. Modeling of eating pathology and social reinforcement of the thin-ideal predict onset of bulimic symptoms. *Behaviour Research and Therapy* 36, no. 10 (1998): 931–944.

Stice, E, and Agras WS. Predicting onset and cessation of bulimic behaviors during adolescence: A longitudinal grouping analyses. *Behavior Therapy* 29, no. 2 (1998): 257–276.

Stice, E, Becker CB, and Yokum S. Eating disorder prevention: Current evidence-base and future directions. *International Journal of Eating Disorders* 46, no. 5 (2013a): 478–485.

Stice, E, Marti CN, Spoor S, Presnell K, and Shaw H. Dissonance and healthy weight eating disorder prevention programs: Long-term effects from a randomized efficacy trial. *Journal of Consulting and Clinical Psychology* 76, no. 2 (2008): 329–340.

Stice, E, Rohde P, Durant S, Shaw H, and Wade E. Effectiveness of peer-led dissonance-based eating disorder prevention groups: Results from two randomized pilot trials. *Behaviour Research and Therapy* 51 (2013b): 197–206.

Stice, E, Rohde P, Shaw H, and Marti CN. Efficacy trial of a selective prevention program targeting both eating disorder symptoms and unhealthy weight gain among female college students. *Journal of Consulting & Clinical Psychology* 80, no. 1 (2012b): 164–170.

Stice, E, Trost A, and Chase A. A healthy weight control and dissonance-based eating disorder prevention programs: Results from a controlled trial. *International Journal of Eating Disorders* 33, no. 1 (2003): 10–21.

Striegel-Moore, RH, Silberstein LR, and Rodin J. Toward an understanding of risk factors for bulimia. *American Psychologist* 41, no. 3 (1986): 246–263.

Tillman, KS, Arbaugh T, and Balaban MS. Campus programming for National Eating Disorders Awareness Week: An investigation of stigma, help-seeking, and resource knowledge. *Eating Behaviors* 13, no. 3 (2012): 281–284.

Tillman, KS, Sell DM, Yates LA, and Mueller N. Effectiveness of one-time psychoeducational programming for students with high levels of eating concerns. *Eating Behaviors* 19 (2015): 133–138.

White, S, Reynolds-Malear JB, and Cordero E. Disordered eating and the use of unhealthy weight control methods in college students: 1995, 2002, and 2008. *Eating Disorders* 19, no. 4 (2011): 323–334.

Yager, Z and O'Dea JA. Prevention programs for body image and eating disorders on university campuses: A review of large, controlled interventions. *Health Promotion International* 23, no. 2 (2008): 173–189.

Zagorsky, JL, and Smith PK. The freshman 25: A critical time for obesity intervention or media myth? *Social Science Quarterly* 92, no. 5 (2011): 1389–1407.

Zhao, Y, and Encinosa W. Hospitalizations for eating disorders from 1999 to 2006, Statistical Brief #70. In *Healthcare Cost and Utilization Project Statistical Briefs (Internet)*. Rockville, MD: Agency for Healthcare Research and Quality, 2009. Available at https://www.ncbi.nlm.nih.gov/books/NBK53970.

7 Eating Disorders in Athletes

Kate Bennett, PsyD

CONTENTS

LEARNING OBJECTIVES

After reading this chapter the reader should be able to do the following:

- Discriminate between eating and exercise behaviors related to the pursuit of athletic goals versus maladaptive behaviors used to engage in eating disorders
- Recognize risk factors unique to athletes
- Understand physical, psychological, and performance concerns related to energy deficiency in athletes
- Be familiar with athletic culture and athletic identity

- Describe unique treatment considerations when supporting athletes recovering from eating disorders

PREVALENCE

Research on the prevalence of eating disorders within the athletic population is equivocal. Prevalence rates vary based on multiple factors including sport type, level of competition, nationality, and screening instrument (Currie 2007). While each of these factors impacts outcome data, current research clearly indicates that eating disorders exist among athletes and may manifest in unique ways compared to the general population.

An eating disorder literature review reported that prevalence rates of disordered eating and eating disorders varied from 6% to 45% among female athletes and 0% to 19% among male athletes across multiple studies demonstrating significant variability in the research (Bratland-Sanda and Sundgot-Borgen 2013). Among elite Norwegian athletes, 70% in weight class sports (i.e., rowing or wrestling) were found to engage in abnormal eating behaviors and diet (Torstveit and Sundgot-Borgen 2005). Additionally, clinical eating disorders increased over time with the largest shift (20%–28%) occurring during the last 5 years of this 1990–2008 study.

Among Norwegian female athletes, 46.7% of lean sport athletes (i.e., running or cycling) and 19.8% of nonlean sport athletes (i.e., soccer or weight lifting) demonstrated clinical eating disorders (Torstveit et al. 2008). In 2015, 13% of female athletes were found to experience clinical or subclinical eating disorders. Interestingly, female lean sport athletes experienced lower levels of body dissatisfaction (24%) compared to nonlean sport athletes (32%) (Coker-Cranney and Reel 2015). This finding suggests that the drive for thinness in leanness sports may originate for performance gains rather than body image concerns as these athletes typically fall among the idealized body types portrayed by the media.

In regards to the prevalence of eating disorders among male athletes, one study found that 3% of national and international level athletes experienced clinical eating disorders while 6% struggled with subclinical eating disorders (Sundgot Borgen and Torstveit 2004). Petrie et al. (2007) reported that 1% of male college student athletes experienced clinical eating disorders and another 16.6% demonstrated maladaptive eating behaviors. Chatterton and Petrie (2013) found that 82.9% of male collegiate athletes were asymptomatic of disordered eating, 16% were symptomatic, and 1.1% suffered from eating disorders. A study of young, elite male athletes demonstrated that 59% of the athletes struggled with body dissatisfaction, 19% dieted, and 11% engaged in clinical eating disorders (Rosendahl et al. 2009). These studies suggest that male athletes may engage in disordered eating behaviors more frequently than nonathletes as a result of sport-specific risk factors discussed later in this chapter. Regardless of numbers, professionals are encouraged to recognize that athletes are not immune to eating disorders and require careful assessment to discern between athletic pursuit and eating disorders.

ASSESSMENT AND EVALUATION

Initially, the assessment and evaluation of this population are similar to the assessment and evaluation of nonathletes. It is important to understand the presenting problems in terms of frequency, intensity, and duration and also identify other comorbid conditions. Exploring presenting problems from a biopsychosocial model helps identify all potential risk factors and also aids in the conceptualization of individual cases.

Most notable among this population is the fact that weight loss enhances performance in some disciplines such as endurance sports (i.e., cycling, running, rowing). In cycling, the concept of power to weight ratio is well-known and based on mathematics. For example, if two cyclists have a lactate threshold of 250 W but one weighs 135 lb. while the other weighs 150 lb. (assuming both cyclists are healthy), the lighter cyclist will perform better uphill because that athlete has less mass to move and more power (per pound) to climb with. However, maximizing the power-to-weight ratio and sustaining *race weight*, require a delicate balance of energy in and energy out. If the lighter cyclist drops below his ideal race weight, he will actually be at an energy deficit and will experience performance decrements for a variety of reasons including fatigue and low glycogen stores. The phenomenon of race weight exists in other endurance sports such as running and rowing as well. In these sports, athletes work to minimize their weight while maximizing their physical output. Typically, athletes employ disordered eating behaviors to manage the delicate balance of energy in/ energy out. When athletes shift from managing weight in the interest of maximizing performance to disordered eating/eating disorders, their performance suffers as a result. Similar to the idea of fueling a car to perform, athletes who under-fuel their bodies will struggle to perform optimally.

There is a very fine line between performance enhancement and eating disorders. The best way to determine whether athletes are truly working to improve performance versus engaging in an eating disorder is to explore their goals and thought processes. Once athletes step across the line toward eating disorders, they lose sight of athletic pursuits and become obsessed with numbers, rules, and eating disorder behaviors.

To discern whether disordered eating behaviors are pathological, professionals need to examine the behaviors in the context of sport and athletic goals. Sundgot-Borgen and Torstveit (2010) acknowledged that diagnosis of eating disorders among athletes extends beyond the *Diagnostic and Statistical Manual of Mental Disorders* (*DSM*). The authors clarified that low energy availability (i.e., eating what appears to be "normal" for nonathletes may not adequately fuel athletes in training), pathogenic weight control measures, transient behaviors associated with the demands of sport (i.e., weight cycling among rowing and wrestling), and psychological states (i.e., anxiety related to performance and worth as an athlete) present uniquely among this population. Performance concerns, which are discussed in detail in this chapter, are indicative of these symptoms. Oftentimes, athletes seek help when they are under-performing rather than feeling concerned about maladaptive eating and exercise behaviors. With this in mind, it is important to think beyond performance-related concerns and explore underlying issues such as eating disorders.

DSM-5's criteria for anorexia nervosa (AN) require that individuals be at a significantly low body weight within the context of standardized peer group norms (i.e., age, sex, developmental trajectory; American Psychiatric Association 2013). It is important to remember that athletes' body composition frequently differs from the nonathletic population (Sundgot-Borgen 1993). Athletes tend to have lower body fat percentages and more muscular development; therefore, their weights might not reflect *DSM-5*'s criteria despite struggling with clinical eating disorders. Furthermore, body mass index has limited diagnostic validity within the athletic population because athletes typically weigh less than the general population and maintain lower body fat percentages regardless of eating disorder concerns (Bär and Markser 2013).

Screening for menstrual dysfunction in lean sport athletes is helpful in identifying potential eating disorders (Torstveit et al. 2008). While amenorrhea is not a criterion for the diagnosis of AN in *DSM-5*, it is an indicator of low energy availability which may indicate the presence of disordered eating. Reportedly, nonlean sport female athletes are more likely to recognize their eating behaviors as pathogenic and self-report concerns as a result (Sundgot-Borgen 1993). Generally speaking, the authors found that athletes tend to underreport maladaptive eating behaviors because the behaviors are normalized within athletic culture (Torstveit et al. 2008).

In general, male and female athletes respond similarly to treatment; however, males tend to demonstrate subclinical symptoms (Petrie et al. 2007). As a result, it is important to examine males more closely for subclinical features such as restriction, purging, substance abuse (anabolic steroids), over-exercising, and negative affect.

In addition to assessing for disordered eating behaviors, it is also critical to explore whether athletes struggle with compulsive exercise or exercise dependency. Familiarizing oneself with periodization and seasonality of sports is essential for understanding how athletes utilize exercise to maximize performance versus engage in eating disorders. Finally, it is important to note that athletes fear interruption of sport participation, which interferes with self-reporting and pursuit of professional support. Again, performance-related concerns may reflect energy deficiencies and warrant further investigation.

ANOREXIA ATHLETICA

In 1983, health professionals introduced the construct of anorexia athletica in response to sport-specific subclinical eating disorders (Bär and Markser 2013). While anorexia athletica is not recognized by *DSM-5* as a psychiatric disorder, the term is commonly used among professionals who work with this population. The following criteria were identified to categorize this clinical presentation:

- Intense fear of gaining weight despite being lean or underweight
- Decreased caloric intake
- Excessive and/or compulsive exercise
- Body image distortion
- Presence of menstrual irregularities or amenorrhea
- Presence of purging behaviors (Sundgot-Borgen 1993)

When compared to AN, the criteria for anorexia athletica are similar but exist subclinically. Athletes struggling with anorexia athletica may be medically sound and able to participate in sports despite struggling with disordered eating behaviors and cognitions. As with all subclinical disordered eating presentations, early intervention is essential to prevent escalation of anorexia athletica into clinical AN.

PATHOLOGICAL BEHAVIORS

Athletes face multiple risk factors that nonathletes are not exposed to. In addition to weight and shape concerns, athletes participate in a culture that sanctions maladaptive eating behaviors to gain a competitive edge. Clearly stated, athletes can be psychologically healthy but may appear as though they have an eating disorder as a result of intentional behaviors to manipulate food and weight (Currie 2007). For individuals not closely associated with the world of athletics, it may sound absurd that behaviors such as meticulous attention to diet and weight, frequent weigh-ins and body composition measurements, weighing food, following a rigid diet, careful meal planning, and dietary tracking are considered "normal" within the world of sport. This may be particularly difficult to comprehend because mental health professionals consider these very same behaviors maladaptive in the nonathletic population. Working with athletes requires a radical acceptance of the sport culture; however, that does not include condoning eating disorders. A fine line exists between meticulous attention to diet and weight to gain a competitive edge and pathology.

Given the blurry line separating "normal" behaviors in sport from pathology, it is crucial for professionals to not only understand and appreciate the sport environment but also to develop a skill set for discerning between adaptive and pathological behaviors. When assessing at-risk athletes, it is critical to explore athletes' goals related to food and exercise. In addition to typical eating disorder behaviors (restriction, purging via vomiting, and abuse of diet pills, diuretics, and stimulants), athletes struggling with an eating disorder may extend exercise beyond the normal training load to manipulate body shape and size (Currie 2007). Athletes are at a high risk for the development of exercise dependence as both compensatory and compulsive behaviors (Holland et al. 2013). Evidence of pathogenic exercise includes a sudden increase in load (volume or intensity), exercising without clear athletically based goals, and secretive training. Athletes may also engage in extreme diets, compromising vital nutrients, without a clear performance goal. It is important to remember that dietary intake for athletes varies from the nonathletic population. What seems like a "normal" intake for the average person may not account for the caloric needs of elite athletes training several hours per day. Similar to nonathletes, once athletes cross the eating disorder threshold, they become preoccupied with food, weight, and/or exercise. They are no longer focused on performance. Instead, athletes struggling with eating disorders obsess about their bodies at the expense of performance.

BODY IMAGE

Whether athletes struggle with AN, BN, or anorexia athletica, body image distortion is a key factor. Research sheds interesting light on athletes' experience of body image, revealing that athletes experience their bodies in two contexts, the athletic body image and social body image (de Bruin et al. 2011). Athletic body image refers to athletes' evaluation of their bodies within the context of their sport whereas social body image refers to athletes' evaluation of their bodies in daily life. De Bruin et al. explained this concept using female runners and rugby players. Rugby players value their strength and size on the field, where it is an asset to be strong and sturdy.

However, the ideal body type for female rugby players does not correspond with westernized social ideals; therefore, while rugby players feel confident on the field, they may feel self-conscious about their bodies in daily life. Runners, on the other hand, tend to be lean. Their body type fits well within the social ideals for females; therefore, they likely feel confident in their daily life. Contrary to rugby players, though, they view excess weight as detrimental to performance and may seek to alter their body type in effort to gain a competitive edge in competition. With this concept of body image in mind, it is important to consider how athletes perceive themselves both in sport and in daily life as either source of body dissatisfaction can fuel the development of eating disorders.

RISK FACTORS

Risk factor differences between athletes and nonathletes present with ambiguity, similar in nature to the equivocal prevalence rates findings. While athletes are commonly thought to be at greater risk for developing eating disorders than nonathletes, a review of 22 studies, 11,000 women, 68 sports, and 11 countries revealed that athletes and nonathletes are at similar risk for the development of an eating disorder (de Oliveira Coelho et al. 2010). This supported an earlier finding that no statistical difference exists between athletes and the control group when controlled for age (Torstveit et al. 2008).

A recent survey of female Norwegian athletes revealed 14% of athletes experienced eating disorders compared to 5% of nonathletic controls (Martinsen and Sundgot-Borgen 2013). In contrast, another study of female collegiate athletes found zero cases of eating disorders compared to 5.9% of the nonathlete control group (DiPasquale and Petrie 2013; Voekler et al. 2014). Another study focused on female figure skaters revealed that 13% of the athletes reported problematic eating attitudes and behaviors; however, they were no more symptomatic than age-group peers. Interestingly, the level of disordered eating did not vary significantly between elite and subelite athletes. This finding suggests that competitive level may not influence the development of disordered eating. Importantly, it was found that athletes were more medically compromised when diagnosed with an eating disorder as evidenced by higher levels of menstrual dysfunction (de Oliveira Coelho et al. 2010). This finding may be explained by the fact that sport culture normalizes disordered eating and menstrual dysfunction as part of high-level training and competing.

Regardless of whether athletes report higher levels of eating disorders compared to age-group controls, these individuals face numerous factors that increase their risk of developing eating disorders. Similar to nonathletic peers, athletes face risk factors such as social media content, relationship problems, cultural influences, body dissatisfaction, pressure to diet, maturational fears, identity concerns, personality characteristics, genetic predisposition, traumatic life events, and negative affect.

Unfortunately, athletes face multiple unique factors that may contribute to the onset of an eating disorder. Athletes experience increased risk of developing an eating disorder as they transition from high school athletics to the elite level (Smolak et al. 2000). This is not surprising, given an increased pressure to win at the elite level to secure scholarships, sponsorships, and professional contracts. Research has also linked seasonal status, uniforms, and injury to the development of eating disorders. One study reported that athletes who struggled with maladaptive eating behaviors tended to experience a decrease in eating disorder symptomology during the competitive season and engaged in pathological behaviors during the off-season (Duffy-Paiement 2010). Additionally, a survey of college female athletes indicated that coaches, teammates, and revealing uniforms influenced the development of maladaptive eating behaviors (Reel et al. 2010). Newer research identified the coach–athlete relationship as a mediating factor in the development of eating disorders in regards to weight-related pressure (Coker-Cranney and Reel 2015) and coach–athlete conflict (Shanmugam et al. 2014). Finally, overtraining, injuries, weight-cycling, sport rules and regulations, and an early start in the sport were also linked to the development of eating disorders among athletes (Bratland-Sanda and Sundgot-Borgen 2013; Sundgot-Borgen and Torstveit 2010).

The "Ideal Athlete" persona is both a protective and risk factor. This cluster of personality traits, such as obsessive–compulsive tendencies, perfectionism, and high-achieving aspirations, leads to athletic success as well as drives tendencies to excessively exercise and be overly compliant (Sundgot-Borgen and Torstveit 2010). Researchers explored the impact of different types of perfectionism on the development of eating disorders. The two types of perfectionism included conscientious perfectionism (high standards) and self-evaluative perfectionism (self-criticism) (Goodwin et al. 2014; Shanmugam et al. 2014). Interestingly, both studies linked self-evaluative perfectionism to disordered eating but not conscientious perfectionism.

Athletes can be described as self-sacrificing, comfortable with pain/discomfort, accepting of risk, willing to push limits, and in pursuit of distinction (Coker-Cranney and Reel 2015). This group of individuals is also known to be driven, hard-working, goal-oriented, and resilient. The very traits that support athletic success may also contribute to the development of an eating disorder. However, athletes' history of success serves as a protective factor (and, if needed, a motivating factor for recovery) as athletes desire to be successful again.

Sport Type

Aesthetic sports—sports that are judged subjectively—are most commonly associated with the development of eating disorders among athletes. While aesthetic sports put athletes most at risk for the development of eating disorders, many other sports also pose risks to athletes. The perception of the sport ideal and the perception of performance-enhancing behaviors contribute to the development of eating disorders (Sundgot-Borgen and Torstveit 2010). Sports correlated with the use of pathogenic weight-control measures include aesthetic sports (i.e., gymnastics, figure skating, diving, dance, body building), power to weight sports (i.e., cycling), weight category sports (i.e., wrestling, rowing, jockeying), high-intensity sports (i.e., alpine skiing, squash, speed skating), endurance sports (i.e., track and field, running, swimming, Nordic skiing), antigravity sports (i.e., ski jumping), and martial arts (i.e., judo, kick boxing, karate) (Baum 2006; Chatterton and Petrie 2013; Currie 2007; Pietrowsky and Straub 2008; Sundgot-Borgen and Torstveit 2010).

GENDER

When comparing male and female athletes (Baum 2006), females struggled more frequently with eating disorders than males, similar to outcome data for the general population. In comparison to females, male athletes tend to report subclinical eating disturbances and weight-class athletes are the most likely to be symptomatic of disordered eating (Chatterton and Petrie 2013). Males feel less pressure from coaches and teammates to modify physical appearances but experience increased pressure from the media to display the ideal body type for their respective sport (Petrie et al. 2007). As a result of the pressure from the media, athletes may engage in maladaptive eating behaviors for fear of being scrutinized by the public. Male athletes often present with a drive for muscularity known as muscle dysmorphia. In fact, the drive for muscularity may outweigh the drive for thinness in male athletes (Bratland-Sanda and Sundgot-Borgen 2013). Muscle dysmorphia is characterized by preoccupation with muscle mass and predisposes individuals to the use of anabolic steroids (Petrie et al. 2007; Pope et al. 1997). Male athletes most frequently use dieting and exercise to manage their weight and increase muscle mass (Chatterton and Petrie 2013). Despite these differences, male and female athletes respond similarly to treatment.

CULTURAL CONSIDERATIONS

The world of athletics is a unique subpopulation that developed a culture within itself. In addition to the culture of sport, athletes bring their own cultural experiences into sport. The risk of eating disorders among athletes may be best represented as a combination of cultural values, the athletic environment, and personal variables (Hulley et al. 2007). With this in mind, it is important to conceptualize cases through a multicultural lens that incorporates the unique influences of sport on athlete development and values.

Unfortunately, very little data are available about the interactions between sport culture and individual diversity factors. However, two studies began to explore this facet of sport and diversity. A study conducted among high school female athletes revealed that Caucasian and Latina athletes were at greater risk for the development of eating disorders when compared to African American peers (Pernick et al. 2006). Latina athletes were at the greatest risk for the development of binge eating disorder.

A study on the effect of culture on the development of eating disorders among elite athletes compared the prevalence of eating disorders between elite female distance runners from the United Kingdom and Kenya (Hulley et al. 2007). The UK runners demonstrated significantly higher levels of eating disorder pathology as compared to the Kenyan runners. The UK runners were considered to be high achievers who experienced increased body awareness as a result of internalized sport ideals, that is, the UK runners may have idealized lean bodies because that type of body is associated with successful distance runners. As a result of idealizing the lean body type, the UK runners may have been more prone to use disordered eating behaviors to achieve an "ideal" body in hopes of improved performance. On the contrary, Kenyan runners viewed running as a career and used sport to achieve success, which subsequently lead to improvements in self-esteem and performance (compared to the UK runners who may have experienced a decrease in self-esteem due to body dissatisfaction as a result of body comparisons). The Kenyan runners correlated with the lowest proportion of probable eating disorder cases when compared to UK athletes as well as controls in both countries. Furthermore, the onset of dieting began 2 years later in Kenyan athletes and occurred only after being exposed to the Western ideal at elite levels of competition.

HEALTH CONSEQUENCES

PHYSICAL CONCERNS

The Female Athlete Triad links low energy availability, menstrual dysfunction, and bone mineral density as a health concern for female athletes (Bär and Markser 2013; De Souza et al. 2014; Javed et al. 2013; Melin et al. 2015). Female athletes may suffer from one or all three of these health concerns. The cluster of symptoms exists on a continuum ranging from healthy energy consumption, menstruation, and bone density to eating disorders, hypothalamic amenorrhea, and osteoporosis (Javed et al. 2013; Melin et al. 2015). Forty female athletes on national and competitive teams had normal body mass index measurements. Of those 40 athletes, 63% reported low or reduced energy availability, 25% had eating disorders, 60% experienced menstrual dysfunction, 45% suffered from impaired bone health, and 23% met criteria for the Female Athlete Triad (Melin et al. 2015). In addition to these symptoms, the athletes also suffered from decreased resting metabolic rates, hypotension, hypoglycemia, and hypercholesterolemia.

In regards to the relationship of symptoms in the Female Athlete Triad, energy deficits alter hormones involved in menstrual function and bone metabolism (Bär and Markser 2013). This is particularly concerning for adolescents whose bodies are still developing. Low energy availability can result from restricting and/or increased energy expenditure through training (Javed et al. 2013). Athletes participating in leanness-based sports including aesthetics, endurance, and weight-based categorization (e.g., rowing) are at greatest risk. Red flags for this syndrome include decrements in performance, negative mood shifts, frequent illness or injuries, fractures, body dissatisfaction, and weight loss (Javed et al. 2013). Importantly, athletes can be energy deficient, despite being at a healthy weight and in the absence of menstrual or bone health concerns (Javed et al. 2013). Early intervention is essential to protect athletes' health.

The International Olympic Committee (IOC) revised their original consensus statement on the Female Athlete Triad to account for male athletes. The IOC coined the term "Relative Energy Deficiency in Sport" (RED-S) to include male athletes and emphasize the complexity of health concerns related to energy deficiencies in athletes (Mountjoy et al. 2014). In addition to symptoms associated with the Female Athlete Triad (energy availability, menstrual functioning, bone mineral density), RED-S addresses other physiological concerns including metabolism, immunity, protein synthesis, and cardiovascular functioning and the impact of those health issues on psychological health and performance (Mountjoy et al. 2014).

While male athletes do not have a natural "red flag" (such as amenorrhea in female athletes) to indicate physical consequences of an eating disorder, they are subject to health consequences as the introduction of RED-S indicates. In addition to the already mentioned concerns that can be generalized across sexes, male athletes are also susceptible to low testosterone levels (Sundgot-Borgen and Torstveit 2010). Nonweight bearing sports, such as cycling, increase the risk of osteopenia and osteoporosis among males. Furthermore, as discussed earlier, male athletes are more susceptible to anabolic steroid abuse. Use of these performance enhancing substances may result in premature closure of the epiphyses (growth plates), increased blood pressure, liver tumors, and sterility (Baum 2006). Premature closure of the epiphyses is of particular concern among adolescents. Anabolic steroids cause bones to mature too quickly and inhibit development which results in stunted growth.

PSYCHOLOGICAL CONCERNS

In general, athletes as a group are psychologically healthy (Petrie et al. 2007). Resiliency and adaptive coping factors developed through sport often serve as protective factors against negative moods. However, as with any population, psychopathology certainly exists within sport culture. Eating disorders may be the result of other psychological concerns or the foundation for issues such as depression and anxiety. Athletes with eating disorders may experience low self-esteem, depression, anxiety, and mental exhaustion (Petrie et al. 2007). Furthermore, constant denial of food despite feeling hungry, obsessions about food, agonizing about body shape, and fear of weight gain may result in severe psychological distress. Suicidal ideation and suicide attempts are correlated with the presence of eating disorders among athletes (Petrie et al. 2007). Finally, anabolic steroids are linked to depression, psychosis, and suicidal ideation (Baum 2006).

PERFORMANCE CONCERNS

In addition to physical and psychological health concerns, athletes struggling with eating disorders may experience performance issues. Numerous performance issues might arise as a result of intense dieting, inadequate carbohydrate and protein intake, and dehydration such as decreases in maximal oxygen uptake (VO_2 max) and running speed as well as increases in fatigue, muscle weakness, muscle wasting, and injury (Thompson and Sherman 2010). Furthermore, malnourished athletes might become irritable, struggle with concentration, and/or be emotionally flat, depressed, or anxious. RED-S may lead to decreased glycogen stores, decreased muscle strength, impaired endurance, increased risk of injury, diminished training response, impaired judgment, decreased coordination, and concentration, as well as negative shifts in mood such as irritability and depression (Mountjoy et al. 2014).

Reportedly, once engaged in the recovery process, athletes often feel motivated to challenge their eating disorders as a result of performance improvements related to refueling and positive energy balances (Arthur-Cameselle and Quatromoni 2014). While some performance concerns (i.e., decreases in physical strength, endurance, mood, and concentration) may be easily mitigated by refueling, the long-term effects of sustained energy deficits on other aspects of physiology, such as bone mineral density and reproductive functioning, may respond more slowly to refueling. For athletes concerned about renewing scholarships, professional contracts, and sponsorships, the recovery process may feel burdensome as they seek to return to sport as quickly as possible regardless of overall health and progress.

The concept of "bonking" provides a helpful analogy to understand maladaptive thinking and performance concerns that occur with disordered eating. Bonking occurs when an athlete is under-fueled during a workout. As nutrients are depleted, the athlete feels light-headed, lethargic, and weak and becomes preoccupied with eating instead of focusing on the workout. As a result of these symptoms, the athlete focuses on finding something to eat at the expense of the training quality. Once the athlete refuels, the obsession with consuming food is alleviated. Athletes with eating disorders are in a constant state of denial; therefore, they are constantly obsessing about the next meal time but never allowing themselves to refuel appropriately. The constant state of denial creates an obsession that begins to perpetuate itself. These athletes essentially find themselves in a continuous state of bonking, which not only affects physical performance but also deters from focus and concentration. Healthy athletes (those not struggling with eating disorders) refuel their bodies and resume training. Athletes struggling with eating disorders agonize over eating: what to eat, how much to eat, when to eat, and how to burn extra calories if they break a "food rule."

TREATMENT CONSIDERATIONS

This section focuses specifically on athletes who engage in sport at an elite level and receive some form of compensation (scholarship, sponsorship, endorsements, or salary) for their athletic endeavors or participate in NCAA sports. Overall treatment goals are outlined in Table 7.1. Currently, there is also a population of people who struggle with exercise dependence as a complication of an eating disorder. While some of the material in this chapter may be relevant to clients struggling with exercise dependence, the following treatment recommendations are specific to athletes as described above.

TABLE 7.1

Treatment Goals for Elite Athletes

Restore weight

Resume a healthy meal plan

Interrupt the pattern of maladaptive eating and weight control behaviors

Maintain or resume healthy levels of sport participation

Reconnect with or develop an identity separate from the eating disorder

Develop emotional awareness

Develop healthy coping alternatives

Develop or utilize existing support networks

Note: If athletes are medically compromised, unable to interrupt the eating disorder at an outpatient level of care, or enmeshed in an unhealthy relationship dynamic, a higher level of care may be warranted.

ATHLETIC CULTURE

When working with athletes, it is imperative that professionals appreciate the athletic culture and temperament as well as recognize sport culture as a facet of diversity. Similar to other unique cultures, it is important to understand the values, ideals, stressors, and influences that exist within sport culture. Values within sport include performance (winning), strength (physical and mental), and relationships (sponsors, employers, coaches, and teammates). Athletes typically have a public persona that depicts an ideal self. They are always expected to be "on" (performing in sport and in public). Weakness, whether a physical injury or emotional struggle, is frowned upon. Athletes may train through injuries to avoid losing a starting spot on the roster. Likewise, athletes may feign a physical problem to avoid disclosing a psychological struggle to team directors and coaches. Perhaps the greatest stressor other than performing well is losing a contract to injury. Professional athletes, in particular, excel through their bodies. It is also their bodies that make them money. This means athletes train hard, zero in on nutrition, and internalize strength to the best of their abilities. In order to ensure successful treatment outcomes for athletes recovering from eating disorders, psychiatric care must adapt to the athletic context (Bär and Markser 2013). Furthermore, acceptance of and respect for this culture is paramount in regards to athletes accepting and welcoming new professionals into their environment.

ATHLETIC IDENTITY

Athletes positively correlate athletic identity with disordered eating behaviors and attitudes (Dunn 2010). In fact, professional cyclists often joke to this author that cyclists "have to have some sort of eating disorder to be successful." Not only do athletes see disordered eating behaviors as a crucial aspect to their performance, they also struggle to disclose pathology for fear of the stigma that mental illness creates (Papathomas and Lavallee 2010). Mental illness contradicts athletic identity. Elaborating on this idea, athletic identity is associated with a sense of strength, confidence, and self-efficacy. Mental illness is the antithesis of these traits. Athletes correlate mental illness with mental weakness and fear being viewed as weak by competitors (Papathomas and Lavallee 2010); mental illness is stigmatized in the sport culture (Bär and Markser 2013). Athletes often struggle to integrate eating disorders (disordered self) with their athletic identities (strong, confident, resilient self; Papathomas and Lavallee 2010). Furthermore, athletes often avoid seeking professional help as a result of questioning whether professionals are competent at working with athletes. For these reasons, athletes often resist professional treatment for their eating disorders. However, athletes may seek treatment when negative consequences arise from disordered eating behaviors, such as being pulled from sport participation, in hopes of restoring their health and being successful in sport again (Arthur-Cameselle and Quatromoni 2014).

SPORT PARTICIPATION

As just indicated, athletic identities are strongly tied to athletes' sense of self; therefore, continued involvement in sport is important for two primary reasons:

maintaining connections to athletic identities and social networks. However, sport participation is contraindicated when athletes are medically compromised or are noncompliant with treatment recommendations (Baum 2006; Sundgot-Borgen and Torstveit 2010). To determine medical stability, a medical history, physical exam, blood tests, and bone scans need to be conducted (Currie 2007; Sundgot-Borgen and Torstveit 2010). It is important to remember that BMI is not a reliable source of information in this population. Athletes tend to carry more muscle mass compared to nonathletes; therefore, their BMI scores may be skewed indicating an athlete is at a healthy size despite having too little body fat, suffering from energy deficiencies, or experiencing other medical concerns.

If athletes are pulled from sport participation, it is recommended that they return to sport once they are medically stable as demonstrated by normalized lab results, cardiovascular tests, and bone scans. Additionally, readiness for return to training is evidenced by active participation in treatment, absence of using training to alter body shape or size, compliance with meal plan, willingness to restore and restoration of body weight, and healthy levels of body fat (which is dependent on body type but a general guideline is >6% for males and >12% for females) (Sundgot-Borgen and Torstveit 2010). Ideally, athletes will also demonstrate the use of healthy coping alternatives as participation in sport increases. Athletes are ready to return to competition once those criteria are met in addition to achieving their treatment goal weight. If athletes struggle to maintain gains, lose weight, or return to maladaptive behaviors after returning to sport, all activity should be withdrawn.

Compromising athletic identities in sport may be difficult for athletes as they pursue health and interrupt eating disorders. Additionally, potential career termination may create grief and loss issues among athletes and needs to be addressed on an individual basis (Baum 2006).

TREATMENT TEAM

As discussed above, acknowledgement, appreciation, and acceptance of sport culture are crucial for the development of rapport with athletes. Additionally, it is imperative to work with a treatment team. A typical treatment team includes a psychotherapist, a nutritionist, a psychiatrist, and a medical doctor. It is also important when working with athletes to involve athletic support staff such as the coach and athletic trainer. In some cases, the team coach provides crucial information in regards to athletes' participation in treatment including meal completion during team meals, willingness to comply with exercise restrictions, changes in mood, ability to focus, and engagement with teammates. Furthermore, the coach–athlete relationship may be used to facilitate recovery (Currie 2007). It is important to note that not all coaches are supportive of recovery and some may encourage disordered eating behaviors among a team. When bringing a coach on board, be mindful of the coach's beliefs about food and weight as they relate to performance and overall health. Finally, process groups and family therapy are options for treatment as well.

Over the past few years, coaches and athletic staff have become increasingly more informed about the presence of eating disorders among athletes. The

National Collegiate Athletic Association (NCAA) recommends screening for eating disorders and other interventions as part of a wider effort to address mental health issues among college athletes (National Collegiate Athletic Association 2016). Institutions such as the NCAA created informational handouts and online resources for coaches. Despite these efforts to raise awareness and prevent eating disorders, recognition of eating disorders and appropriate treatment for athletes continues to be a problem. Psychoeducation is an important aspect of the treatment process. Therefore, it is crucial to disseminate education to coaches and support staff as they make efforts to support athletes interrupting eating disorders while pursuing athletic goals.

PSYCHIATRIC CONSIDERATIONS

When working with competitive athletes, it is important to consider the rules of the sport's governing bodies. Specifically, prior to prescribing psychotropic medications, a professional should refer to online resources to determine whether potential medications are a banned substance for that sport. The following agencies govern the use of substances in sports:

- United States Anti-Doping Agency (USADA)
- Global Drug Reference Online
- World Anti-Doping Agency (WADA)

PREVENTION

The majority of this chapter was dedicated to intervention at the secondary and tertiary levels of care: intervening once a problem is identified. Professionals also have the opportunity to intervene at the primary level of care, working to prevent the development of eating disorders. Given the prevalence of eating disorders among athletes and risk factors associated with sport culture, prevention is an important aspect of promoting health and well-being among this population. It involves two aspects: awareness and education.

Creating awareness of the prevalence of eating disorders among athletes is crucial to early identification, implementation of support, and triage of care. Education coincides with awareness. Once athletes and athletic staff are aware of the potential for eating disorders to thrive within the athletic culture, they need resources for responding. Education includes educating athletes and team staff on signs, symptoms, and treatment options in addition to providing information about how staff–athlete relationships can influence and deter the onset of eating disorders. Additionally, it is imperative for athletes to understand how athletic pursuit may morph into eating disorders, how eating disorders impact performance, and how sport culture covertly encourages the development of maladaptive thoughts and behaviors related to food and weight.

CASE STUDY 7.1

Hans

A professional cyclist schedules an appointment to discuss his lack of motivation to train midway through his race season. Hans, a 23-year-old Caucasian male, reports that he started racing professionally this year and spent the past 2 months away from home while training and racing. He indicates that he feels frustrated by his lack of motivation because racing professionally is his dream. He states that he has very little motivation to train despite his biggest race of the season being weeks away. During your evaluation, you discover that Hans is very weight-conscious. He describes himself as a "clean eater," elaborating that he does not eat processed foods and eliminated gluten from his diet this year. Hans also states that he counts calories as well as weighs everything he eats. He indicates that he would like to lose another 5 lb. for his biggest race of the season and already shed 10 lb. over the past 3 months.

QUESTIONS

1. What additional information is needed to assess the possibility of an eating disorder diagnosis?
   a. Weight History: Hans' height and current weight, highest and lowest adult weights, weight trend in-season compared to off-season, "race" weight versus current goal weight, and recent weight loss patterns
   b. Restriction: Nature of "new" diet in regards to being a "clean eater" and having a gluten-free diet, typical daily intake, caloric intake compared to caloric expenditure
   c. Bingeing: Presence of bingeing–assess for behavior during training and racing
   d. Purging: Vomiting, exercising, laxatives, enemas, diuretics, fasting, and/or diet pills
   e. Bone Density: Osteopenia (particularly of concern given Hans participates in a nonweight-bearing sport)
   f. Blood Draw/Hormone Levels: Indicator of low energy availability
   g. Training: Typical training day, presence of any extra training outside coach's prescribed workouts
   h. Body Image: Perception of body as it relates to sport and society
2. How would you proceed with treatment?
   a. Step 1: Schedule a medical evaluation with a physician.
   b. Step 2: Assuming Hans is medically stable, set up an outpatient treatment team.
   c. Step 3: Educate Hans on his diagnosis, potential medical concerns, and the impact of an eating disorder on athletics, health, and relationships.

(Continued)

CASE STUDY 7.1 *(CONTINUED)*

    d. Step 4: Agree upon treatment goals, expectations, and conse-
quences of noncompliance (removal of sport, higher level of
care, etc.).

3. Would you recommend that Hans continue to race this season?

Yes: Assuming Hans is medically stable and willing to engage
in treatment, outpatient treatment with clear goals and expectations while allowing Hans to continue to engage with his team
(maintaining his athletic identity and social network) is ideal. If
Hans is unwilling to engage in treatment or unable to demonstrate progress toward his goals, removal of sport would be an
important consideration in order to support restoration of Hans'
physical and mental health.

4. Who would you include on the treatment team?

Individual therapist and/or sport psychologist trained in the
treatment of eating disorders, sport nutritionist or registered dietician, team physician, psychiatrist (at least for an initial evaluation),
and possibly his coach.

Support network: While not part of the treatment team, it is
important for Hans to identify friends and family members who he
can use as support during his treatment.

REFERENCES

American Psychiatric Association. *Diagnostic and Statistical Manual of Mental Disorders* (5th ed.). Washington, DC: Author, 2013.

Arthur-Cameselle, JN, and Quatromoni PA. A qualitative analysis of female collegiate athletes' eating disorder recovery experiences. *Sport Psychologist* 28, no. 4 (2014): 334–346.

Bär, KJ, and Markser VZ. Sport specificity of mental disorders. *European Archives of Psychiatry and Clinical Neurosciences* 263, no. 2 (2013): S205–S210.

Baum, A. Eating disorders in the male athlete. *Sports Medicine*, 36, no. 1 (2006): 1–6.

Bratland-Sanda, S, and Sundgot-Borgen J. Eating disorders in athletes: Overview of preva-lence, risk factors and recommendations for prevention and treatment. *European Journal of Sport Science*, 13, no. 5 (2013): 499–508.

Chatterton, JM, and Petrie TA. Prevalence of disordered eating and pathogenic weight control measures among male collegiate athletes. *Eating Disorders* 21, no. 4 (2013): 328–341.

Coker-Cranney, A, and Reel JJ. Coach pressure and disordered eating in female collegiate athletes: Is the coach–athlete relationship a mediating factor? *Journal of Clinical Sport Psychology* 9, no. 3 (2015): 213–231.

Currie, A. A psychiatric perspective on athletes with eating disorders. *Journal of Clinical Sport Psychology* 1, no. 4 (2007): 329–339.

de Bruin, AP, Oudejans RR, Bakker FC, and Woertman L. Contextual body image and ath-letes' disordered eating: The contribution of athletic body image to disordered eating in high performance women athletes. *European Eating Disorders Review* 19, no. 3 (2011): 201–215.

de Oliveira Coelho, GM, de Abreu Soares E, and Gonçalves Ribeiro B. Are female athletes at increased risk for disordered eating and its complications? *Appetite* 55, no. 3 (2010): 379–387.

De Souza, MJ, Nattiv A, Joy E, Misra M, Williams NI, Mallinson RJ, Gibbs JC, Olmsted M, Goolsby M, and Matheson G. 2014 Female Athlete Triad Coalition consensus statement on the treatment and return to play of the female athlete triad. *British Journal of Sports Medicine* 48, no. 4 (2014): 289–309.

DiPasquale, LD, and Petrie TA. Prevalence of disordered eating: A comparison of male and female collegiate athletes and non-athletes. *Journal of Clinical Sports Psychology* 7, no. 3 (2013): 186–197.

Duffy-Paiement, C. Disordered eating among female collegiate athletes: The role of athletic seasonal status and self-objectification. *Dissertation Abstracts International: ProQuest Information and Learning*, 70, no. 12-B (2010): 7876.

Dunn, A. The effects of athletic identity, perceived sport competence, and self-esteem on disordered eating among female collegiate athletes. *Dissertation Abstracts International: ProQuest Information and Learning*, 70–10, Section: B (2010): 6546.

Goodwin, H, Arcelus J, Geach N, and Meyer C. Perfectionism and eating psychopathology among Dancers: The role of high standards and self-criticism. *European Eating Disorders Review* 22, no. 5 (2014): 346–351.

Holland, LA, Brown TA, and Keel PK. Defining features of unhealthy exercise associated with disordered eating and eating disorder diagnoses. *Psychology of Sport and Exercise* 15 (2013): 116–123.

Hulley, A, Currie A, Njenga F, and Hill A. Effects of eating disorders in elite female distance runners: Effects of nationality and running environment. *Psychology of Sport and Exercise* 8, no. 4 (2007): 521–533.

Javed, A, Tebben PJ, Fischer PR, and Lteif AN. Female athlete triad and its components: Toward improved screening and management. *Mayo Clinic Proceedings* 88, no. 9 (2013): 996–1010.

Martinsen, M, and Sundgot-Borgen J. Higher prevalence of eating disorders among adolescent elite athletes than controls. *Medicine and Science in Sports and Exercise* 45, no. 6 (2013): 1188–1197.

Melin, A, Tornberg AB, Skouby S, Møller SS, Sungot-Borgen J, Faber, Jakobsen Sidelmann J, Aziz M, and Sjödin A. Energy availability and the female athlete triad in elite endurance athletes. *Scandinavian Journal of Medicine and Science in Sports* 25, no. 5 (2015): 610–622.

Mountjoy, M, Sundgot-Borgen J, Burke L, Carter S, Constantini N, Lebrun C, Meyer N, Sherman R, Steffin K, Budgett R, and Ljungqvist A. The IOC consensus statement: Beyond the female athlete triad–Relative energy deficiency in sport (red-S). *British Journal of Sports Medicine* 48 (2014): 491–497.

National Collegiate Athletic Association. *Mental Health Best Practices: Inter-Association Consensus Document: Best Practices for Understanding and Supporting Student-Athlete Mental Wellness.* NCAA Sport Science Institute, Indianapolis, IN, 2016.

Papathomas, A, and Lavallee D. Athletes' experiences of disordered eating in sport. *Qualitative Research in Sport and Exercise* 2, no. 3 (2010): 354–370.

Pernick, Y, Nichols JF, Rauh MJ, Kern M, Ji M, Lawson MJ, and Wilfley D. Disordered eating among multi-racial/ethnic sample of female high-school athletes. *Journal of Adolescent Health* 38, no. 6 (2006): 689–695.

Petrie, TA, Greenleaf C, Carter JE, and Reel JJ. Psychosocial correlates of disordered eating among male collegiate athletes. *Journal of Clinical Sport Psychology* 1, no. 4 (2007): 340–357.

Pietrowsky, R, and Straub K. Body dissatisfaction and restrained eating in male juvenile and adult athletes. *Eating and Weight Disorders* 13, no. 1 (2008): 14–21.

Pope, HG Jr, Gruber AJ, Choi P, Olivardia R, and Phillips KA. Muscle dysmorphia: An under-recognized form of body dysmorphic disorder. *Psychosomatics: Journal of Consultation Liaison Psychiatry* 38, no. 6 (1997): 548–557.

Reel, JJ, Soohoo S, Petrie TA, Greenleaf C, and Carter JE. Slimming down for sport: Developing a weight pressures in sport measure for female athletes. *Journal of Clinical Sport Psychology* 4 (2010): 99–111.

Rosendahl, JB, Aschenbrenner BK, Aschenbrenner F, and Strauss B. Dieting and disordered eating in German high school athletes and non-athletes. *Scandinavian Journal of Medicine and Science in Sports* 19, no. 5 (2009): 731–739.

Shanmugam, V, Jowett S, and Meyer C. Interpersonal difficulties as a risk factor for athletes eating psychopathology. *Scandinavian Journal for Medicine and Science in Sports* 24, no. 2 (2014): 469–476.

Smolak, L, Murnen, SK, and Ruble, AE. Female athletes and eating problems: A meta-analysis. *International Journal of Eating Disorders* 27, no. 4 (2000): 371–380.

Sundgot-Borgen, J. Prevalence of eating disorders in elite female athletes. *International Journal of Sport Nutrition* 3, no. 1 (1993): 29–40.

Sundgot-Borgen, J, and Torstveit MK. Aspects of disordered eating continuum in elite high-intensity sports. *Scandinavian Journal of Medicine and Science in Sports* 20, no. S2 (2010): 112–121.

Sundgot-Borgen, J, and Torstveit MK. Prevalence of eating disorders in elite athletes is higher than in the general population. *Clinical Journal of Sports Medicine* 14 (2004): 25–32.

Thompson, RA, and Sherman RT. *Eating Disorders in Sport*. New York, NY: Taylor & Francis Group, 2010.

Thompson, RA, and Sherman RT. Reflections on athletes and eating disorders. *Psychology of Sport and Exercise* 15 (2014): 729–734.

Torstveit, MK, Rosenvinge JH, and Sundgot-Borgen J. Prevalence of eating disorders and the predictive power of risk models in female athletes: A controlled study. *Scandinavian Journal of Medicine and Science in Sports* 18, no. 1 (2008): 108–118.

Torstveit, MK, and Sundgot-Borgen J. The female athlete triad exists in both elite athletes and controls. *Medicine and Science in Sport and Exercise* 37, no. 9 (2005): 1449–1459.

Voekler, DK, Gould D, and Reel JJ. Prevalence and correlates of disordered eating in female figure skaters. *Psychology of Sport and Exercise* 15, (2014): 696–704.

8 Eating Disorders during Pregnancy and Postpartum

Maggie Baumann, LMFT, CEDS and
Jessica Setnick, MS, RD, CEDRD

CONTENTS

LEARNING OBJECTIVES

After reading this chapter the reader should be able do the following:

- Describe the assessment and evaluation of women with eating disorders who are pregnant
- Identify risk factors and prevalence rates in pregnant women with eating disorders
- Recognize medical and mental health consequences with eating disorders in pregnant women
- Plan psychological treatment goals/interventions for pregnant women with eating disorders during pregnancy and postpartum
- Understand recommended nutritional needs for pregnant women with eating disorders and nutritional needs for the postpartum mom
- Examine a case study of treatment of one pregnant woman with an eating disorder

INTRODUCTION

Eating disorders on the surface level focus on controlling behaviors and attitudes related to food, body size, and weight. It is reasonable that a pregnancy, requiring increased caloric needs and body weight, may be difficult for women suffering from eating disorders. For some, it can evoke a sense of extreme loss of control, potentially alluding to the deeper levels of the eating disorder's conception.

During pregnancy, all four subtypes of eating disorders can occur in women including (1) anorexia nervosa (AN), (2) bulimia nervosa (BN), (3) binge eating disorder (BED), and (4) other specified feeding eating disorder (OSFED). Outlined in the updated 5th edition *Diagnostic and Statistical Manual of Mental Disorders; DSM-5* (American Psychiatric Association, 2013), OSFED recently replaced the formerly noted diagnosis eating disorder not otherwise specified (EDNOS), thus much of the research cited in this chapter is based on *DSM-IV-Text Revision (TR)* classifications (Crow et al. 2015).

The harmful and sometimes deadly impact of the eating disorders on those who suffer can significantly impair physical and mental health as well as psychosocial functioning. What happens if the suffering is simultaneously doubled?

Twenty million females, primarily within the childbearing years, struggle with eating disorders at some point in their lives (National Eating Disorders Association 2015). A woman struggling with an eating disorder during pregnancy is relatively common, with an estimate between 5% and 7.5% of pregnant women meeting diagnostic criteria for an eating disorder. Through large cohort studies on eating disorders during pregnancy, findings appear to show health risks to mother and her baby related to sleep, maternal nutrition, birth outcomes, and child feeding and eating behaviors. (Watson et al. 2014a).

In 2008, a new buzzword called pregorexia, an informal term coined by the media, described eating disorder behaviors such as calorie restriction, excessive exercise, and bingeing and purging experienced by women while pregnant (Mathieu 2009). Eating disorders in women become even more complex to understand and treat if these women are also pregnant. Two lives are at stake, mom and fetus. Health risks are associated with negative birth outcomes, maternal nutrition, as well as child feeding and eating. Even though negative health consequences on both mother and baby can last a lifetime, the denial, guilt, and shame pregnant mothers with eating disorders . Through large cohort studies on eating disorders during pregnancy, findings appear to show health risks to mother and her baby related to sleep, maternal nutrition, birth outcomes, and child feeding, and eating behaviors. often feel keep them hiding in silence, fearful of reaching out for help (Crow et al. 2015).

This chapter features diverse components of this complex mental and physical illness and how it affects this unique population of pregnant women and their unborn children. It is important for health-care professionals, the general public, and pregnant women with eating disorders to understand a common misconception that this disease is of pure vanity (Watson et al. 2014a). Eating disorders are not a choice. They are serious, biologically based mental illnesses affecting emotional and physical health with life-threatening consequences. Eating disorders during pregnancy are dangerous combinations as the lives of both the expectant mom and her fetus are at stake.

SCREENING AND ASSESSMENT

Having an eating disorder prior to and during pregnancy increases the risk of pregnancy complications and negative birth outcomes (Watson et al. 2014a). Only 44% of women report their eating disorder to their doctor due to the shame and secrecy that is associated with the disorder. This statistic indicates eating disorder prevalence is underestimated in the obstetrics office, and data reveals only about 20% of obstetricians/gynecologists (OB/GYNs) feel comfortable in successfully diagnosing eating disorders, making this condition even more underreported. Despite the risks associated with eating disorders and pregnancy, one study found that less than half of OB/GYNs assess their patients for eating disorder history, body image concerns, weight loss practices, or current eating disorder symptoms (Leddy et al. 2009).

Getting on the scale for an eating disorder patient, pregnant or not, can be a frightening experience. In some OB/GYN offices, there is very little sensitivity to weight issues at precisely the time when most women need it. One solution to help these patients is to include an evaluation for eating disorders on the routine history form offices provide before the patient sees the OB/GYN or nurse the first time. This will set the stage for safety (Bulik 2015).

From the obstetricians to the nursing staff, OB/GYN offices can take a proactive patient approach with participation in sensitivity trainings on eating disorder and body image issues. A simple modification of weight assessments to include blind weigh-ins (stepping on the scale backward) can improve the patient's experience, with office staff mindful that stepping on the scale without talk about the body or weight can offer sensitivity to the needs of the expectant mom at that time.

The SCOFF questionnaire, developed in the United Kingdom, is a screening and assessment tool clinicians and health professionals use to detect a possible eating disorder in anorexic and bulimic populations. It includes five questions designed to raise the suspicion that an eating disorder may be present. Setting the threshold at two or more "yes" questions provides 100% sensitivity for AN and BN. The SCOFF questionnaire is to be used as a screening tool, not as a diagnosis (Hill et al. 2010).

The SCOFF questions are

1. Do you make yourself Sick because you feel uncomfortably full?
2. Do you worry that you have lost Control over how much you eat?
3. Have you recently lost more than One stone (14 lb.) in a 3-month period?
4. Do you believe yourself to be Fat when others say you are too thin?
5. Would you say that Food dominates your life? (Hill et al. 2010)

The SCOFF screening improves detection of a possible eating disorder and follow-up treatment (Perry et al. 2002). One study looked at the reliability of the SCOFF screening tool with a written questionnaire versus oral delivery of the questionnaire. The results showed that participants feel freer to disclose symptoms in the written as opposed to oral form. Noting this improvement with written versus verbal questioning, clinicians and health professionals may gain valuable information by including these assessment questions in their initial intake form. The treatment provider can then follow up on questions or concerns verbally with the patient.

In addition to screening for eating disorders, women seeking prenatal care should also be evaluated for other mental health issues, including anxiety, depression, and trauma (Meltzer-Brody et al. 2011). These types of conditions can exacerbate during pregnancy causing increased stress to the expectant mom, correspondingly causing increased stress to her fetus. Potential devastating developmental complications can occur when the fetus is exposed to prebirth stress (Monk et al. 2012). During routine prenatal care, it is important for obstetrical providers to screen for mental health conditions, asking questions about eating disorders, abuse, and symptoms of anxiety or depression. If at-risk patients are identified, referrals to collaborating clinicians should be established so appropriate mental health treatment is provided during pregnancy and after childbirth. Of course, if the provider can screen for eating disorders before a pregnancy occurs, this is optimal. It is optimal to first treat the patient's eating disorder and restore her recovery prior to a pregnancy to ensure mother and baby's health are best protected (Meltzer-Brody et al. 2011).

RISK FACTORS

Women with a history of an eating disorder, including AN, BN, or BED, face distinct challenges during pregnancy (Meltzer-Brody et al. 2011). Predisposing factors for eating disorders during pregnancy are generally the same as for other eating disorders occurring during other periods of life. Research supports a correlation between early history of developing eating disorders and the disruption of early attachment relationships (Maine and McGilley 2010). Factors such as the genetic heritability, unhealthy family dynamics, excessive exercise, distinct personality types including those with traits of perfectionism, and obsessive–compulsive behaviors, as well as comorbid psychiatric disorders including depression and anxiety, can all play a part in an eating disorder during pregnancy.

However, sometimes a pregnancy perceived by the woman as a stressful or traumatic event can trigger the development of an eating disorder for the first time (Larsson and Andersson-Ellstrom 2003). Generally, most eating disorders occur during pregnancy in women, with a history of the disorder or in women who are currently active in their disorder. Pregnancy can also exacerbate subthreshold eating disorder behaviors in some untreated women, causing a shift from mild disordered eating behaviors to an increased level of restriction and purging that can have serious consequences for the mother and the baby in utero. On the contrary, some women with active eating disorders report a temporary and sometimes permanent cessation of these behaviors during pregnancy. Usually, this occurs when the pregnant mother desires to protect her baby from any harm the eating disorder could inflict (Mitchell-Gieleghem et al. 2012).

When a pregnant mother with an eating disorder can sacrifice her own issues with food for the safety of the baby, this is a step forward in her dealing with some deep psychological issues. As she begins to focus more on the health of her baby, her eating disorder diminishes in importance (Zauderer 2012). Whether the pregnant mother reduces her eating disorder behaviors or continues performing the behaviors, she should be working with a collaborative team of professionals joining her OB/GYN in managing her medical and psychological care.

In general, when a pregnant woman with an eating disorder is asked what her biggest pregnancy fear is, a likely response may be, "I feel a complete loss of control." This may relate to loss of control over body size, loss of control over weight gain, and in some cases loss of control over her identity.

SEXUAL ABUSE AND OTHER TRAUMA HISTORY

Women with a history of chronic eating disorders are more likely to report a history of childhood sexual abuse and physical abuse when compared to women with no history of an eating disorder. It has been estimated that 30% of those with an eating disorder have been sexually abused. Also at high risk for eating disorders related to trauma are victims/observers of domestic violence and those who suffer from post-traumatic stress disorder (National Eating Disorders Association 2015). It has been shown that trauma and abuse histories increase risk to perinatal depression, postpartum depression, as well as other psychiatric disorders. Traumatic life incidences are also associated with complications during pregnancy, including miscarriages, higher rate of pregnancy hyperemesis (vomiting), preterm contractions, and delivery complications (Meltzer-Brody et al. 2011).

Trauma is at the core of many eating disorders and why some eating disorders become so complex to treat and so difficult to resolve. Underneath the eating disorder is an attempt to take back control that was taken away from the trauma survivor. Until the trauma is addressed and treated, the person may never truly recover from the eating disorder and continued relapses may prevent treatment advancement. To better understand trauma in pregnant women with eating disorders, expert clinical trauma psychologist Curtis C. Rouanzoin, PhD, was interviewed (Rouanzoin 2015). Irvine, California–based Rouanzoin has been treating trauma clients, many with eating disorders, for over 25 years. He uses a variety of trauma modalities to treat his clients, including Eye Movement Desensitization Reprocessing (EMDR) therapy.

MB: **It has been established that trauma/abuse/neglect can put someone at a higher risk of developing an eating disorder. What can happen to pregnant women who have eating disorders with a history of unresolved trauma?**

CR: One of the ways that unresolved trauma can get expressed is when the pregnancy itself becomes a trigger. The feelings inside the body of the pregnant woman may trigger earlier nonconscious somatosensory (body) memories so that the woman's psychological reaction to the pregnancy is different from one who has not been traumatized.

MB: **How would you define unresolved trauma?**

CR: Unresolved trauma is defined not by the magnitude of the event but by how it is stored in the nervous system and in the brain. What makes trauma unresolved is that memory is stored as a state-specific, negatively charged emotion with all the sounds, smells, and other senses relating to the trauma—and it is developmentally specific, meaning that it exists at the age at which the abuse occurred. In other words, unresolved trauma memory is frozen as if it were suspended in time and space.

MB: **Is experiencing one type of trauma (sexual, physical, verbal, or emotional) more harmful to a pregnant mom with an eating disorder and her baby?**

CR: Physical abuse to the mother while she's pregnant definitely is the most traumatic thing a mother and her unborn child can go through. In regard to the mother's past history, all abuse is horrible. Sexual trauma is seen in a high rate of clients with eating disorders. If the trauma is not resolved, the pregnant mom can bring her eating disorder and unresolved sexual trauma into her pregnancy. Because of the reproductive system, the woman's genitalia itself can be a trigger in the mother because of her earlier sexual abuse.

Verbal and emotional abuse also create a psychologically violent environment for the pregnant mother. Research suggests that mothers who are pregnant and are exposed to a violent physical or emotionally abusive environment experience the release of adrenaline into their bloodstreams. This trauma reaction is a survival response in the body known as the flight, fight, or freeze response. Most often the adrenaline dissipates in the pregnant mother within a few minutes after the trauma stimulus has been removed. This corresponds to the release of cortisol in the bloodstream that deactivates the adrenaline in the mother. However, in the unborn fetus the adrenaline that is passed through the placenta remains active for hours due to the fetus' underdeveloped brain in utero. The fetus' brain does not have the ability to release cortisol to deactivate the adrenaline flowing through the fetus and its environment.

This impacts the unborn baby by causing an increased and prolonged arousal state due to this adrenaline. So the baby goes into a fight-or-flight response within the mother. This turbulent fetal environment may result in low birthweight and other neurological difficulties once the child is born. If the pregnant mother has experienced severe neglect when she was an infant or child this can impact (if trauma is unresolved) her ability as an adult to bond with both the fetus inside her womb and the newborn baby once it is born. This unconscious disconnection makes it difficult for her to feel connected to the fetus and her own body because of the neglect that she has experienced. Her own neglect experiences make it impossible on many biological levels to bond sufficiently with that unborn child. Without the bonding experience, the baby's mirror neurons in the brain are not activated, causing distress in the baby and the missed opportunity to bond with the mother.

MB: **Some women with eating disorders who become pregnant are able to cease/reduce eating disorder behaviors during pregnancy for the health of the baby, and other women continue their eating disorder behaviors knowing they may be risking the baby's health. Society would look at this as one pregnant mom caring and loving, and the other pregnant mom as selfish and unloving. How do you see these two sets of pregnant women in eating disorder populations?**

CR: Different women respond to trauma differently. One pregnant woman may be able to suspend her eating disorder during her pregnancy while another may not. I would hypothesize that the one who was unable to suspend her eating disorder was probably traumatized at an earlier age developmentally than the time the other pregnant woman experienced trauma who is able to suspend her eating disorder during pregnancy.

Because such an early trauma is stored in the sensorimotor system, the traumatized mother will be more apt to be triggered by the sensorimotor sensations of the baby within her body. And these reactions will be nonconscious reactions over which intellect and rationalization have no control or influence. She engages in unhealthy activities, such as excessive exercise, food restriction, or bingeing and purging, and doesn't know why she practices them. These women can dissociate the baby inside them during the pregnancy because they have already dissociated from their bodies as a result of having been traumatized. The function of eating disorders is to separate the body from awareness of the trauma. The fetus becomes part of the body.

Therefore, to the mother, the fetus does not exist just as the body does not exist. Society and clinicians often characterize the mother as bad, uncaring, weak, selfish … when the truth is … the trauma is speaking and they cannot help their reactions. A dissociated pregnant mother can simply go about her life ignoring the fact that she's getting bigger, eating or not eating, as though nothing is inside of her. Denying the pregnancy allows her to deny the changes in her growing body. She feels totally disconnected from any change or growth within her body. This is not a baby. The fetus is a growth. To the mother, the fetus is simply an extension of this horrible thing called a body.

MB: One thing many women feel when they are pregnant is the sense of losing control over their bodies. What types of behaviors might be common in a pregnant eating disorder mom with history of unresolved trauma?

CR: Many pregnant women with unresolved trauma do engage in a lot of unhealthy and excessive behaviors in an effort to gain control trying to compensate for the time they did not have control during their own traumatization. Some new mothers with eating disorders will choose not to breastfeed because the subjective experience of a baby draining something from her body, in this case the breast milk, is unimaginable. To the mother, food is a nonconscious trigger that she has taken a great deal of time and effort to control. Food (breast milk) is now being removed from her outside of her control by this new life. Rather than lovingly breastfeeding her baby, the mother, out of her own trauma "eyes," sees the act as taking away her control.

MB: If a pregnant woman with an eating disorder has unresolved trauma, is it appropriate to do intense trauma work, like EMDR, while the woman is pregnant, or wait until after the baby is born?

CR: It depends. If the trauma is related to a previous pregnancy and childbirth, then resolving the fear of giving birth may help the mother be a much better vehicle through which her next baby is born. So the answer may be yes in this situation. Again if we look at the issue of adrenaline being released into her body, it is better if a mother's pregnancy trauma be targeted and completed quickly to protect the fetus inside. If you're dealing with long-term chronic trauma issues, it is better for the pregnant mother to give birth and then do the trauma work after the delivery.

MB: You mentioned how traumatized pregnant mothers can dissociate and completely leave their bodies. Explain the meaning of dissociation. And why do people dissociate? Is all dissociation bad?

CR: Dissociation is simply the splitting off of awareness. As was once said by internationally known dissociation/trauma psychiatrist Dr. Colin Ross, "Dissociation is a little girl who is being so overwhelmed and traumatized that she separates herself from the trauma and looks at it as though it is happening to someone else." It is a splitting off of streams of consciousness. Dissociation is not bad—it is necessary. We all dissociate, every one of us. It's a biological built-in phenomena for survival. Trauma may require one person to utilize it more than another. But as a wise woman once said, "Dissociation is God's gift to abused children."

MB: Anything that you'd like to add about your expertise in trauma and how it might relate to pregnant women with eating disorders in regard to how clinicians relate to them?

CR: The professionals in the community need to understand that a severely traumatized pregnant mother who is unable to connect to her baby in the womb, or to her baby once born, doesn't mean she is a bad or cruel person. Her trauma isn't a character defect in her personality. She just needs the appropriate time to heal and be nurtured through her trauma experience that will enable her to reach out to nurture others, like her own children. It's our jobs as treating professionals to help move our clients past the trauma so they can be present for their own children. In most cases, I have seen with my own eyes very traumatized women become the most amazing nurturing parents, not necessarily because of any specific mentoring, but because of the inherent nature of wanting to give her child something she never had … love (Rouanzoin 2015).

INFERTILITY AND UNPLANNED PREGNANCIES

Reproductive health is compromised in women with a history of all types of eating disorders (Linna et al. 2013). For those women with AN, BN, BED, or what was formerly called EDNOS-purging only type (EDNOS-P), becoming pregnant is often difficult due to the erratic hormonal imbalances and poor nutrition from the disorders that affect the menstrual cycle where some women become amenorrheic (lack of ovulation) or oligomenorrheic (menstrual irregularity). Similarly, women with BED who have a higher body mass index (BMI) and who are more likely to be obese have increased difficulty conceiving due to the higher fat ratio in their body (Mitchell and Bulik 2006).

In a study looking at reproductive outcomes with eating disorders, remaining childless was common for women with lifetime eating disorders. In women with lifetime eating disorders who did get pregnant, the rates of pregnancy and childbirth were lower compared to those without eating disorders. For women with lifetime AN, pregnancy rates were less than half of the rates of the reference group. Elective abortions were most common in women with a lifetime of BN, whereas a surprisingly high rate of miscarriages, almost 50%, were seen in women with a lifetime of BED (Linna et al. 2013).

A longitudinal birth cohort of more than 14,000 women in the United Kingdom was enrolled in the Avon Longitudinal Study of Parents and Children (ALSPAC). The women with lifetime eating disorders AN ($n = 171$), BN ($n = 199$), and those with both AN + BN ($n = 82$) were found to struggle with fertility problems, unplanned pregnancies, and more negative attitudes to pregnancy than those women without eating disorders in the general population group ($n = 10,636$).

The results showed that women with a history of eating disorders were no more likely than women without eating disorders in the population study to take longer than 1 year to conceive. However, a higher percentage of the eating disorder groups did take more than 6 months to conceive compared with control group (39.5% vs. 25%). Additionally, the eating disorder population was more than twice as likely as the general population to use fertility treatment to conceive (6.2% vs. 2.7%). Importantly, the study found 41% of AN women within the eating disorder group reported that their pregnancies were unplanned, compared to 28% of women with no eating disorder history. Women with the eating disorders showed increased reporting of negative feelings upon discovery of their pregnancies than the general population group (Linna et al. 2013).

Another population-based birth cohort based in the Netherlands included women with history of AN ($n = 160$), BN ($n = 265$), or both AN + BN ($n = 130$) and a general population of women of more than 4300 with no histories of eating disorders. Similarly, study results showed all lifetime eating disorder groups to have increased odds of receiving fertility treatment, increased prevalence of unplanned pregnancies with AN women having the highest percentage, and more mixed feelings about being pregnant than the general population group. Another outcome measured was likelihood of twin births. Results showed all eating disorder groups to have increased odds of twin births compared to the general population group (Micali et al. 2014).

Pregnancy can occur in the absence of menstruation and it is important that amenorrheic and oligomenorrheic women and teens realize that they are not protected from pregnancy. If there is no menstruation, one might consider it impossible for conception. However, when ovulation occurs for the first time after a period of amenorrhea, it is possible for the first egg ovulated to become fertilized if the woman is not taking any birth control measures. In other words, a woman with AN and amenorrhea may become pregnant without having experienced a return of menstruation (Hoffman et al. 2011).

As clinicians, it is important to educate women with AN and BN that becoming pregnant is a possibility with irregular menstruation or lack of menstruation. The old myths of the anorexic woman as infertile and not sexually active need to be debunked. Women with AN are sexually active and can conceive. Clinicians must talk openly to the eating disorder population about contraception, sexuality, sexually transmitted diseases, and pregnancy (Bulik et al. 2010).

Alarming Trend of Pregnancy through Fertility Clinics

With the high-technology fertility treatments available today, there is a risk of underweight or malnourished women to conceive. An undiagnosed, undisclosed, or untreated eating disorder may interfere with the outcome of infertility treatment and place the mother and baby at risk of negative health outcomes (Franko and Walton 1993).

Two infertility studies revealed between 16% and 20% of women seeking fertility treatment have eating disorders, which is significantly higher than the U.S. prevalence of eating disorders in the general population that has been estimated between 1% and 4% in women with lifetime eating disorders (Bulik 2013). One of these studies revealed that not one of the participants who met the eating disorder criteria disclosed their past or current diagnosis. Of participants diagnosed with menstrual complications, 58% met the criteria for an eating disorder. As the trend is showing, women with past or current eating disorder history (including BED) are likely to seek assistance with treatment for conception from fertility clinics across the nation. The study investigators suggest an eating disorder screening assessment should be included in the initial intake at infertility clinics because these patients may be at an increased risk of maternal and fetal negative outcomes relative to those patients without a history of an eating disorder. Since patients with a past or current eating disorder may not disclose their history to their reproductive health-care providers, this silence, in turn, may limit providers' ability to offer essential medical and psychological referrals these patients need for their health and their babies' (Freizinger et al. 2010).

Body Image

Body image is the picture of your body you see in your mind. Body image starts developing in childhood. Negative body comments from a parent, teacher, coach, a peer, and exposure to the media displaying ideals of a "perfect body" (that coincidently only 2% of American women can achieve) bear long-lasting effects on a person's viewpoint of his or her body. It is no wonder so many woman and men develop negative body image. One significant risk factor for developing an eating disorder is having a negative body image (Maternal, Child and Adolescent Health Division Center for Family Health California Department of Public Health 2015).

What happens to the body image of a pregnant woman with an eating disorder? The answer is it depends. Many pregnant women with eating disorders are terrified of gaining weight during pregnancy. More than 400 women were interviewed regarding fears of pregnancy, and weight gain is one of the most common fears in women with or without eating disorders (Mysko 2009).

On an optimistic note, approximately one-third of women struggling with eating disorders believe that pregnancy could offer them a time to recover, even though they fear they will feel out of control with their gestational weight gain. Many view that having a bigger body size during pregnancy is more acceptable than at other times (Hoffman et al. 2011).

They may see their bodies at this time as more functional, as they are creating another human being. They may feel a boost in self-esteem that they are putting the well-being of their baby over the appearance of their body. The connection to the baby, such as when the baby kicks, starts that important bonding process necessary for the mother with her baby, even in utero (Clark et al. 2009).

However, for some pregnant women with eating disorders, the change in their body shape or size may trigger anxiety and restrictive behaviors regarding weight gain (Ward and Waller 2008). These women are at high risk of engaging in their eating disorder behaviors throughout their pregnancy. This can increase the chance of depression as they struggle with weight gain and body image issues, as well as increase the potential of medical complications for them and their babies (National Eating Disorder Association 2005).

The body image and weight gain issues can continue through postpartum. Women with histories of eating disorders have an increased risk of postpartum depression, even if they were in remission of the eating disorder during the pregnancy. Also, a mother with an eating disorder in the postpartum period is often preoccupied with body size and weight loss rather than placing her attention on ensuring her best physical and emotional health and connecting to her baby (Mysko 2009).

Researchers on a body image study concluded body dissatisfaction does not improve during pregnancy in women with or without eating disorders. For women with eating disorders during pregnancy, body weight dissatisfaction remained unchanged, before a decrease at 6 and 12 months postpartum. For pregnant women without eating disorders, body weight dissatisfaction increased and remained elevated until 6 months postpartum. This information suggests all pregnant women need additional support regarding body image during pregnancy and postpartum (Coker and Abraham 2015).

MEDIA INFLUENCES

There is a dangerous dichotomy in today's culture as it is sending a message of positive reinforcement to pregnant women struggling with eating disorders to lose postpartum weight in unhealthy ways in order to quickly regain prepregnancy body size (HuffPost Live 2015). The media continues to praise celebrities who achieve the "baby bump" followed by rapid postpregnancy weight loss; in turn, expectant mothers internalize the unrealistic pressure and concern accentuated in our culture valuing thinness over health. This mentality inhibits the critical moments in which new life and new mother are meant to weave together to form a precious, life-affirming bond (Orbach and Rubin 2014). There is a cultural insinuation that a mother's job is to present her body physically as though nothing as momentously life-changing or body-changing as having a baby has occurred (Abraham 2004).

When there is a media focus on pregnant celebrities' weight this can affect how "regular" pregnant women see their bodies and weight. Women increasingly feel the pressure to have the "perfect" pregnancy and quickly lose weight to achieve back their prepregnancy body. Claire Mysko, coauthor of the book *Does This Pregnancy Make Me Look Fat?* and 2015 spokeswoman for the National Eating Disorders Association remarked,

> Between 2003 and 2005, the number of baby-related, baby weight-related covers on the tabloids doubled and since then, it's almost become an expectation now that if a celebrity is pregnant, there will be a mention of her body during pregnancy and then there's the countdown to how fast she's going to get the weight off ...[The media] has an effect on women and it absolutely fuels... and validates this obsession with weight during pregnancy and after.... We can't necessarily make a direct connection between whether that has increased the rate or the incidence of eating disorders, but certainly it has amped up this anxiety that women feel. (Wallace 2013)

LIFE TRANSITIONS

Puberty, going away to college, getting married, and having a baby are huge life transitions, especially for individuals who have trouble coping with transitional life periods. Sometimes individuals cope in an unhealthy way by developing an eating disorder to manage the stress.

Whether a pregnancy is planned or unexpected, it can evoke a lot of conflicting feelings in women. Pregnancy can particularly affect women with eating disorders as the disorder disconnects them from themselves, their babies, and others in life. Entering the pregnancy phase can bring up the ambivalent feelings similar to other major life transitions. It is also stressful during the preparation to motherhood depending on if this is the first pregnancy, whether the pregnancy was planned, the outcome of any previous pregnancies, or the supportive relationship with the father of the child (Müldner-Nieckowski et al. 2014). Pregnancy heralds a period of change in partner relationships. The strength of the relationship weighs heavily on the mood and self-esteem of a pregnant woman, as well as the gratification of having a child. Pregnant women often become much more focused on their child than their partner, which may result in them feeling misunderstood. Sometimes, partners can make careless remarks about the expanding body, triggering a cascade of negative emotions about their pregnant bodies. It is common for a mother to begin to perceive her partner as intrusive, childish, or uninvolved (Müldner-Nieckowski et al. 2014). Changes in sex life are common during and after pregnancy. Approximately 86% of couples continue to have sexual problems well after birth. This may be related to the partner feeling rejected because the mother may be feeling unattractive after birth or preoccupied with the newborn and the resurgence of eating disorder symptoms.

The transition to the role of motherhood can be overwhelming to new moms with eating disorders. Life typically becomes very chaotic and unstructured which can cause a lot of stress. There is disruption in daily routine and sleep schedule, making it more difficult to maintain proper eating habits. With the chaos, stress, and feelings of loss of control, some mothers may be triggered to engage in binge eating episodes or severe caloric restriction. All of the above contribute to an increase in eating disorder behaviors during the postpartum period (Astrachan-Fletcher et al. 2008; Patel et al. 2005). A study following women with a history of AN or BN found that more than 90% of these first-time moms reported problems regarding their maternal adjustment at 3 months postpartum compared to 13% of the control group (Koubaa et al. 2008).

Some women with eating disorders have trouble adjusting to the bodily changes that occur during pregnancy while others embrace it with a sense of value that they have a baby growing inside them. It is common for women with eating disorders to restrict their diets due to fear of weight gain, while other may eat an excessive amount of calories. Even with the best intent for a healthy pregnancy, many women with eating disorders lack the knowledge of how to properly nourish themselves and the baby. Many women rely on their eating disorders as a coping mechanism during pregnancy. Some women with eating disorders also engage in self-harm during pregnancy. "One woman cut her abdomen several times during pregnancy as she struggled with her changing body" (Pekar 2013). For many women with eating disorders there is a "conflict between doing the best for their child and heeding to the demands of their eating disorder" (Pekar 2013).

HEALTH CONSEQUENCES DURING PREGNANCY

Health consequences for a pregnant woman with an eating disorder can impact expectant mother and her fetus concomitantly with potentially serious, even life-threatening, medical complications and increased risks for negative mental health outcomes. In fact, the health consequences affecting the fetus can persist into infancy and through its lifespan. In this section, research-driven insights are summarized on the medical and mental health complications in pregnancy that can endanger a mom with an eating disorder and her unborn child.

PATTERNS OF REMISSION, CONTINUATION, AND INCIDENCE OF EATING DISORDERS DURING PREGNANCY

Large population-based birth cohort studies have found the most common course of eating disorders during pregnancy is toward remission, yet complete remission is rare. Although some women can continue to engage in eating disorder behaviors during pregnancy, the vast majority of pregnant women reflect a decrease in eating disorder symptoms.

Pregnancy and the transition into motherhood can be an influential opportunity for remission to occur in women with eating disorders. For some pregnant women, the responsibilities for caring for themselves for the sake of the health of their unborn babies can be strong motivators to decrease or remit symptoms of the eating disorder. However, after birth, "eating for the baby" is no longer seen as a priority for many women and the return of eating disorder symptoms can increase to prepregnancy rates (Barnes 2015).

A large Norwegian-based pregnancy cohort study examining remission, continuation, and new onset eating disorder during pregnancy found about 5% of pregnant women (in sample size of 95,000) were affected by eating disorders, similar to the prevalence in the general population. Another population-based birth cohort study, the ALSPAC in the United Kingdom, has estimated that the prevalence rate of eating disorders in pregnant women was up to 7.5%; however, they used a smaller sample size (about 14,000) and participating women were from a clinical setting where the eating disorder cases are often more medically severe compared to a general population study (e.g., the Norwegian Mother and Child Cohort [MoBa] study). Results showed that EDNOS-P women tended to enter remission during pregnancy at a rate of 78%; BN outcomes varied with 34% entering remission, another 34% entering partial remission, and the remaining 29% continuing to engage in eating disorder behaviors. For those with prepregnancy BED, the most common course of the illness was continuation during pregnancy at 61%. A surprising study observation revealed that pregnancy can be a high-risk period for first-time onset BED in those women who previously did not have a history of eating disorders. Estimates for AN during pregnancy were not assessed in this study due to the weight criterion being deemed unreliable as it was based on self-reports of weight gain (Bulik et al. 2007).

Few women with eating disorders report complete symptom relief and abstinence from all behaviors during pregnancy. One study revealed 30% of women with a recent and lifetime eating disorder reported to participating in at least one eating disorder behavior during the second and third trimester of pregnancy (Micali et al. 2007). Even with most pregnant women experiencing recovery improvements with eating disorder behaviors, weight, body size, and body dissatisfaction can remain high or even get worse (Crow et al. 2008). Although past research has mixed results, there is some evidence that pregnancy can trigger a relapse in previously recovered women with a history of eating disorders. One study followed 49 women during pregnancy who at conception had recovered from past eating disorders. During the course of pregnancy, 22% of women relapsed and required treatment (Koubaa et al. 2005).

Pregnancy can be a time eating disorder symptoms improve for many women. However, evidence to date suggests the symptoms' improvements are temporary, and most women with current or past eating disorders are at risk of relapse in the postpartum period (Easter et al. 2015).

MEDICAL COMPLICATIONS AND CONSEQUENCES IN BABIES AND MOTHERS

Collectively, researchers assert that pregnant women with past or active eating disorders should be recognized and treated as at-risk patients during pregnancy (Koubaa et al. 2005). As the baby grows in the womb, it receives all its nourishments from the mother. If the pregnant mother is not nourishing herself properly with adequate food intake, the baby takes its nourishment of carbohydrates, proteins, fats, vitamins, minerals, and other nutrients directly from the mother's body, depleting her own nutrition stores she requires for her own optimal health and the ability to sustain a pregnancy. This can cause severe malnourishment for the mother and complications including depression, fatigue, and other serious health conditions. Similarly, the fetus' physical and mental health will also be compromised by existing in the womb of a malnourished mother (National Eating Disorder Association 2005).

Hormonal changes in pregnant women without an eating disorder are dramatic. However, in the eating disorder pregnant population, hormonal changes shift from the norm with a higher chance of low hormone levels, especially estrogen and progesterone. These hormonal changes can affect the baby with a higher chance of fetal growth restriction, premature birth, low birthweight, and miscarriage. The hormonal imbalance also puts the pregnant mom at a more medically compromised position (Dennis 2015).

The baby's brain is in a crucial period of accelerated growth from late pregnancy (in utero) through the third year of life. During this time, higher amounts of energy are consumed than any other stage in the lifespan of the brain development. This process requires sufficient amounts of nutrients, especially long-chain polyunsaturated fatty acids. The human brain begins forming by 3 weeks after conception. It now appears that at least 5/6 of the human brain growth spurt is postnatal (Schore 2011). With this information, the negative impacts on brain development begin when the baby is still in the pregnant mother's womb. Poor nutrition, in particular with restriction of protein, in the mother during pregnancy interacts with the maternal hypothalamic–pituitary–adrenal axis causing increased fetal exposure to maternal cortisol. Cortisol is also known as the stress hormone, in that, in stressful situations, it helps with the "fight-or-flight" response, increasing energy levels. Maternal cortisol passes through the placenta to the fetus and the hormone puts the fetus into a stressful "fight-or-flight" response. As mentioned in the section "Sexual Abuse and Other Trauma History," the cortisol stays in the fetus' system for hours as the fetus is unable to deactivate the cortisol like the mother can in a matter of minutes. This increased exposure to maternal cortisol can have long-lasting effects. At birth, the baby has a potential for low birthweight. As the baby grows up, an impaired central nervous system can develop and an increased risk of obesity can occur (Hoffman et al. 2011).

Let's now look more specifically at the medical and the associated consequences that can occur in pregnancy within the three main eating disorder types—AN, BN, and BED—and the effects on mother and baby.

RESEARCH SUMMARY ON PREGNANCY AND BIRTH OUTCOMES FOR AN, BN, AND BED

AN, BN, and BED can present a range of potential risks to the expectant mother and baby that may compromise a successful pregnancy outcome. The reported medical complications and birth outcomes for mother and baby for these three eating disorder subtypes have shifted over the years. Why the ambiguity of medical complications?

There are a number of factors that come into play. In general, in regard to study findings, more severe outcomes are seen in clinical studies simply because these studies may reflect the more severe cases of eating disorders that are active during pregnancy, compared with population-based studies that are not set within a treatment or clinical setting. The results of these population-based studies often report fewer complications and healthier delivery outcomes than clinical studies.

In presenting the medical complications section, data was collected (unless noted otherwise) from a peer review literature research study on "Eating Disorders in Pregnancy" in October 2015. What follows is a summary of outcomes for pregnancies in mothers with AN, BN, or BED and the effects on their fetuses (Crow et al. 2015).

Consequences Associated with AN during Pregnancy

Researchers have found estimating the prevalence of AN in pregnant women is complicated by the difficulty in accurately determining low body weight in women who are gaining weight due to pregnancy. Community population-based studies of pregnant women in Norway and the Netherlands provide the best estimates, finding that in the 6–12 months prior to becoming pregnant, the prevalence of AN was 0.1%–0.3%. The actual prevalence is actually higher as many patients often conceal their illness from their health providers due to shame and guilt.

Although amenorrhea in women/teens with AN was exhibited in up to 90% of patients, fertility rates in women with a history of AN were comparable to women in the general population without a history of eating disorders. However, many AN patients seek treatment for infertility.

In one observational study, smoking appeared to be more common in women with a history of AN ($n = 35$) than in women with no history of eating disorders ($n > 33,000$; 37% vs. 9%). Another observational study by ALSPAC found smoking during pregnancy (for women with or without eating disorders) can change certain "marks" on a child's "genome" (set of genetic instructions) when it is developing in the womb. These changes are radical and cannot be reversed. The study found that these marks—known as *epigenetic* marks—are still apparent almost two decades later (Molloy 2015).

Gestational weight gain in AN patients varies. Using weight recommendations from the Health and Medicine Division of the National Academies of Sciences, Engineering, and Medicine, a prospective study of pregnant women with AN ($n = 32$) found at delivery, weight gain was as follows:

- Inadequate: 22% ($n = 7$)
- Adequate: 28% ($n = 9$)
- Excessive: 50% ($n = 16$)

Although prepregnancy weight in patients was low, the "excessive" weight gain during pregnancy was appropriate and most likely the body's innate survival mechanism to protect the baby and mom. Gestational weight gain appeared to be greater at delivery in women with AN than women without the history of the disorder (Crow et al. 2015).

Course of illness: The course of AN during and after pregnancy varies across patients. Although active AN may diminish during pregnancy, patients can relapse postpartum. A prospective study ($n = 72$ patients with prepregnancy AN) found the following outcomes at 36 months postpartum:

- Persistence or recurrence of AN: 29%
- Crossover to a different eating disorder (e.g., BN): 12%
- Remission: 59%

Pregnancy and delivery outcomes: Adverse pregnancy outcomes that are observed more often in pregnant women with AN than in women without include the following:

- Antepartum hemorrhage: One retrospective study found that antepartum hemorrhage occurred in more mothers with a history of AN ($n = 230$ births) than in mothers without AN ($n = 1144$ births; Eagles et al. 2012).
- Lower birth weight babies: A meta-analysis of nine observational studies examined birth weight in babies of mothers with AN (active or past history; $n > 4000$) and babies of mothers without the disorder ($n > 2,000,000$). Birth weight was lower in children of AN mothers than controls; however, the standardized mean difference was small (190 g). Yet, results from across some of the studies were inconsistent, so the standardized mean difference in weight may be inconclusive and actually higher than predicted (Solmi et al. 2014). Due to conflicting study results, it is unclear if AN in pregnant women is associated with stillbirth and neonatal death.

Pregnant women with a history of AN do not appear to be at risk for the following:

- Miscarriage
- Preeclampsia
- Preterm delivery
- Cesarean delivery
- Small for gestational age babies
- Large for gestational age babies

Cesarean delivery is one birth outcome for women with AN with conflicted study results. Renowned eating disorder researcher and author Cynthia Bulik, PhD, summarizes why different study results for Cesarean deliveries may vary: "Some studies suggested that they had a higher rate of Cesarean sections, while other studies did not. Women with more severe, active symptoms of AN during pregnancy may be viewed as high-risk by their obstetricians, resulting in more frequent Cesarean sections" (Bulik 2013).

One fact that is not refuted is that AN has the highest mortality rate of any mental illness. A recent study looking at the relationship between childbearing and mortality from AN found that childbearing among women with AN was associated with a 65% lower mortality rate than for those with AN who have never been pregnant. This suggests childbearing is a positive factor associated with lower mortality among women with AN compared to women with AN who never become pregnant.

Consequences Associated with BN during Pregnancy

The estimated prevalence of BN during pregnancy in a large community study in Norway ($n > 77,000$) was 0.2%. Initial onset of BN during pregnancy is rare. Pregnant women with BN were more distressed with changes in body shape and the concerns of weight gain than pregnant woman without an eating disorder. Smoking during pregnancy occurred in more mothers with BN ($n > 300$) than mothers without eating disorders ($n > 33,000$; 15% vs. 9%). However, pregnant mothers with AN smoke more than twice as much as pregnant mothers with BN.

Gestational weight gain in mothers with BN is frequently excessive. Using weight recommendations from the Institute of Medicine, a prospective study of pregnant women with BN ($n = 275$) found at delivery, weight gain was as follows:

- Inadequate: 20%
- Adequate: 20%
- Excessive: 60%

The study also reported the average total weight gain at delivery was greater in women with BN than in women with no history of eating disorders ($n > 30,000$; 37.5 lb. vs. 11 lb.).

Pregnancy and delivery outcomes: BN is associated with an increased rate of miscarriages. Pregnant women with a history of BN do not appear to be at risk for the following:

- Preeclampsia
- Preterm delivery
- Cesarean delivery
- Small for gestational age babies
- Large for gestational age babies

A prospective study observed pregnancy-related nausea and vomiting (distinguished from self-induced vomiting) in pregnant women with BN whose illness included purging (e.g., self-induced vomiting or laxative abuse; $n = 100$), and pregnant women with no eating disorders ($n > 37,000$). Pregnancy-related nausea and vomiting in the first gestational month occurred in more women with BN who purged, compared to women with no eating disorders (29% vs. 21%).

Course of illness: Pregnant women with BN typically find remission or partial remission during pregnancy. However, a prospective study ($n = 672$ patients with prepregnancy BN) reported the following outcomes at 36 months:

- Full relapse of BN symptoms: 18.7%
- Subthreshold symptoms of BN: 32.5%
- Crossover to a different eating disorder (e.g., BED): 19.3%
- Remission of BN: 29.5%

Consequences Associated with BED during Pregnancy

BED is characterized by recurrent binge eating without the use of any compensatory measures (such as vomiting, exercise, or laxatives) to counter the binge. The estimated prevalence of BED during pregnancy reported in a community study in Norway ($n > 77,000$ pregnant women) was 5%. Many of these cases were new onset of BED during pregnancy. Like pregnant women with BN, those women with BED also experienced more distress with body shape and weight concerns than women without an eating disorder. Expectant mothers with BED ($n > 1800$) smoked during pregnancy more than mothers with no eating disorders ($n > 33,000$) (14% vs. 9%).

Gestational weight gain in pregnant women with BED is usually excessive. Using weight recommendations from the Institute of Medicine, a prospective study of pregnant women with BED ($n > 1700$) found at delivery, weight gain was as follows:

- Inadequate: 18%
- Adequate: 17%
- Excessive: 65%

The study also reported the average total weight gain at delivery was greater in women with BED than women with no history of eating disorders ($n > 30,000$; 37.5 lb. vs. 11 lb.).

Pregnancy and delivery outcomes: BED may be associated with an increased rate of miscarriages. A registry study found miscarriages occurred three times more often in women with BED ($n = 149$) than in a matched control group ($n = 596$).

Pregnant women with a history of BED do not appear to be at risk for

- Preeclampsia
- Preterm delivery
- Cesarean delivery
- Small for gestational age babies

It is not clear if a pregnant mother with BED has an increased risk of giving birth to an infant who is large for gestational age due to conflicting results across studies.

Course of illness: Pregnant women with BED typically persist in their BED behaviors during pregnancy. A prospective study ($n > 2600$ patients with prepregnancy BED) reported the following outcomes at 36 months:

- Full relapse of BED symptoms: 21%
- Subthreshold symptoms of BED: 23%
- Crossover to a different eating disorder (e.g., BN): 14%
- Remission of BED: 42%

COMPLICATIONS DURING CHILDBIRTH FOR WOMEN WITH AN, BN, OR BED

The presence of an eating disorder during pregnancy can increase labor complications including an increase in Cesarean section deliveries (Knoph et al. 2013). Insight into the increase in Cesarean rates for the eating disorder population comes from the perspective of obstetrician Sherry A. Ross, MD, of Santa Monica, California, whose 24-year practice specializes in treating pregnant women with eating disorders. Dr. Ross states persistent malnutrition leads to placental insufficiency that ultimately affects fetal growth and fetal well-being, especially during labor. Placental insufficiency and severe fetal growth restrictions often affect the pregnant mom's ability to attempt a successful vaginal birth. These fetuses have more difficulties enduring the stress of a vaginal birth and are more prone to fetal distress during labor. As a result, women with eating disorders during pregnancy are more likely to deliver via Cesarean section (Ross 2015).

It has been well-documented: women with eating disorders have an increased history of past sexual abuse. When pregnant women with eating disorders also have a history of early sexual abuse, birth complications can occur as part of their traumatic response to the situational and physical feelings of not being in control. Being "in control" is very important for many childhood survivors of sexual abuse because the opposite feeling, "out of control," can trigger a cascade of body feelings and memories of the early abuse that in her mind makes her feel helpless. The bodily process of labor is outside one's conscious control. For a survivor, the crisis may hit when she realizes in labor she is helpless to control this natural birthing process (Simkin and Klaus 2004).

Traumatic births are much more likely in women with eating disorders who have a history of childhood sexual abuse. An obstetrician might explain a traumatic birth as a complication that can cause serious physical damage to the mother or baby. For example, a baby is in fetal distress, causing the need for an emergency Cesarean section for the mother, perhaps with inadequate anesthesia; shoulder dystonia; severe perineal damage; fetal asphyxia, vacuum extractor or forceps injuries; severe hemorrhage; newborn disabilities; or death. Even psychological distress can impact childbirth if the woman has previously suffered trauma that was never resolved and during childbirth experiences the symptoms of posttraumatic stress. Examples include invasive interventions that the woman perceives as physically damaging her body; a fear she or her baby is dying; lack of privacy; nakedness; and unwanted exposure. Women may carry with them the aftermath of a traumatic birth, perhaps leading to posttraumatic stress disorder. These types of complications of traumatic births are times the mother may need the support of her treatment team more than ever. Counseling by the eating disorder therapist who has experience with sexual trauma during the postpartum time is crucial for the new mom to heal any childbirth traumas (Simkin and Klaus 2004).

Obstetric complications can play a role in the later development of a first-time eating disorder in a mom who has given birth with no prior eating disorder history. A birth cohort study published in 2015 found a significant relationship between specific obstetric complications and the later development of AN and BN. Signs of retarded fetal growth found in the babies of the moms who later developed BN was a distinguishing factor from the babies of the moms who later developed AN. The study reported a significantly higher number of obstetric complications in moms who later developed binge-eating/purging AN in comparison with restricting AN (Tenconi et al. 2015).

MENTAL HEALTH CONSEQUENCES

The focus of a pregnant woman's perspective on motherhood, self-image, and self-esteem can be significantly impacted if she has a history of an eating disorder or is struggling with one during her pregnancy (Müldner-Nieckowski et al. 2014). There is an increased risk of perinatal depression and anxiety in women with current or past eating disorders compared to women with no history of an eating disorder (Easter et al. 2015).

Perinatal depression is a frequent mental health consequence among women during pregnancy. From a population-based study, researchers reported 39.1%–66.7% of women with a diagnosis of a lifetime eating disorder revealed experiencing depression during the pregnancy period as well as 45.5%–70% experiencing postpartum depression. The comparison group that included women with no history of an eating disorder but a history of major depression reported 36.8% experience perinatal depression and 41.2% postpartum depression (Meltzer-Brody et al. 2011). Another more current study supports data that women with current and past eating disorders have higher depressive and anxiety symptoms during prenatal and postpartum periods, compared with women without an eating disorder history (Easter et al. 2015). Past childhood sexual abuse and physical abuse are reported more often in women with a lifetime history of an eating disorder in comparison to women with no eating disorder history. Similarly, an increased risk of perinatal depression, postpartum depression, and other psychiatric conditions align with trauma and abuse histories (Meltzer-Brody et al. 2011).

Pregnancy can be a motivation for recovery for some women with active eating disorders. However, pregnancy can also be a time for the first onset of an eating disorder or relapse for women who have past histories of eating disorders (Watson et al. 2014b). In those who relapse, the physical and emotional changes associated with pregnancy can trigger old behaviors to resurface in fear of excessive weight gain and increased body size in a culture, like Western society, where the small baby bump is sadly applauded. Externalizing the pregnant self to a number on a scale and an accepted body size can push vulnerable women to restrict calories, binge and purge, and exercise excessively in an attempt to control the natural changes the body embraces to create new life. Motherhood is also a transitional phase in life that can bring up other fears of change where one's psychological control can feel threatened (Müldner-Nieckowski et al. 2014).

Many women with active eating disorders have a diminished sense of identity as a woman, decreased connectedness to other women, and impaired social/spiritual development. One core component of spirituality is a sense of connectedness to something bigger than oneself. This happens naturally for many women during pregnancy, even for those who do not experience it before pregnancy. When a woman is very sick physically, emotionally, and spiritually, this connection does not happen and the woman remains primarily attached to her eating disorder (Dennis 2015).

Impact of Prenatal Maternal Distress to Fetal Development Can Span a Lifetime

"The developing brain of the baby adapts itself, on a neurobiological level, to the quality of the caregiving environment. The first 'caregiving environment' is the womb" (Music 2013).

Eating disorders during pregnancy can negatively affect intrauterine growth of the fetus. This concept that links in utero environmental conditions during fetal development with risk of physical and psychiatric illnesses later in life is called fetal programming (Music 2013). Potentially harmful environmental influences on fetal development can significantly affect the structure and function of the developing fetus' organs and can produce negative long-term physical and mental health outcomes of the offspring. Fetal undernutrition and overexposure to stress hormones are thought to be the two main processes that are involved in fetal programming (Hoffman et al. 2011).

Maternal malnutrition of the fetus during pregnancy is associated with increased risk for obesity, heart disease, metabolic disease, and stroke in the adult. Infants born under the effects of in utero malnourishment are also at increased risk throughout their lifespan for lower cognitive function, behavioral issues, stress reactivity, and psychopathology. Poor nutrition combined with insufficient protein intake during pregnancy interacts with the maternal hypothalamic–pituitary–adrenal axis, which causes an increased fetal exposure to maternal cortisol (Hoffman et al. 2011).

The negative effects of maternal stress, anxiety, and depression during pregnancy can be passed through the placenta influencing the distress level of the fetus. The consequences of the exposure of maternal mental health transmitted to the growing fetus can persist into infancy and through the lifespan of the adult. Research indicates that prenatal distress exposure predicts an increased likelihood to future poor emotional regulation, symptoms of attention deficit hyperactivity disorder (ADHD), and other psychopathology (Monk et al. 2012).

A mother's state of mind influences the prenatal environment in one pathway via the release of hormones. Cortisol is a hormone with a very important role in helping the body respond to stress. During pregnancy, the expectant mother naturally produces a higher level of cortisol and it passes through the placenta to the fetus. In an unstressed fetal environment, cortisol helps regulate the growth of the fetus. In one prenatal maternal stress study, researchers observed pregnant women with consistently higher than normal pregnancy cortisol levels deliver infants who displayed a significantly higher sensitivity to stress than infants born to pregnant mothers with normal pregnancy cortisol levels. These inherently stressed infants were monitored as they grew older and they exhibited higher levels of anxiety compared to other children. At approximately 7 years of age, magnetic resonance imaging (MRI) scans were performed on these children and revealed larger than normal sizes of the amygdala, the section of the brain associated with human flight, fight, or freeze response. A larger amygdala can be associated with a higher anxiety state, which these children exhibited (Buss et al. 2012).

The potential lifelong effects of fetal programming can also affect a fetus' development through exposure to cigarette smoke, alcohol consumption, and drug use by the expectant mom during pregnancy (Music 2013).

ASSEMBLING A TREATMENT TEAM

Detection of eating disorders in pregnant women in the clinical setting can be a challenge. While a woman with severe AN might be visibly detectable, detecting someone with BN visibly is not obvious, as many of these women are of normal or slightly above normal weight. Someone with BED (who can be at normal, above, or obese weight range) is another group that clinicians cannot detect easily without exploration into the patient's eating history (Mitchell-Gieleghem et al. 2012).

Once identified, a collaborative team approach should be initiated to care for a pregnant mother with an eating disorder. Each professional on the team will have his or her own respective treatment goals. The attending obstetrician/gynecologist (OB/GYN) oversees the medical management of the health of the mom and fetus. In more complex medical cases, a perinatologist, an obstetrical subspecialist, may join the team to care for the mom and fetus who both have higher-than-normal risks for medical complications. An experienced eating disorder therapist with expertise in treating pregnant women will work on the psychological dynamics of how the pregnant mother is adjusting to the pregnancy as well as the body image changes, weight gain, and transition into motherhood. Another important team member is the eating disorder dietitian who monitors the patient on nutritional intake, body image, and weight gain.

If necessary, a psychiatrist with expertise in treating eating disorders may also join the team. Adding a lactation consultant to the team in the last trimester is helpful to assist the mom with breastfeeding education prior to delivery and offer personal support once the baby is born and the mom starts breastfeeding. Also, selecting a pediatrician 1 month or more prior to delivery is recommended so the baby is connected to a doctor at birth to monitor closely the infant's health and growth. The team works together to provide the highest level of care to the pregnant woman and her baby in utero (Zauderer 2012).

Having an established team in place during the prenatal period offers a vital opportunity to provide education and support that can positively alter fetal and maternal outcome (Mitchell-Gieleghem et al. 2012). If the expectant mother is identified with an eating disorder that is severe and medically unstable for outpatient care, a referral to a specialized eating disorder residential treatment center may be required (Crow et al. 2015).

For mental or medical health professionals treating pregnant women with eating disorders, it is important to address any area of denial of the disorder as well as ongoing discussions on the negative impacts restrictive eating, bingeing, or purging can have on the mom and fetus. Also helpful is mentioning the importance early on in the pregnancy to make the fetus as "real" as possible so the mother can connect her feeding behaviors directly to her unborn child (Franko and Walton 1993). The attachment between the pregnant woman and her fetus starts during pregnancy; it is the first important relationship to the baby and has been strongly associated with having a stronger mother–baby attachment after birth (Öhman 2011). A pregnant mother's concern for her fetus' well-being is thought to be the primary motivating force behind positive behavioral change as it pertains to an eating disorder. Thus, if the pregnant mother can find a direct connection to the fetus early on, the likelihood of her commitment and desire to protect her baby increases. This protective factor, along with monitoring by the entire treatment team, helps in the success of the treatment goals during pregnancy (Newton and Chizawsky 2006).

SUPPORT GROUPS

The team can provide additional support to patients by offering them resources to free eating disorder support groups, such as Anorexia Nervosa and Associated Disorders (ANAD) or Overeaters Anonymous. These support groups, offered free throughout the United States, can be valuable as well, so the pregnant mother has a place to openly talk and gain support from others struggling with eating disorders. There is also a free online support group created just for pregnant women and mothers who have eating disorders. The group is called "Lift the Shame" and it is a supportive place pregnant women with eating disorders can connect in a confidential setting to other pregnant group members from all over the United States. A professional group facilitator leads the hour-long session where the women can share and receive support. To protect confidentiality, group members join the conversation via audio and/or a chat board. The group was cofounded by chapter author Maggie Baumann, LMFT, psychotherapist, and CEDS certified by iaedp, in partnership with the Chicago-based Timberline Knolls Residential Treatment Center in March 2014. In the first 2 years following the launch date, the support group's membership base grew to nearly 100 pregnant women and/or moms with eating disorders from locations throughout the United States. (Please see the resource section at the end of the chapter for registration and contact information.)

PREGNANCY TREATMENT GOALS

Ideally, professionals recommend women with eating disorders be in healthy recovery in terms of best resolutions for disordered eating, weight, and behavioral symptoms before attempting to become pregnant (National Eating Disorders Association n.d.). Researchers indicate the importance of diagnosis and treatment of the eating disorder before conception or during early prenatal care to reduce the occurrence of eating disorders during pregnancy and potential negative outcomes to the mother and baby (Fornari et al. 2014).

EDUCATING OBSTETRIC TEAMS: EATING DISORDERS IN PREGNANCY

Unplanned pregnancies happen to those with and without eating disorders, and planned pregnancies can happen in the eating disorder population, usually to those in denial of their illness or its severity. Given the stigma and shame associated with eating disorders, many women withhold information regarding their history or may believe they do not have a problem. It is crucial for current and resident OB/GYNs to understand their role in assessing signs and symptoms of disordered eating in order to avoid medical consequences that may jeopardize the developing fetus or pregnant mom (Fornari et al. 2014).

Unfortunately, many obstetricians' and gynecologists' lack of follow-through on screening for eating disorders in their patient populations is alarming. In one study, a survey of OB/GYNs suggest most physicians assess patient's body weight, exercise, dietary habits, and BMI, yet less than half screen for history of eating disorders or body image concerns. Even more significant, approximately 90% of respondents reported their residency training was "barely adequate" in diagnosing and treating

eating disorders. Although these OB/GYNs understood that eating disorders during pregnancy can negatively impact mother and fetus, only half considered eating disorder assessment as their responsibility due to low confidence in their medical training programs on how to assess and treat eating disorders (Fornari et al. 2014).

The lack of adequate education in eating disorders for medical doctors in training programs is apparent. Advocacy is necessary to promote improved and more comprehensive curriculum in assessing and treating eating disorders for physicians across all medical training programs as well as in the general physician practicing population. The Academy for Eating Disorders (AED) (n.d.) offers a free medical guide for health professionals on early recognition and medical management in treating patients with eating disorders. AED is an international professional association committed to leadership in eating disorders research, education, treatment, and prevention.

Warning Signs

In terms of obstetric care of a pregnant mother with an eating disorder and her baby, obstetricians need to be aware of red flags that indicate an eating disorder may be interfering with the pregnancy progress (Table 8.1). Some pregnant women with eating disorders may require high-risk obstetrical care (Crow et al. 2015).

Need for Hospitalization

In working with pregnant patients with eating disorders, a pregnancy population considered to be at high risk for medical complications, close monitoring of the growing fetus, and frequent communication by the entire treatment team is necessary. Often a perinatologist, who has expertise in treating high-risk pregnancies, leads the obstetrician and entire treatment team in supporting the mother and fetus to ensure a healthy outcome.

TABLE 8.1
Warning Signs ED May Be Present in Pregnant Women

Lack of weight gain in second trimester over two consecutive prenatal visits

History of eating disorder

Hyperemesis gravidarum (severe vomiting)

Unexplained high levels of potassium or other electrolyte abnormalities from use of laxatives

Presence of a depression or anxiety disorder

Dangerously low levels of potassium that may be related to excessive vomiting

Dental problems indicative of poor dental enamel from excessive vomiting

Abnormal body mass index (BMI), either too low (indicating possible AN/BN) or too high (indicating possible BED)

Excessive worries of gestational weight gain

Detection of any cardiac irregularities or arrhythmias that would require an immediate EKG screening

Difficulties with eating due to lack of hunger, no nausea symptoms

Sources: Crow, SJ et al., Eating Disorders in Pregnancy, 2015, available at http://www. uptodate.com/contents/eating-disorders-in-pregnancy (accessed 5 December 2015); Setnick, J., Interview by M Baumann, 1 December 2015.

In some high-risk cases, hospitalization of the pregnant mother may be warranted. Hospitalization in pregnant women with eating disorders is indicated in the first trimester if hyperemesis gravidarum becomes a significant problem. This condition is considered the severe end of the spectrum of nausea and vomiting during the first trimester and is seen more frequently in patients with a history of an eating disorder. Hyperemesis gravidarum is persistent nausea and vomiting which leads to weight loss, low blood pressure, electrolyte imbalances, and dehydration creating a starvation state for the mom and growing fetus. Hospitalization includes electrolyte replacement, hydration, and the use of anti-nausea medication. In severe cases, intravenous nutrition may be necessary. Other indications of hospitalization for this high-risk patient population include fetal monitoring for delayed fetal growth issues and dehydration due to poor nutrition that can lead to preterm labor (Ross 2015).

NUTRITIONAL NEEDS OF PREGNANCY FOR WOMEN WITH EATING DISORDERS

Weight Gain during Pregnancy: Recommendations and Monitoring

Weight gain associated with pregnancy triggers a wide variety of thoughts and reactions in women in weight-conscious cultures. It can be especially challenging for a woman with an eating disorder who has previous or current experience with dysfunctional eating patterns, distorted body image, or difficulty sustaining adequate nutrition and weight. Pregnancy can be traumatic since patients with eating disorders have often had a lifetime of significant disturbances in normal eating patterns, body image dysmorphia, and sustaining normal weight. It is incorrect to presume that only underweight women are weight-conscious or that a woman of normal or above normal weight is comfortable with pregnancy weight gain. After a lifelong, culturally indoctrinated fear of weight gain, some women do experience relief during pregnancy via their perception that society's (or their personal or familial) thin ideal is relaxed during pregnancy. In some cases, this results in an improvement in overall nutrition, comfort with eating, decrease or cessation of purging behaviors, and an appreciation of food for the growing fetus. In fact, some women report an improvement in their sense of well-being and ability to eat without purging prior to their knowledge that they are pregnant, suggesting a possible beneficial physiological impact of pregnancy on eating disorder symptoms.

For other women, pregnancy and the associated expectation of weight gain trigger a worsening of eating disorder symptoms and negative body image, and exacerbation of existing fears of "losing control" and "getting fat." Pregnancy can add an extra dimension to weight issues for women who are in the process of losing or trying to lose weight and women who become unexpectedly pregnant after bariatric surgery.

Sometimes an explanation of the components of pregnancy weight gain (e.g., blood volume, placenta and fluids, etc.) can allay the misconception that pregnancy "will make me fat." In other cases, no logical explanation can successfully counteract a woman's fears associated with eating and weight gain. The authors have heard women comment that they hope not to gain any weight during pregnancy, as the fetus can "live off my body"; a woman who intended to gain only 8 lb. with the goal of delivering an 8 lb. baby; and others who eat what they have read are the increased nutritional needs of pregnancy, for example, 500 kcal/day, believing that this will be adequate to nourish the fetus while the woman continues eating little or nothing "for myself." If a woman is unable to meet the nutritional needs of herself and her pregnancy, hospitalization and nutrition support in the form of tube or intravenous (IV) feeding may be necessary to support a healthy pregnancy outcome.

Standard recommended weight gain during pregnancy is based on a woman's pre-pregnancy weight and whether she is expecting more than one baby (Table 8.2). These standards may not be appropriate across the board and should be individualized as needed until more evidence-based standards are published (Hutcheon and Bodnar 2014).

Weight gain and the experience of being weighed can create shame and retrau-matization for an individual with an eating disorder, to the point that a pregnant woman may avoid prenatal appointments entirely simply to avoid being weighed. In clinics where every patient is weighed by a technician prior to her appointment, instructions should be given to forgo this at the first appointment until the following information has been gathered. The professional responsible for monitoring weight should initiate a discussion on weight expectations and the procedures for weighing with each patient individually. Although this may seem to take a substantial amount of time at first, it is essential to building trust with each patient, demonstrating your understanding of the issues related to eating disorders and pregnancy, and maintain-ing a relationship that will allow the patient to manage her anxiety about appoint-ments. Ultimately, this one conversation can have a significant impact on a healthy pregnancy outcome.

- What is your understanding of your need for weight gain during this pregnancy?
- What are your concerns about pregnancy weight gain?
- What are your concerns about the process of being weighed?
- Is there anything I can do that would help you feel safer during or after the weighing process? (e.g., weighing you in a gown each time rather than in your street clothes; weighing you backward and not saying your weight out

---

TABLE 8.2
Recommended Weight Gain during Pregnancy

Prepregnancy Body Mass Index	Single Pregnancy	Twin Pregnancy	Triplet Pregnancy
<18.5	28–40 lb.	No specific guideline available	No specific guideline available
18.5–24.9	25–35 lb.	37–54 lb.	50–60 lb.
>25.0–29.9	15–25 lb.	31–50 lb.	No specific guideline available
>30.0	11–20 lb.	25–42 lb.	No specific guideline available

Sources: Rasmussen, KM, and Yaktine AL, *Weight Gain during Pregnancy Reexamining the Guidelines,* National Academies Press, Washington, 2009; Fornari, V et al., *Open Journal of Obstetrics and Gynecology,* 4, 90–94, 2014.

---

loud or leaving it out where you can see it; saying "You are right on track," rather than "You have gained x number of pounds.")
- Are you currently being weighed elsewhere, either at another provider's office or on your own?
- Which is the one place you feel the most comfortable weighing? I will instruct all other providers that this is the only place you will weigh and ask that provider (or my own office) to share your weight information with the others so that they do not ask to weigh you.

From a medical point of view pregnancy weight gain is "good" and "the right thing to do," a woman with an eating disorder may experience it as wrong, bad, or physically and emotionally painful. The impact of ongoing support and reassurance cannot be overestimated because for some women, even saying, "your weight is on the right track" may be triggering as it indicates that weight gain has occurred. For these women, simply weighing with no comments at all may be best, and you will only address weight if there is a problem. Some women may feel proud of their lack of weight gain, even if you phrase it as a danger, and when the eating disorder pathology is this strong, hospitalization for purposes of feeding may be the only option for a healthy outcome.

In the literature review, pregnancy weight gain, birth outcomes, and other measures for women with a history of active eating disorders vary depending on the population sample studied. In clinical/medical settings, the severity of the study participants' eating disorder symptoms is greater. A pregnant woman with severe AN and extreme fear of weight gain is going to have a poorer response to gaining adequate weight for the health of her fetus, not to mention for the health of herself. In studies including pregnant women within a community setting, generally less critical symptoms emerged in the pregnant women who had a history of or who had active eating disorders. Pregnant women with AN who start at a baseline lower pregnancy weight than the control group are able to gain more weight during the pregnancy. This could be a mechanism of the body's own protective nature to reduce any negative pregnancy-related outcomes and safeguard the fetus to ensure adequate nutrients for optimal growth (Bulik 2013).

Results from a community-based gestational weight gain study in pregnant women with eating disorders showed mothers with AN, BN, BED, and EDNOS had greater increases in BMI during pregnancy (Zerwas et al. 2014). Whereas the higher weight gain in women with AN was a protective outcome factor, the higher weight gain observed in women with BN and BED was seen as unprotective for potential negative maternal and fetal outcomes (Watson et al. 2014a).

The attitudes associated with weight gain are more distressed during early pregnancy among women with all types of eating disorders than women with no history of eating disorders. Cynthia Bulik (2013), in her book *Midlife Eating Disorders: Your Journey to Recovery*, noted that some women with gestational eating disorders found their pregnancies to be "an out-of-control experience, and whether you have a history of AN, BN, BED, or another variation on the theme, when weight is out of your control, anxiety follows on its heels."

An increase in body dissatisfaction can be seen in some women with restrictive eating behaviors during late pregnancy. In more freedom from the rigid controls, some pregnant women with history of eating disorders can shift the focus on their growing bodies from "appearance" to "function" in terms of housing a healthy environment for their babies to grow and survive (Watson et al. 2014a).

Energy (Caloric) Needs

In the context of eating disorders, numbers and guidelines can become inflexible and punitive. To mitigate this, professionals should translate numerical data (such as caloric needs) into functional and practical goals that mesh with the abilities of each individual patient. Phrasing nutrition recommendations as beneficial for the fetus may ameliorate fear or guilt that may be related to eating more than usual.

Not ideal: "In the second trimester, you need 350 more calories a day."

Better: "Now that you are in your second trimester, your baby needs you to eat a granola bar and a cup of yogurt each day in addition to what you are already eating. Where would it be easiest for you to add those into your schedule?"

An exception would be when a woman is using calorie counting as a method to ensure that she eats enough, rather than the more typical method to control and limit food intake. In this circumstance, asking a woman to add 350 kcal/day to her usual daily intake is appropriate, along with assisting her in determining when and with which foods to do so.

Recommended energy intake during pregnancy:

1st trimester: Normal (prepregnancy) energy needs—no additional caloric intake needed

2nd trimester: Normal (prepregnancy) energy needs + 350 calories/day

3rd trimester: Normal (prepregnancy) energy needs + 450 calories/day (Otten 2006)

To calculate normal (prepregnancy) energy needs, an interactive calculator is available at https://fnic.nal.usda.gov/fnic/interactiveDRI/. However, general nutrition guidelines should not be used in lieu of personalized nutrition counseling and guidance.

Food and Fluid Intake

Ideally every pregnant woman, with or without an eating disorder, has access to a registered dietitian for nutrition and eating guidance. Balancing the nutritional needs of supporting a healthy pregnancy while attempting an eating disorder recovery is not a do-it-yourself project. The information provided in this section is therefore generalized for educational purposes and must be individualized to each patient.

A woman who restricts certain foods or beverages from her diet, whether due to preferences, a medical or postsurgical condition, mistaken beliefs about food, aversions, or for purposes of weight loss will need a thorough nutrition assessment to determine if she is meeting the macro- and micronutrient needs of pregnancy. This nutrition assessment may combine an oral report of typical food intake with written documentation and blood tests. Nutritional deficiencies are not always detectable in blood tests until they are very severe, so normal lab results should not be misinterpreted as adequate nutrition intake.

Vegetarian, vegan, gluten-free, renal, diabetic, and postbariatric surgery eating, depending on how they are implemented, can lack essential nutrients. Some women may be willing to reincorporate previously excluded foods for the purpose of a healthy pregnancy. The dietitian can identify whether individual nutritional supplements are needed, or if nutritional supplement beverages, whether purchased pre-prepared or home blended with or without a protein supplement, would be helpful.

Pregnancy requires approximately 10 cups of free fluids/day (i.e., separate from the fluids contained in foods; Kaiser and Campbell 2014). This may be an adjustment for a woman who restricts fluid intake due to a fear of weight gain, and the intake may need to be increased gradually and with a specific plan for when and how much to drink. Although weight gain will result, the explanation that it is an increase in blood volume rather than body mass is factual if not completely reassuring. Fluid intake is also an issue for women who have had bariatric surgery and are limited in the amount of fluids and fluid-containing foods, like soups, that they can consume.

Some women with eating disorders overconsume fluids, sometimes excessive amounts of warm beverages, in an effort to feel warm or feel full, nonnutritive beverages such as high-caffeine drinks and other stimulant beverages ("energy" drinks) in order to stay alert or diminish hunger pangs, or carbonated beverages as a way to induce purging. Binge drinking and alcohol dependence also occur. Nutrition counseling should address the issues pertinent to each individual and encourage more appropriate fluid intake.

Pregnancy cravings for formerly restricted foods or binge foods can be very upsetting to a woman with an eating disorder. They can lead to temptations or episodes of binge eating, purging, restriction, overexercise, and self-harm. Provide education that such cravings and aversions are normal and do not require "penance" in the form of purging and offer assistance incorporating craved foods appropriately without binge eating.

In all cases, the dietitian should share nutrition recommendations with all other providers so that they can convey consistent messages about weight, food, and nutrition that are accurate and appropriate for each patient and within the scope of each professional's domain. Any concerns that other providers have regarding a patient's eating should be referred back to the dietitian to avoid miscommunication. What may seem to the average person as a casual comment, such as, "I didn't think pregnant women were supposed to be eating that," can send a woman with an eating disorder into a spiral of shame, binge eating, restricting, or any number of destructive behaviors. Therefore, providers who are not experts in nutrition counseling should refrain from engaging in conversations about what a pregnant patient is eating.

PRENATAL DEPRESSION AND ANXIETY: IS MEDICATION USE ADVISED?

Women with active eating disorder symptoms during pregnancy and a past history of depression experienced the highest levels of depression and anxiety during pregnancy. Some pharmacological and nonpharmacological treatments are associated with positive and negative outcomes for perinatal depression, a common condition many pregnant women with eating disorders experience. One population-based study with 7696 pregnant women found 570 of them (7.4%) had clinically significant depressive symptoms and used no selective serotonin reuptake inhibitor (SSRI) antidepressants during the pregnancy, while 99 pregnant mothers (1.3%) used SSRIs. Untreated maternal depression was associated with slower rates of fetal body and head growth. Pregnant mothers using the SSRIs had fewer depressive symptoms and their fetuses had no delay in body growth but had delayed head growth and were at increased risk for preterm birth (El Marroun et al. 2012). No treatment is risk free, and leaving maternal mental illness untreated has consequences for the mother, the fetus, and for the infant as it grows into a child and adolescent. The obstetrician or psychiatrist needs to carefully weigh the risks and benefits of using pharmacological treatment of perinatal mood and anxiety disorders in all pregnant women (Misri and Kendrick 2007).

In the United States, approximately four million babies are born every year and close to one-half of all new moms choose to breastfeed their infants. Since postpartum depression is common in new mothers with a current or history of an eating disorder, some of these moms may be taking antidepressants that can be passed onto their infants during breastfeeding (Misri and Kendrick 2007).

It is very common for women with depression and anxiety to not take their medications during pregnancy based on myth, fear, stigma, and shame rather than scientific support of the actual risks and benefits of being on antidepressants during pregnancy (Dennis 2015). Many women and health-care physicians do not take into consideration the health risks for mother and fetus when women stop taking antidepressants.

Although health risks have been reported for mother and fetus using antidepressants during pregnancy, it is important to note there can be significant health risks for mother and fetus without use of antidepressants. Lupatelli et al. (2015) stated that pharmacotherapy with psychotropics may reduce pregnancy-related exacerbation of eating disorder symptoms such as dieting or vomiting, which is beneficial for both mother and fetus rather than detrimental. Untreated depression during pregnancy can have a negative impact on the mother and fetus, including poor maternal–fetal bonding, maternal–fetus malnutrition, and increased risk of premature birth (Robinson 2015).

While there is generally no use for antidepressants in the treatment of AN (Aigner et al. 2011), the use of an antidepressant, such as the SSRI fluoxetine, may be useful in treating depression to improve outcome and prevent relapse in patients with AN after weight restoration. Since most women with AN achieve weight restoration during the course of pregnancy, SSRI antidepressants may be more beneficial during pregnancy than before conception (Lupattelli et al. 2015).

Besides the increase in potential for depressive symptoms to return, other harmful consequences of discontinuing antidepressants on mother and fetus can include:

- Increased use of cigarettes, alcohol, or other substances
- Deteriorating social function, emotional withdrawal, worry related to pregnancy, and excessive concern about the future ability to parent
- Impaired ability to attend regular obstetric visits and comply with prenatal advice

- Malnutrition which can lead to low birth weight
- Increase in risky behavior and impaired capacity to avoid dangerous behavior
- Heightened risk of self-injurious, psychotic, impulsive, and harmful behaviors
- Increased risk of postpartum depression
- Difficulty carrying out maternal duties and bonding with their children (Dennis 2015)

In addition to monitoring psychotropic medications such as antidepressants, the obstetrician should assess the patient during pregnancy for use of other prescribed medications as well as over-the-counter (OTC) medicines. In the study conducted by Lupattelli et al., they found the use of gastrointestinal medication, such as the OTC Gas-X, was high across all pregnant women with eating disorders, with the use in the BED population the highest. The medications included in the study were antacids, laxatives, and drugs for gastroesophageal reflux disease (GERD). Use of these medications in women with BED during pregnancy suggests the need for symptom relief related to possible bingeing episodes (Dennis 2015).

EXERCISE

Exercise during pregnancy is advised with great caution for pregnant women with eating disorders. If a patient has a history of an eating disorder and is not showing any signs of problems in her pregnancy, this patient can exercise with her OB/GYNs approval. However, if the patient is actively using her eating disorder behaviors, exercise may be restricted. For example, if she has problems gaining weight or the fetus shows growth deficits then exercise would be contraindicated. In fact, this patient's activity would overall be limited or she could be at complete bed rest, if conditions are severe. Pregnancy yoga or stretching exercises could be allowed depending on the patient's appropriate weight gain and adequate fetal growth.

In patients who are in remission from an eating disorder, moderate exercise is generally recommended. Regular exercise at least 30–45 minutes approximately four times a week can benefit a patient's physical and mental health through the 9 months of body changes as shown in Table 8.3.

Pregnancy affects joint stability, balance and coordination, and heart rate fluctuations. Most forms of exercise are safe during pregnancy. Brisk walking, swimming, recumbent cycling, and strength training are excellent sources of exercises in healthy patients. Exercises that should be avoided include snow skiing, contact sports such as soccer and basketball, and scuba diving. A patient should not start any new exercises during pregnancy unless she speaks to her doctor (American Pregnancy Association 2012).

If a patient is able to talk normally while exercising, her heart rate is at an acceptable rate. Currently there is no specific recommendation for heart rates during exercise for pregnant women. A patient should stop exercising and call her doctor if she gets any of these symptoms: vaginal bleeding, dizziness or feeling faint, increased shortness of breath, headache, muscle weakness, calf pain or swelling, uterine contractions, decreased fetal movement, or fluid leaking from the vagina.

TABLE 8.3
Exercise Benefits to Pregnant Women in ED Recovery

Helps reduce backaches, constipation, bloating, and swelling

May help prevent or treat gestational diabetes

Increases energy

Improves mood

Improves posture

Improves sleep

Improves ability to cope with the pain of labor

Increases ability to get back in shape after baby is born

Promotes muscle tone, strength, and endurance

Source: American College of Obstetrics and Gynecologists, Exercise during Pregnancy: Frequently Asked Questions, May 2015, available at http://www.acog.org/Patients/FAQs/ Exercise-During-Pregnancy

Prenatal yoga classes, upon approval of the patient's OB/GYN, can be beneficial to physical and emotional stress accompanying pregnancy (Zauderer 2012). The University of Michigan conducted a study to show the first evidence that mindfulness yoga can offer effective treatment for pregnant mothers who are depressed. Pregnant women identified as psychiatrically high risk with no mention of having an eating disorder participated in a 10-week mindfulness yoga program. The study reported the women had a significant reduction in depressive symptoms and the added benefit of feeling a stronger attachment to their babies in the womb (Muzik et al. 2012).

IMPACT OF POSTPARTUM PERIOD ON MOTHERS AND INFANTS

Although most eating disorders can improve during pregnancy, such as weight restoration, and cessation or decrease in binge-purge cycle, often the cognitive and emotional symptoms of the eating disorder persist during pregnancy. Without resolution of the negative thoughts and emotions interlaced with the eating disorder as well as the absence of fears of harming her unborn child during pregnancy—eating disorders may persist and follow the new mother as she transitions into the postpartum period (Zerwas et al. 2014).

For any new mother, the postpartum period is a challenge from adjusting to sleep deprivation and feeding her newborn to adjusting to her post-baby body and trying to balance her emotional and hormonal shifts. New mothers with a history of or active eating disorders find the transition into motherhood especially difficult (Easter et al. 2011). In one ALSPAC study, pregnant women with eating disorders were two times more likely than women with no history of eating disorders to believe that motherhood entailed giving up part of their lives as a personal sacrifice. One study found that over 90% of first-time mothers with a history of AN or BN reported difficulties with maternal adjustment and parenting during the first 3 months after childbirth, compared to 13% of women in the control group without histories of eating of an eating disorder (Koubaa et al. 2008).

Many women are overly focused on the time it takes to shed pregnancy pounds and this can affect the mother's attention to the task of breastfeeding and bonding with her infant. It has been documented that 80% of women with eating disorders who suffered a behavior relapse during the postpartum period felt compelled to lose the weight gained during pregnancy. Obsessive dieting can also play a role in taking off the pounds and the combination of the exercise demands and inadequate nutrient intake can directly affect the mother's ability to produce enough milk for breastfeeding (Carwell and Spatz 2011).

POSTPARTUM NUTRITIONAL NEEDS

After delivery it is essential that the mother takes in enough food and nutrients to heal from the delivery process, replenish nutrient stores, and have energy to care for her infant. Although her temptation may be to restrict her intake and diet for weight loss, advise her that this is not the appropriate focus at this time. Although it may be a relief to have delivered a (hopefully) healthy baby, this is not the time for the treatment team to take a break.

Even if a woman tolerates her pregnancy weight gain without difficulty, after delivery the "thin" ideal may return with a vengeance. The resulting eating disorder symptoms together with the higher risk of postpartum depression can cause a relapse of restrictive eating, purging, pathological exercise, refusal of fluids, and so on, in an effort to return immediately to a prepregnancy weight and shape. Here again an explanation of the physiological results of pregnancy and delivery, including the fact that an empty uterus takes weeks to contract, can possibly help the mother accept and tolerate her postpartum weight and shape.

Breastfeeding does have an energy cost associated with it, approximately 300 kcal/day above normal (prepregnancy) needs. If a new mother is struggling to eat and drink enough for her own nutritional needs, she may not be able to produce breast milk in a quantity that her baby requires. The decision to try to eat more in order to breastfeed is one that the patient will need to work on with the treatment team. If she is unable to improve her intake, breastfeeding may cost more energy than the mother can spare.

Keep in mind that breast milk fortifier only adds a few nutrients to breast milk and does not add calories. If breastfeeding is successful but the milk quantity is inadequate, consult with a dietitian for supplementation recommendations.

POSTPARTUM DEPRESSION AND ANXIETY

After a mother successfully delivers her baby, it is vital for the treatment team to provide close postpartum monitoring. The linking of eating disorders with other psychiatric disorders, including depression and anxiety, can produce serious postpartum complications. Women with a history of eating disorders have been shown to have increased levels of anxiety and depression prenatally and in the postnatal period (Easter et al. 2015). Women with a lifetime or recent history of an eating disorder are at greater risk for postpartum depression than the general population, and the risk of relapse and difficulties with breastfeeding are significant concerns.

As shown in Table 8.4, postpartum mothers with BED and BN have the highest correlation of developing postpartum depression with approximately a three-time greater risk than women without eating disorders. Postpartum mothers with AN are also at a greater risk for postpartum depression. Irrespective of the eating disorder subtype, one of the trademark characteristics of AN, perfectionism, appears to play a function in the severity of postpartum depression (Mazzeo et al. 2006).

However, it is common for most women giving birth, including those without eating disorders, to have an increased dissatisfaction with body shape and weight in the first 6 months of the postpartum period. By 4 months postpartum, 70% of women are attempting weight loss (Carter et al. 2000). However, research has shown that women with AN, BN, EDNOS, and BED lose pregnancy weight quicker during this period. This suggests women with eating disorders are resorting to familiar disordered behaviors such as calorie restriction, compensatory actions (such as excessive exercise or vomiting), or other extreme weight control behaviors (Stein and Fairburn 1996).

Although the data indicates many pregnant mothers can relinquish their eating disorder behaviors during pregnancy from a desire to protect their baby, once the baby is born and postpartum hits, many of these same patients find a resurgence of eating disorder symptoms. What is alarming is the severity of the symptoms is oftentimes worse than the symptoms presented prior to the pregnancy. Research from different studies show approximately 50%–57% of bulimic mothers experience this increase in symptomatology postpartum. As for

---

TABLE 8.4
Remission of Eating Disorders Following Childbirth

Remission from a diagnosis of prepregnancy AN was
- 50% at 18 months following childbirth
- 30% at 36 months following childbirth

Remission from a diagnosis of prepregnancy BN was
- 39% at 18 months following childbirth
- 59% at 36 months following childbirth

Remission from a diagnosis of prepregnancy EDNOS was
- 46% at 18 months following childbirth
- 57% at 36 months following childbirth

Remission from prepregnancy BED was
- 45% at 18 months following childbirth
- 42% at 36 months following childbirth

Source: Knoph, C et al. *International Journal of Eating Disorders,* 46, 355–368, 2013.

---

symptoms in anorexic mothers during the postpartum period, similar patterns were discovered. The severity of the postpartum eating disorder was connected to the initial symptom severity of the prenatal eating disorder, severity of post-partum depression, weak infant–mother relationship, and poor spousal support (Astrachan-Fletcher et al. 2008).

The eating disorder and obsession with thinness may become acute in the post-partum period. And if mood disorders exist, such as postpartum depression, this can cause serious disruption to a mother's ability to care for herself and her baby, preventing a smooth transition in parenthood (Mitchell-Gieleghem et al. 2012).

It has been well-documented that postpartum depression and anxiety affects child development. A population-based birth cohort study conducted in 18 U.S. cities revealed maternal anxiety and depression in the first year of the postpartum period were associated with problems in child behaviors at age 3 years including symptoms of aggression, anxious-depressed behavior, and/or inattention hyperactivity. These risks increased 50% in mothers who had comorbid substance abuse and/or were victims of domestic violence (Lusskin et al. 2007).

BREASTFEEDING

When a new mother chooses to breastfeed her baby she is providing numerous preventive benefits to her baby and herself, and potentially improving the bonding of their relationship together. Breastfed infants are less likely to develop diabetes, infectious diseases, leukemia, gastrointestinal and respiratory diseases, and sudden infant death syndrome (SIDS). Breastfeeding mothers are at lower risk of diabetes, and breast and ovarian cancer. The act of breastfeeding between mother and infant is one of the most intimate bonding experiences they share in during the postpartum period (Watson et al. 2014a).

Limited studies have been dedicated to understanding the practice of breastfeed-ing in mothers with eating disorders. The large-scale MoBa study conducted at the Norwegian Institute of Public Health questioned 39,355 women for information on eating disorders and breastfeeding. The study's purpose was to compare the preva-lence of breastfeeding in women with AN, BN, BED, and EDNOS-P with moth-ers with no history of eating disorders during the first 6 months postbirth. The study looked at the risk of cessation of breastfeeding practice in the women studied (Torgersen et al. 2010).

The results found nearly all Norwegian women (98%) initially breastfed their infants and there was no significant difference between the eating disorder group of women and the women with no history of eating disorders. However, what was discovered was a significant risk of early breastfeeding cessation and shift to bottle-feeding in the first 6 months in all groups of mothers with eating disorders, compared with mothers with no history of an eating disorder. Another significant difference was mothers with AN and EDNOS-P had a profoundly higher risk of early cessa-tion of breastfeeding within the eating disorder groups (Torgersen et al. 2010). The ALSPAC study found the results to be opposite that of the MoBa study—that women with eating disorders were less likely to discontinue breastfeeding compared to the control group of women with no history of eating disorders. One of the discrepancies between these study results may relate to the sociocultural differences between the two different countries; fewer women in the United Kingdom, at 76%, breastfed compared to Norway, where 98% breastfed. In the United States, it's estimated about 60% of new mothers initially breastfeed (Watson et al. 2014a).

"Can I trust myself to adequately feed my child, if I struggle to feed myself?" This is a common question mothers with a history of eating disorders or those with active eating disorders may come into conflict with internally as they strive to be nurturing, attentive mothers. This conflict often begins during pregnancy as they are deciding whether to breastfeed or bottle-feed their infants. Women with eating disorders were found to be less likely to breastfeed; if they do, they discontinue breastfeeding sooner than women without eating disorders (Bulik 2013). There are a number of reasons women with eating disorders choose to forego or discontinue breastfeeding, as shown in Table 8.5..

Many mothers with eating disorders are anxious about whether they know how to feed their children. They do not know how they will be able to recognize hunger or fullness and they doubt their own maternal instincts around feeding. Feeding on schedule and from the bottle seems less anxiety provoking because they can see how much is being consumed and not have to worry about whether the baby is getting enough. It seems to take the judgment out of the process for them (Bulik 2015).

Bingeing, purging, or excessive restriction of calories has a direct negative impact on the mother's health and also on the quality of the breast milk produced (Carwell and Spatz 2011). Studies have indicated that mothers with AN weaned off of breastfeeding early due to low or no milk supply or difficulty with breastfeeding (Torgersen et al. 2010). Also, breastfeeding moms should be assessed for use of laxatives, diuretics, and weight loss products as these can cross over to the infant through the breast milk, which can be medically compromised and dangerous to the feeding baby (Ward and Waller 2008).

Women with a history of an eating disorder and early sexual abuse may have great challenges in the postpartum period with breastfeeding. Breastfeeding itself entails exposure, nakedness, secretions and drippings from the breast, strong sensations

---

TABLE 8.5

Reasons Why Women with Eating Disorders May Choose Not to Breastfeed

Concerns of producing enough breast milk supply

Ability to consume adequate calories to maintain breastfeeding

Strong drive to return to prepregnancy weight; exercising or dieting may interfere with breastfeeding

Women with deeply ingrained body dissatisfaction may find intimate contact of breastfeeding too overwhelming

Some mothers not prepared to sacrifice their body appearance for breastfeeding, which often leads to drooping breasts

Increased anxiety of not knowing how much milk their infants get during breastfeeding

Source: Bulik (2015)

from the baby's suckling, stroking, and fondling in addition to the ongoing demands by the baby. Early sexual abuse survivors may connect some of these sensations with the past abuser. If she has repressed the abuse, she may experience terrifying body memories and not understand where they come from. The baby's suckling on her breast may present too strong of an association with the abuse, and because of this psychological and physical discomfort, the new mom may discontinue breastfeeding (Simkin and Klaus 2004). Other risks associated with breastfeeding difficulty in women with eating disorders include postpartum depression, maternal age/weight, education level, and negative birth outcomes (Watson et al. 2014a).

Treatment during the breastfeeding period can be achieved through education of the new mother by her team regarding the numerous benefits of breastfeeding to the infant and its natural bonding benefits for securing a healthy attachment for both of them. It is often helpful to seek support from a lactation consultant, one with expertise in working with patients with eating disorders, who can also provide education and support of learning how to properly breastfeed, overcome breastfeeding obstacles, and address the increased anxiety of breastfeeding seen in women with eating disorders. In the case of a mom with early history of unresolved sexual abuse, breastfeeding may not be the best option for her or the baby. Treatment would include trauma counseling for the mom and bottle-feeding for the baby (Watson et al. 2014a).

Infant Feeding Difficulties

Additionally, negative medical consequences can continue in the baby if a mother with an eating disorder has difficulties in the feeding process after the baby is born.

The studies on breastfeeding suggest that there is already a difference in feeding practices of infants born to mothers with eating disorders. Researchers have found an increased risk of feeding difficulties in the first year of life in infants who have mothers with a lifetime eating disorder.

Another contributing factor to feeding difficulties is if the mother (with or without an eating disorder) shows maternal distress in the form of anxiety and depression during feeding (Micali et al. 2010).

In one study on maternal eating disorders, early and late feeding difficulties in their infants were examined. Early feeding difficulties occurring in infants at 1 month of life were observed and included any feeding problems such as weak sucking, drinking too fast, exhaustion with feeding, small quantity feeds, slow feeding, being unsatisfied, or hungry after feeding. Late feeding difficulties occurring in infants at 6 months were observed and included small quantity feeding, refusal of solids, and no feeding routine established. A previous study had already predicted early and late feeding difficulties cause low weight of infants at age 9 months (Micali et al. 2010).

Limited research has been done on feeding difficulties. Patterns of restrictive feeding were more common in mothers with eating disorders symptoms of BED and BN (Reba-Harrelson et al. 2010). Additionally, in this study BN and BED were associated with greater reports of child eating problems relative to those mothers with no eating disorder. One limitation to this study was the unbalanced group size with a small AN group for comparisons (Reba-Harrelson et al. 2010).

In other studies, feeding difficulties were fairly common in all groups of eating disorder categories during the infant's first year. Most studies have shown shorter duration of breastfeeding, faster suckling, and lower weight. Mothers with AN reported early-onset and persistent feeding difficulties with their babies, except with refusal to take solid foods compared with control group. Also, AN mothers tend to be more controlling around feeding and playing time with their babies (iaedp 2009).

Caregiver mood and behavior during infant feeding function as mirrors, imprinting the child with experiences that may be associated with food for a lifetime. Caregiver–infant interactions during feeding can have long-lasting effects on the child's ongoing development, sense of self-worth, nutrition, and health. For example, a mother (with or without an eating disorder) who is anxious about her postpregnancy weight and eating may unwittingly convey anxiety around food to the infant through her body language and other nonverbal cues. If the infant becomes agitated and refuses the breast or bottle, the mother's anxiety increases, the child's ability to nurse calmly decreases, and a detrimental cycle occurs. A parent or other caregiver consciously trying to avoid passing on his or her eating disorder behaviors may accidentally overcompensate and under- or overfeed the child. Consulting a pediatric dietitian, lactation consultant, and/or appropriate mental health professional for support early on is the best strategy to promote a healthy feeding relationship before the child's growth and development are impacted (Setnick 2015).

MATERNAL–INFANT ATTACHMENT

The maternal–fetus bonding stage in utero is significant and can be negatively affected by perinatal depression and anxiety. Similarly, a study found that the influence of poor maternal–fetus bond often forecasted a poor maternal–infant bond. The women who showed stronger fetal attachment were less likely to suffer from impaired bonding with their infants after birth (Dubber et al. 2014). In the presence of postpartum depression, this too can considerably affect the attachment and bonding connection between a mother and her baby. In the most severe cases, especially when the mother is active in her eating disorder and absent physically or emotionally, this can lead to child abuse or neglect. Even in "milder" cases, it can cause an increase in poor attachment with long-lasting effects detrimental to the child's development and to the child–mother relationship, even after maternal depression has been treated (Lusskin et al. 2007).

A secure attachment is the bonding process that not only creates a strong emotional link between a mom and her infant that serves to protect the infant's life but also the process that instills in the baby the ability to self-regulate its own arousal. The loving actions of holding, hugging, bathing, and helping the baby to sleep, along with the emotional interchange of the feeding relationship, help the mom build an internal security for her baby (Orbach and Rubin 2014). The importance of skin-to-skin contact for mother and baby is well-documented. One study found that skin-to-skin contact for 25–120 minutes after birth was linked with a more positive later maternal–infant interaction than those between mothers and babies who have been separated at birth (Lefkovics et al. 2014).

A distraction in the mother, due to postpartum depression or anxiety, her maternal eating disorder, or body image problems, inhibits her ability to reliably attune to her baby's needs, including teaching the baby how to self-soothe and regulate emotions. This misattunement creates an insecure maternal attachment for the baby who experiences the environment as unsafe and is fearful his or her survival needs may go unmet. With a distant or avoidant mom, this compromises the baby's capacity to self-regulate, which underlies the development of future insecure relationships and many forms of mental illnesses, including eating disorders later in life (Maine and McGilley 2010).

Maternal eating disorders disrupt the maternal–infant bonding relationship. This rupture in the attachment process with her child can continue long into the future. The bonding wounds can be repaired if the child is still young enough and can gain a secure attachment with a healthy mother. Professional treatment will likely be needed for both mother and baby/child to help achieve a healthy attachment.

GENETIC INFLUENCES

Children of mothers with eating disorders are at risk for the future development of an eating disorder. Two important factors that can increase this risk are the genetic influences that have established eating disorders run in families and play a role in the dynamics of family interactions as well as the environmental/maternal factors the infant is exposed to early in life (Reba-Harrelson et al. 2010).

OPTIMIZING OUTCOMES

The most important piece of the puzzle is bringing the subject of pregnancy and eating disorders out in the open, so that no woman goes without professional guidance because she is ashamed to speak about her eating issues. Bringing a new life into the world is a profound and life-altering responsibility, and it can create every kind of stress imaginable. For a pregnant woman with an eating disorder to go without support, because of someone else's lack of compassion or understanding is tragic. The responsibility for identifying eating and feeding issues belongs to all the clinicians involved. In doing so, we can provide her the the best medical care and emotional support, allowing her the optimal opportunity for a healthy pregnancy and birth of a healthy baby.

CASE STUDY 8.1

Anna

Twenty-two-year-old Anna found out that she was pregnant with her first child while she was in psychotherapy for the treatment of AN and BN. Her eating disorder began at 11 years old with AN. She would eat only carrot sticks and drink alcohol. Anna says the alcohol abuse and a friend giving her tips on how to throw up led her into BN. Anna flip-flopped between the disorders over the years. However, her diagnosis during outpatient treatment was AN, purging-type.

Anna comes from a divorced family and has two younger siblings. She is married with a 4-year-old stepson who lives with her and her husband.

(Continued)

She acknowledges she has experienced a lot of trauma in her life, including sexual, physical, emotional, and verbal abuse. At age 10, her babysitter's boyfriend sexually molested her. This trauma was followed by an older girl abusing her sexually, physically, and emotionally for several years. Anna remembers the girl stripping her down naked and showing her how fat she was in the mirror. The trauma continued with a date rape and other abusive relationships with boyfriends. Along with the alcohol, Anna also abused drugs, mostly cocaine, to help her stay thin. Eventually, she entered treatment for her drug/alcohol abuse and got that under control; however, the eating disorder remained active.

When she started therapy, Anna was amenorrheic with lack of menstruation for several years. During therapy, she was surprised to find out that she was pregnant, not knowing that her body ovulated at least once to fertilize her egg. Her eating disorder behaviors were active and she restricted, binged and purged, overexercised, and used large amounts of laxatives daily. On hearing of her pregnancy news, she immediately made an appointment with her obstetrician who knew about Anna's eating disorder.

With permission from Anna, the therapist contacted her obstetrician to discuss Anna's case. An eating disorder dietitian was brought on the team, and the three professionals worked with Anna through her pregnancy up to the delivery of her baby. Anna met with the dietitian to set up a pregnancy meal plan. The dietitian and the obstetrician collaboratively worked out a plan to wean Anna off her 60-laxative-a-day regime. It took several weeks to wean totally off the laxatives but Anna did it. She had also met with a psychiatrist before she knew she was pregnant and was going to start a medication for her depression. She met again with her psychiatrist and revealed she was pregnant and they discussed the pros and cons of taking an antidepressant during her pregnancy. In specific cases, such as when a patient has a history of chronic and/or severe depression, continuing on an antidepressant dosage prescribed by the patient's doctor during pregnancy may be the best option to avoid other negative side effects. By discontinuing use of an antidepressant, depressive symptoms can return during pregnancy and have negative effects on both mom and fetus. The stress effects of the expectant mom's depression pass through the placenta and can have negative effects on fetus' stress response. Since Anna's symptoms of depression were mild, she chose not to take the antidepressant to avoid any medication-influenced potential fetal side effects.

Anna had very positive feelings with her pregnancy in regard to her connection to the baby inside. "I knew my baby would be a perfect little being and have a better chance of doing great things in the world," she stated. However, she felt a lot of guilt and shame inside of herself, which is understandable considering the traumatic life she had endured. Anna had a lot of unresolved trauma to heal. The therapist knew deep trauma work was not advised during pregnancy due to the increased stress it can cause to the pregnant mother and her baby. So the therapist and Anna dealt with how she was managing her pregnancy and her feelings of guilt if she acted on her eating disorder by restricting, and worked to increase general coping skills to deal with family issues. She did have morning sickness at the beginning

(Continued)

CASE STUDY 8.1 *(CONTINUED)*

and threw up but was unsure if it was truly morning sickness because when she threw up she said, "I didn't mind it since it was a way to get rid of food." Anna was very hungry in the early months of her pregnancy and knew that instead of fighting it, she needed to let the baby win and increased her calories up to 2000 a day.

Anna stopped using laxatives, decreased her exercise, increased her food intake, and was happy for her growing baby inside but felt horrible about herself. The eating disorder thoughts were still upsetting her. During the pregnancy, she started to binge eat. This caused her to feel depressed, sad, and "fat." Yet at her check-ins with the obstetrician she was gaining an appropriate amount of weight and the baby was healthy. Anna said she might have purged a couple times but that it was not a regular occurrence.

Although Anna struggled a lot mentally with negative self-talk and eating disorder thoughts, she knew her pregnancy would have been a lot harder if not for the support of her team —her medical doctor, therapist, and dietitian. She tried to take 1 day at a time and do the best she knew by not giving up and letting herself be upset and cry. She didn't drink alcohol through her pregnancy or starve through it; she felt the excitement about having a baby but also the pain of what created her eating disorder. She said, "There was nowhere to run but be with the pain."

By the delivery date, Anna had gained 40 lbs. and delivered a healthy baby girl with no medical issues. Her weight gain was the amount recommended for women with eating disorders who are underweight before starting a pregnancy. Today Anna is still working on her recovery, and feels mostly recovered but knows she still has work ahead of her to completely heal. She is a wonderful, loving mom and if she could see herself through the eyes of her daughter now who loves her mom so much, and through the eyes of her therapist who holds a deep respect for the effort it has taken to heal, Anna would be filled with adoring, unconditional love for herself—something she undoubtedly deserves.

PREGNANCY AND EATING DISORDER RESOURCES

Free Online Support Group for Pregnant Women and Moms with Eating Disorders

"Lift the Shame" is the first web-based support group of its kind specifically targeted to offer support and resources to pregnant women and moms with eating disorders. This support group is a free, confidential online group hosted the third Sunday of each month: **4–5 PM Pacific, 6–7 PM Central, 7–8 PM Eastern.** Registration for "Lift the Shame" is available online at **www.timberlineknolls.com/ information/support-groups**.

For questions regarding the group, please call Timberline Knolls at (877) 257–9611.

The Lift the Shame *online support group was cofounded in 2014 by certified eating disorder and trauma therapist Maggie Baumann, LMFT, CEDS, in partnership with the Chicago-based Timberline Knolls Residential Treatment Center and the National Association of Anorexia Nervosa and Associated Disorders (ANAD).*

Books

Mysko, Claire, and Magali Amadei. *Does This Pregnancy Make Me Look Fat? The Essential Guide to Loving Your Body before and after Baby.* Deerfield Beach, FL: Health Communications, 2009.

Does This Pregnancy Make Me Look Fat? Body image activists Claire Mysko and Magali Amadei forewarn you on what to expect from your changing body, as well as offer a reality check for each stage of your pregnancy, exposing the myths, challenges, and insecurities you'll face throughout pregnancy and beyond. Learn how you can trust your changing, growing body shape and appreciate it—and how to take the focus *off* the scale. The book also addresses why you should be wary of the Hollywood "bump watch" and post-baby weight-loss stories.

Bulik, Cynthia M. *Midlife Eating Disorders: Your Journey to Recovery.* New York, NY: Walker and Company.

Midlife Eating Disorders guides adults in understanding "Why me?" and "Why now?" It shows a connection between the rise in midlife eating disorders and certain industries that foster discontent with the natural aging process. It also gives readers renewed hope by explaining how to overcome symptoms and access resources and support.

Bulik, Cynthia M. *The Woman in the Mirror: How to Stop Confusing What You Look Like with Who You Are.* New York, NY: Walker & Company, 2012.

The Woman in the Mirror goes beyond typical self-esteem books to dig deep into the origins of women's problems with body image. Psychologist Cynthia Bulik, PhD, guides readers in the challenging task of disentangling self-esteem from body esteem and provides us the tools to reclaim our self-confidence and to respect and love who we are.

Simkin, Penny, and Phyllis H. Klaus. *When Survivors Give Birth: Understanding and Healing the Effects of Early Sexual Abuse on Childbearing Women.* Seattle, Washington: Classic Day, 2004. 75, 91–92, 98.

When Survivors Give Birth is written for a mixed audience of maternity care professionals and mental health professionals as well as for women survivors and their families. The authors expertly and compassionately address the unusual and distressing challenges that arise for abuse survivors during the childbirth experience.

Cabrera, Dena, and Emily T. Wierenga. *Mom in the Mirror: Body Image, Beauty, and Life after Pregnancy.* Lanham, Maryland: Rowman & Littlefield Publishers, 2013.

Mom in the Mirror is for every woman who has ever doubted herself or her self-worth after the birth of a child. Because most women spend much of their lives attempting to change their bodies, it is not surprising that the weight gain that comes along with pregnancy (and postpregnancy), coupled with the challenges of parenting, only exacerbates issues with weight, body image, disordered eating, and self-esteem.

Websites

The Academy for Eating Disorders (AED) is a global professional association committed to leadership in eating disorders research, education, treatment, and prevention. To find out more visit www.aedweb.org.

CynthiaBulik.com. Dr. Cynthia Bulik, Founding Director of the University of North Carolina (UNC) Center of Excellence for Eating Disorders, holds the first endowed professorship in eating disorders in the United States and has her own site in which you can browse through her articles, familiarize yourself with her recovery-driven books and research, and stay connected with e-mail updates. Much of her research has been focused on pregnant women with eating disorders.

Edreferrral.com is dedicated to the prevention and treatment of eating disorders and is the most comprehensive database to search for AN, BN, and other eating disorder treatment professionals in the world.

Eatingdisorderhope.com offers education, support, and inspiration to eating disorder sufferers, their loved ones, and eating disorders treatment providers. This website includes articles on eating disorder treatment options, support groups, treatment providers, recovery tools, and more.

The International Association of Eating Disorders Professionals (iaedp) is a leader in providing its members with excellence in education and training in the treatment of eating disorders to a multidisciplinary group of health-care treatment providers and helping professions. iaedp.com offers a highly respected certification process for those who wish to receive specialized credentials in their work with people with eating disorders.

The National Eating Disorders Association (NEDA) supports individuals and families affected by eating disorders, and serves as a catalyst for prevention, cures, and access to quality care. Visit www.nationaleatingdisorders.org for help and hope to those affected by eating disorders.

The National Association of Anorexia Nervosa and Associated Disorders (ANAD) is a nonprofit organization dedicated to the prevention and alleviation of eating disorders. At www.anad.org you will find treatment centers, support organization groups, conferences, and recovery information.

Edcatalogue.com is an excellent website for publications of a wide variety of book titles dealing with eating and body image issues.

Pregnancy.org offers information covering a wide range of topics related to pregnancy, including articles on eating disorders.

The American College of Obstetricians & Gynecologists (ACOG) website (www .acog.org/Patients) is nationally leading website for women's health. Although it is geared to its members that include OB/GYNs, it has vital patient education information on the site available for free, including information on eating disorders during pregnancy.

www.findingbalance.com/category/40weeks/. Finding Balance is a nonprofit Christian health and wellness organization website with an emphasis on eating and body image issues. Its "40 Weeks blog" allows women to post their experiences during pregnancy. The blog offers inspiration and encouragement for moms and moms-to-be with help to navigate pregnancy, body image, eating, and identity in a way that gives life to the mom's soul, and the little life growing inside.

REFERENCES

Abraham, L. The perfect little bump. New York Magazine. 2004.

Academy for Eating Disorders. Available at http://www.aedweb.org (accessed 3 December 2015).

Aigner, M, Treasure J, Kaye W, and Kasper S. The WFSBP task force on eating disorders. World Federation of Societies of Biological Psychiatry (WFSBP) guidelines for the pharmacological treatment of eating disorders. *World Journal of Biological Psychiatry* 12 (2011): 400–443.

American College of Obstetrics and Gynecologists. Exercise during Pregnancy: Frequently Asked Questions. May 2015. Available at http://www.acog.org/Patients/FAQs/Exercise-During-Pregnancy

American Pregnancy Association. Exercise and Pregnancy. 30 April 2012. Available at http://americanpregnancy.org/pregnancy-health/exercise-and-pregnancy/ (accessed 3 January 2016).

American Psychiatric Association. *Diagnostic and Statistical Manual of Mental Disorders* (5th ed.). Washington, DC: Author, 2013.

Astrachan-Fletcher, E, Veldhuis C, Lively N, Fowler C, and Marcks B. The reciprocal effects of eating disorders and the postpartum period: A review of the literature and recommendations for clinical care. *Journal of Women's Health* 17, no. 2 (2008): 227–239.

Barnes, D. *Women's Reproductive Mental Health across the Lifespan.* Switzerland: Springer International Publishing, 2015.

Bulik, C. M. (2015, December 7). [E-mail interview by M Baumann].

Bulik, CM. *Midlife Eating Disorders: Your Journey to Recovery.* New York, NY: Walker & Company, 2013.

Bulik, CM. *The Woman in the Mirror: How to Stop Confusing What You Look Like with Who You Are.* New York, NY: Walker & Company, 2011.

Bulik, CM, Hoffman ER, Von Holle A, Torgersen L, Stoltenberg C, and Reichborn-Kjennerud T. Unplanned pregnancy in women with anorexia nervosa. *Obstetrics and Gynecology* 116, no. 5 (2010): 1136–1140.

Bulik, CM, Von Holle A, Hamer R, Knoph Berg C, Torgersen L, Magnus P, Stoltenberg C, Siega-Riz AM, Sullivan P, and Reichborn-Kjennerud T. Patterns of remission, continuation and incidence of broadly defined eating disorders during early pregnancy in the Norwegian mother and child cohort study (MoBa). *Psychological Medicine* 37, no. 8 (2007): 1109–1118.

Buss, C, Davis EP, Shahbaba B, Pruessner JC, Head K, and Sandman CA. Maternal cortisol over the course of pregnancy and subsequent child amygdala and hippocampus volumes and affective problems. *Proceedings of the National Academy of Sciences* 109, no. 20 (2012): E1312–E1319.

Carter, AS, Baker CW, and Brownell KD. Body mass index, eating attitudes, and symptoms of depression and anxiety in pregnancy and the postpartum period. *Psychosomatic Medicine* 62, no. 2 (2000): 264–270.

Carwell, M, and Spatz D. Eating disorders and breastfeeding. *American Journal of Maternal/ Child Nursing* 36, no. 2 (2011): 117–119.

Clark, A, Skouteris H, Wertheim EH, Paxton SJ, and Milgrom J. My baby body: A qualitative insight into women's body-related experiences and mood during pregnancy and the postpartum. *Journal of Reproductive and Infant Psychology* 27, no. 4 (2009): 330–345.

Coker, E, and Abraham, S. Body weight dissatisfaction before, during and after pregnancy: A comparison of women with and without eating disorders. *Eating and Weight Disorders— Studies on Anorexia, Bulimia and Obesity* 20 (2015): 71–79.

Crow, SJ, Agras WS, Crosby R, Halmi K, and Mitchell JE. Eating disorder symptoms in pregnancy: A prospective study. *International Journal of Eating Disorders* 41, no. 3 (2008): 277–279.

Crow, SJ, Yager J, and Lockwood CJ. Eating Disorders in Pregnancy. 2015. Available at http:// www.uptodate.com/contents/eating-disorders-in-pregnancy (accessed 5 December 2015).

Dennis, K. Abundant Living. 2015. Available at http://drkim.timberlineknolls.com

Dennis, K. (2015, November 30). [E-mail interview by M. Baumann]

Dubber, S, Reck C, Müller M, and Gawlik S. Postpartum bonding: The role of perinatal depression, anxiety and maternal–fetal bonding during pregnancy. *Archives of Women's Mental Health* 18, no. 2 (2014): 187–195.

Eagles, JM, Lee AJ, Raja EA, Millar HR, and Bhattacharya S. Pregnancy outcomes of women with and without a history of anorexia nervosa. *Psychological Medicine* 42, no. 12 (2012): 2651–2660.

Easter, A, Solmi F, Bye A, Taborelli E, Corfield F, Schmidt U, Treasure J, and Micali N. Antenatal and postnatal psychopathology among women with current and past eating disorders: Longitudinal patterns. *European Eating Disorders Review* 23, no. 1 (2015): 19–27.

Easter, A, Treasure J, and Micali N. Fertility and prenatal attitudes towards pregnancy in women with eating disorders: Results from the Avon longitudinal study of parents and children. *BJOG: An International Journal of Obstetrics and Gynaecology* 118, no. 12 (2011): 1491–1499.

El Marroun, H, Jaddoe VW, Hudziak JJ, Roza SJ, Steegers EA, Hofman A, Verhulst FC, White TJ, Stricker BH, and Tiemeier H. Maternal use of selective serotonin reuptake inhibitors, fetal growth, and risk of adverse birth outcomes. *Archives of General Psychiatry* 69, no. 7 (2012): 706–714.

Fornari, V, Dancyger I, Renz J, Skolnick R, and Rochelson B. Eating disorders and pregnancy: Proposed treatment guidelines for obstetricians and gynecologists. *Open Journal of Obstetrics and Gynecology* 4 (2014): 90–94.

Franko, DL, and Walton BE. Pregnancy and eating disorders: A review and clinical implications. *International Journal of Eating Disorders* 13, no. 1 (1993): 41–47.

Freizinger, M, Franko, D, Dacey, M, Okun B, and Domar A. The prevalence of eating disorders in infertile women. *Fertility and Sterility* 93, no. 1 (2010): 72–78.

Hill, LS, Reid F, Morgan JF, and Lacey JH. SCOFF, the development of an eating disorder screening questionnaire. *International Journal of Eating Disorders* 43, no. 4 (2010): 344–351.

Hoffman, ER, Zerwas SC, and Bulik CM. Reproductive issues in anorexia nervosa. *Expert Review of Obstetrics and Gynecology* 6, no. 4 (2011): 403–414.

HuffPost Live. Sized Up: When Pregnant Women Struggle with Food. 23 February 2015. Available at http://live.huffingtonpost.com/r/segment/pregnancy-eating-disorders/54c2 c0c3fe344478c90002a2 (accessed 12 May 2015).

Hutcheon, JA, and Bodnar LM. A systematic approach for establishing the range of recommended weight gain in pregnancy. *American Journal of Clinical Nutrition* 100, no. 2 (2014): 701–707.

International Association of Eating Disorder Professionals. Infants of Mothers with Eating Disorders. (2009, January/February). Available at Retrieved from http://www.eatingdisordersreview.com/nl/nl_edr_20_3_4.html (accessed 29 November 2015).

Kaiser, LL, and Campbell CG. Practice paper of the Academy of Nutrition and Dietetics abstract: Nutrition and lifestyle for a healthy pregnancy outcome. *Journal of the Academy of Nutrition and Dietetics* 114, no. 9 (2014): 1447.

Knoph, C, Von Holle A, Zerwas S, Torgersen L, Tambs K, Stoltenberg C, Bulik CM, and Reichborn-Kjennerud T. Course and predictors of maternal eating disorders in the postpartum period. *International Journal of Eating Disorders* 46, no. 4 (2013): 355–368.

Koubaa, S, Hällström T, and Lindén Hirschberg A. Early maternal adjustment in women with eating disorders. *International Journal of Eating Disorders* 41, no. 5 (2008): 405–410.

Koubaa, S, Hällström T, Lindholm C, and Lindén Hirschberg A. Pregnancy and neonatal outcomes in women with eating disorders. *Obstetrics and Gynecology* 105, no. 2 (2005): 255–260.

Larsson, G, and Andersson-Ellstrom A. Experiences of pregnancy-related body shape changes and of breast-feeding in women with a history of eating disorders. *European Eating Disorders Review* 11, no. 2 (2003): 116–124.

Leddy, MA, Jones C, Morgan MA, and Schulkin J. Eating disorders and obstetric-gynecologic care. *Journal of Women's Health* 18, no. 9 (2009): 1395–1401.

Lefkovics, E, Baji I, and Rigó J. Impact of maternal depression on pregnancies and on early attachment. *Infant Mental Health Journal* 35, no. 4 (2014): 354–365.

Linna, MS, Raevuori A, Haukka J, Suvisaari JM, Suokas JT, and Gissler M. Reproductive health outcomes in eating disorders. *International Journal of Eating Disorders* 46, no. 8 (2013): 826–33.

Lupattelli, A, Spigset O, Torgersen L, Zerwas S, Hatle M5, Reichborn-Kjennerud T, Bulik CM, and Nordeng H. Medication use before, during, and after pregnancy among women with eating disorders: A study from the Norwegian mother and child cohort study. *PLoS ONE* 10, no. 7 (2015): e0133045.

Lusskin, S, Pundiak T, and Habib S. Perinatal depression: Hiding in plain sight. *Canadian Journal of Psychiatry* 52, no. 28 (2007): 479–483.

Müldner-Nieckowski, L, Cyranka K, Smiatek-Mazgaj B, Mielimąka M, Sobański JA, and Rutkowski K. Multiaxial changes in pregnancy: Mental health: A review of the literature. *Ginekologia Polska* 85, no. 10 (2014): 784–787.

Maine, M, and McGilley B. *Treatment of Eating Disorders: Bridging the Research-Practice Gap*. Burlington, MA: Academic Press/Elsevier, 2010.

Maternal, Child and Adolescent Health Division Center for Family Health California Department of Public Health. Body image and disordered eating. In *California Nutrition and Physical Activity Guidelines for Adolescents*. California, MA: Child and Adolescent Health Division Center for Family Health California Department of Public Health Maternal. 2015.

Mathieu, J. What is pregorexia? *Journal of the Academy of Nutrition and Dietetics* 109, no. 6 (2009): 976–979.

Mazzeo, SE, Slof-Op't Landt MC, Jones I, Mitchell K, Kendler KS, Neale MC, Aggen SH, and Bulik CM. Associations among postpartum depression, eating disorders, and perfectionism in a population-based sample of adult women. *International Journal of Eating Disorders* 39, no. 3 (2006): 202–211.

Meltzer-Brody, S, Zerwas S, Leserman J, Holle AV, Regis T, and Bulik C. Eating disorders and trauma history in women with perinatal depression. *Journal of Women's Health* 20, no. 6 (2011): 863–870.

Micali, N, dos Santos Silva I, De Stavola B, Steenweg-de Graaff J, Jaddoe V, Hofman A, Verhulst FC, Steegers E, and Tiemeier H. Fertility treatment, twin births, and unplanned pregnancies in women with eating disorders: Findings from a population-based birth cohort. *British Journal of Obstetrics and Gynaecology: An International Journal of Obstetrics and Gynaecology* 121, no. 4 (2014): 408–416.

Micali, N, Simonoff E, Stahl D, and Treasure J. Maternal eating disorders and infant feeding difficulties: Maternal and child mediators in a longitudinal general population study. *Journal of Child Psychology and Psychiatry* 52, no. 7 (2010): 800–807.

Micali, N, Treasure J, and Simonoff E. Eating disorders symptoms in pregnancy: A longitudinal study of women with recent and past eating disorders and obesity. *Journal of Psychosomatic Research* 63, no. 3 (2007): 297–303.

Misri, S, and Kendrick K. Treatment of perinatal mood and anxiety disorders: A review. *Canadian Journal of Psychiatry* 52, no. 8 (2007): 480–498.

Mitchell, A, and Bulik C. Eating disorders and women's health: An update. *Journal of Midwifery and Women's Health* 51, no. 3 (2006): 193–201.

Mitchell-Gieleghem, A, Mittelstaedt ME, and Bulik CM. Eating disorders and childbearing: Concealment and consequences. *Birth* 29, no. 3 (2012): 182–191.

Molloy, L. 2015 Family Newsletter. University of Bristol. 2015. Available at http://www.bristol.ac.uk/media-library/sites/alspac/documents/ChildrenOfThe90s_FamilyNewsletter_2015.pdf (accessed 2 January 2016).

Monk, C, Spicer J, and Champagne FA. Linking prenatal maternal adversity to developmental outcomes in infants: The role of epigenetic pathways. *Development and Psychopathology* 24, no. 4 (2012): 1361–1376.

Music, G. Stress pre-birth: How the fetus is affected by a mother's state of mind. *International Journal of Birth and Parent Education* 1, no. 1 (2013): 12–15.

Muzik, M, Hamilton SE, Rosenblum LK, Waxler E, and Hadi Z. Mindfulness yoga during pregnancy for psychiatrically at-risk women: Preliminary results from a pilot feasibility study. *Complementary Therapies in Clinical Practice* 18, no. 4 (2012): 235–240.

Mysko, C. *Does This Pregnancy Make Me Look Fat? The Essential Guide to Loving Your Body before and after Baby*. Deerfield Beach, FL: Health Communications, 2009.

National Eating Disorders Association. *Eating Disorders & Pregnancy: Some Facts about Risks*. 2005 (accessed 29 November 2015).

National Eating Disorders Association. Get the Facts on Eating Disorders. 2015. Available at http://www.nationaleatingdisorders.org/get-facts-eating-disorders (accessed 5 December 2015).

National Eating Disorders Association. Pregnancy and Eating Disorders. Available at http://www.nationaleatingdisorders.org/pregnancy-and-eating-disorders (accessed 3 January 2016).

National Eating Disorders Association. Trauma and Eating Disorders. Available at https://www.nationaleatingdisorders.org/trauma-and-eating-disorders (accessed 5 December 2015).

Newton, MS, and Chizawsky LLK. Treating vulnerable populations: The case of eating disorders during pregnancy. *Journal of Psychosomatic Obstetrics and Gynecology* 27, no. 1 (2006): 5–7.

Öhman, SG. Prenatal examinations for down syndrome and possible effects on maternal-fetal attachment. 2011. In *Prenatal Diagnosis and Screening for Down Syndrome*, edited by S Dey. Intech, 2011. Available at http://www.intechopen.com/books/prenatal-diagnosis-and-screening-for-down-syndrome/prenatal-examinations-for-down-syndrome-and-possible-effects-on-maternal-fetal-attachment. (accessed 22 December 2015).

Orbach, S and Rubin H. *Two for the price of one: The impact of body image during pregnancy and after birth*. London: Government Equalities Office, 2014.

Otten, JJ. *Dietary Reference Intakes: The Essential Guide to Nutrient Requirements*. Washington, DC: National Academies Press, 2006.

Patel, P, Lee J, Wheatcroft R, Barnes J, and Stein A. Concerns about body shape and weight in the postpartum period and their relation to women's self-identification. *Journal of Reproductive and Infant Psychology* 23, no. 4 (2005): 347–364.

Pekar, T. *Pregnancy, Motherhood, and Eating Disorders: Women's Experiences* (23 January 2013). Available at http://www.scienceofeds.org/2013/01/23/pregnancy-motherhood-and-eating-disorders-womens-experiences/ (accessed 2016).

Perry, L, Morgan J, Reid F, Brunton J, O'Brien A, Luck A, and Lacey H. Screening for symptoms of eating disorders: Reliability of the SCOFF screening tool with written compared to oral delivery. *International Journal of Eating Disorders* 32, no. 4 (2002): 466–472.

Rasmussen, KM, and Yaktine AL. *Weight Gain during Pregnancy: Reexamining the Guidelines.* Washington, DC: National Academies Press, 2009.

Reba-Harrelson, L, Von Holle A, Hamer RM, Torgersen L, Reichborn-Kjennerud T, and Bulik CM. Patterns of maternal feeding and child eating associated with eating disorders in the Norwegian mother and child cohort study (MoBa). *Eating Behaviors* 11, no. 1 (2010): 54–61.

Robinson, GE. Controversies about use of antidepressants in pregnancy. *Journal of Nervous and Mental Disease* 203, no. 3 (2015): 159–163.

Ross, S. A. (2015, January 12). [E-mail interview by M Baumann].

Rouanzoin, C. (2015, November 17). Trauma in Pregnant Women with Eating Disorders [Personal interview by M Baumann].

Schore, AN. *The Science of the Art of Psychotherapy.* New York, NY: WW Norton and Company, 2011.

Simkin, P, and Klaus, PH. *When Survivors Give Birth: Understanding and Healing the Effects of Early Sexual Abuse on Childbearing Women.* Seattle, WA: Classic Day, 2004.

Solmi, F, Sallis H, Stahl D, Treasure J, Micali N. Low birth weight in the offspring of women with anorexia nervosa. *Epidemiologic Reviews* 36 (2014): 49–56.

Stein, A, Fairburn CG. Eating habits and attitudes in the postpartum period. *Psychosomatic Medicine* 58, no. 4 (1996): 321–325.

Tenconi, E, Santonastaso P, Monaco F, and Favaro A. Obstetric complications and eating disorders: A replication study. *International Journal of Eating Disorders* 48 (2015): 424–430.

Torgersen, L, Ystrom E, Haugen M, Meltzer HM, Von Holle A, Berg CK, Reichborn-Kjennerud T, and Bulik CM. Breastfeeding practice in mothers with eating disorders. *Maternal and Child Nutrition* 6, no. 3 (2010): 243–252.

Wallace, K. Pregorexia: Extreme Dieting by Pregnant Women. CNN. 20 November 2013. Available at http://www.cnn.com/2013/11/20/living/pregnant-dieting-pregorexia-moms / (accessed 10 December 2015).

Ward, VB, and Waller, D. Eating disorders in pregnancy. *British Medical Journal* 336, no. 7635 (2008): 93–96.

Watson, HJ, Torgersen L, Zerwas S, Reichborn-Kjennerud T, Knoph C, Stoltenberg C, Siega-Riz AM, Von Holle A, Hamer RM, Meltzer H, Ferguson EH, Haugen M, Magnus P, Kuhns R, and Bulik CM. Eating disorders, pregnancy, and the postpartum period: Findings from the Norwegian mother and child cohort study (Moba). *Norsk Epidemiologi* 24, no. 1 (2014a): 51–62.

Watson, HJ, Von Holle A, Knoph C, Hamer RM, Torgersen L, Reichborn-Kjennerud T, Stoltenberg C, Magnus P, and Bulik CM. Psychosocial factors associated with bulimia nervosa during pregnancy: An internal validation study. *International Journal of Eating Disorders* 48, no. 6 (2014b): 654–662.

Zauderer, C. Eating disorders and pregnancy: Supporting the anorexic or bulimic expectant mother. *Journal of Obstetric, Gynecologic, & Neonatal Nursing* 37, no. 1 (2012): 48–55.

Zerwas, SC, Von Holle A, Perrin EM, Cockrell Skinner A, Reba-Harrelson L, Hamer RM, Stoltenberg C, Torgersen L, Reichborn-Kjennerud T, and Bulik CM. Gestational and postpartum weight change patterns in mothers with eating disorders. *Eating Disorders Review* 22, no. 6 (2014): 397–404.

9 Eating Disorders in Males

Helen B. Murray, BA and Adelaide S. Robb, MD

CONTENTS

LEARNING OBJECTIVES

After reading this chapter the reader should be able to do the following:

- Realize the prevalence of male eating disorders in the general population
- Recognize risk factors in males
- Understand recommendations for assessment and treatment specific to males
- Consider gaps in the field that need to be addressed with future research

BACKGROUND AND SIGNIFICANCE

The first documented evidence of a male with an eating disorder appeared in Robert Morton's account of an adolescent boy with anorexia nervosa (AN) in the seventeenth century (Morton 1694). Despite the long-term presence of eating disorders in males, there is a paucity of data on the prevalence and treatment of males with eating disorders (Hart et al. 2011). Existing literature shows that males present a clinical picture that is disparate from that of females in some aspects (Carlat et al. 1997). Recent changes in diagnostic criteria in the *Diagnostic and Statistical Manual of Mental Disorders-5 (DSM-5)* may increase access to services and direct research for males with eating disorders (American Psychiatric Association 2013). However, with a long-standing professional and cultural bias toward eating disorders as "female" disorders, men currently are often less likely than women to seek treatment or be correctly diagnosed (Räisänen and Hunt 2014). Increased clinician awareness and training together with better assessment tools will hopefully lead to better detection and treatment implementation in males struggling with eating disorders.

PREVALENCE

Eating disorders typically present between late adolescence and early adulthood and 25% of early detected cases of eating disorders are in males (Carlat et al. 1997; Hudson et al. 2007). This statistic is consistent with a study of a residential treatment facilities' eating disorder unit, which had 25% male admissions over an 18-year period (out of 672 total adult admissions; Zayas et al. 2015). As of 2007, the estimated lifetime prevalence rates in adult males for full-threshold (e.g. meeting all *DSM-IV-TR* diagnostic criteria) AN, bulimia nervosa (BN), and binge-eating disorder (BED) were 0.3%, 0.5%, and 2.0%, respectively (Hudson et al. 2007), while adolescent males were estimated at 0.3%, 0.5%, and 0.8%, respectively (Swanson et al. 2011). Eating disorders other than AN and BN were previously termed "eating disorders not otherwise specified," which accounted for 83% of eating disorder diagnoses in adolescent and adult males, with subthreshold (not meeting full syndrome diagnostic criteria) BED as the most common subtype (Le Grange et al. 2012). Subthreshold BED appears to be more prevalent in males than in females, while subthreshold AN is more prevalent in females than in males (Le Grange et al. 2012). Although full-threshold eating disorders are characteristically a small portion of the population (Hoek and Van Hoeken 2003), the severity of subthreshold eating disorders can be high, often with similar levels of impairment to full spectrum eating disorders. In addition, longitudinal diagnostic crossover is highly likely (based on a female sample; Eddy et al. 2008), thus patients may meet criteria for different diagnostic categories over time.

COMORBIDITY AND MEDICAL MORBIDITY

As chronic conditions that can be life-threatening, eating disorders are severe disorders both psychologically and physically. Eating disorders in males are commonly comorbid with psychiatric disorders, particularly mood disorders and anxiety disorders (Hudson et al. 2007; Ulfvebrand et al. 2015). Substance abuse and dependence also appear to have a relatively high rate of comorbidity with eating disorders in males (Ulfvebrand et al. 2015). Co-occurring disorders can further complicate treatment, mask eating disorder symptoms, and infer a higher risk of relapse of the eating disorder symptoms. Suicidality can also be associated with eating disorders with self-injurious behavior likely correlated with comorbid pathologies (Peebles et al. 2011).

AN UNDERSERVED POPULATION

As disorders that have been historically associated with females, eating disorders hold a cultural bias that has stigmatized men who suffer from disordered eating. The majority of eating disorder treatment research has focused on female clinical populations because females with eating disorders more commonly seek treatment. Fewer than 10% of eating disorder cases in clinics are male (Hoek and Van Hoeken 2003) and many residential and inpatient treatment programs accept only females. Males are less likely to seek out psychiatric services in general (Pollack and Levant 1998) and secrecy and embarrassment could be major barriers (Pope et al. 2001). In addition, many physicians have a lack of awareness of and training in eating disorders (Räisänen and Hunt 2014; Støving et al. 2011) including a low index for being suspicious of eating disorders in men (Flahavan 2006). When young men present with weight loss and eating changes, eating disorder diagnoses are not at the top of the differential and time to appropriately diagnose may take longer in men, delaying the initiation of treatment. In addition to providing more settings for males to seek out treatment, clinicians can aid in the process by becoming more familiar with the presentation of eating disorders in the male population.

RISK FACTORS

A community survey of adolescents (Neumark-Sztainer and Hannan 2000) found approximately half of the boys in the sample were concerned about becoming overweight. With a culture that encourages models of thinness and muscularity, the standard for beauty and attractiveness is set quite high. Biological and environmental conditions can increase the risk of some males for developing an eating disorder. At present, there is a dearth of research focused on the specific risk factors for males and the extent to which they share known risk factors with females. The literature that is available gives us a preliminary understanding of vulnerability in males, but further investigation is needed. Identification of individual factors as well as the environmental factors that put men at risk for eating disorders is of utmost importance, hopefully leading to informed prevention strategies.

INDIVIDUAL FACTORS

Genetic vulnerability for disordered eating exists through pathways such as temperament, personality traits, or related psychopathology (Bulik 2005) interacting with environmental factors. Risk and maintenance factors are then mediated by endophenotype contributions, linking risk from genes and environment with observed symptoms (phenotypes; Gottesman and Gould 2003). Endophenotype research on cognitive processes (i.e., set-shifting, central coherence, impulsivity) and eating disorders is growing, mostly with female samples (Lopez et al. 2009). Males may have some differences that future research should identify, for example, a negative association between set-shifting and focus on muscularity (Griffiths et al. 2013). Similar to females, comorbid pathologies such as obsessive–compulsive disorder, personality disorders, or substance abuse (Fichter and Krenn 2003) may also affect the onset and maintenance of eating disorder behavior.

Depending on these individual contributions, the phenotype (i.e., what a client presents with clinically) is affected. A desire to change one's body may stem from various motivations and may often occur during development with pubertal changes and gender identification. As males age from childhood to adolescence, the risk for weight and shape concerns increases (Calzo et al. 2012). For many males, eating disorder behavior may arise from being overweight. Using dieting strategies in an attempt to lose weight or become more muscular may lead some individuals to start exhibiting disordered eating behaviors, such as restricting or bingeing and purging for weight control. Carlat et al. noted roughly 60% of males with eating disorders had premorbid overweight in youth (Carlat et al. 1997). Thirty-nine percent of males with AN have been found to have higher than average premorbid weights (Gueguen et al. 2012). Higher premorbid weights may also be a predictor of BN in males (Carlat et al. 1997).

Sexual orientation may also be a specific risk factor for eating disorders in males (Carlat et al. 1997; Feldman and Meyer 2007; Russell and Keel 2002). Male homosexuality and bisexuality may correlate with eating disorders due to a desire for muscularity and/or to be physically attractive to other males (Brown and Keel 2013; Calzo et al. 2013; Robb and Dadson 2002).

SOCIOCULTURAL CONSIDERATIONS

Environmental factors can also adversely impact how individuals view themselves and the world. This occurs throughout time, setting the stage for eating disorders during development with continued influence into adulthood. Physically, the ideal masculine figure in the western world tends to be lean and muscular, often with the ideal as a "V-shape" with broad shoulders, narrow waist, and a "six or eight pack" of abdominal muscles (Weltzin et al. 2005; Yang et al. 2014). In the past 30 years, advertising (Pope et al. 2001), the media (Leit et al. 2002), and even male action figures (Pope et al. 1999) have increased the dissemination of an ideal muscular male body type to the community. In turn, males may see these images as vehicles of social comparison, possibly leading to feelings of inadequacy. An "ideal" lean and thin body type is also culturally present, particularly associated with some sports. Exposure to an "ideal" male body type through these modalities can affect internalization of the cultural norm. This can adversely affect some males' self-image, body esteem, or body satisfaction (Barlett et al. 2008). Decreases in body satisfaction may even occur after brief exposures (Lorenzen et al. 2004), but it is still not clear how long these effects last and most likely interact with individual factors that contribute to eating disorder vulnerability.

Peer influence can also contribute to an individual's internalization of these cultural norms for physical appearance (Tremblay and Lariviere 2009). Particularly, the influence of peers may be significant on athletic teams when performance is dependent on weight. This may be especially salient if other team members are engaging in disordered eating behaviors as a means to control weight before a sporting event. Sports such as wrestling, jockeying, gymnastics, or rowing require certain weights for performance and can put some individuals at risk for development of an eating disorder (Mickalide 1990; Robb 2001). Sociocultural influences can place a large pressure on the individual to meet certain standards. Traumatic or negative experiences can also add to vulnerability.

NEGATIVE LIFE EXPERIENCES

Physical and sexual abuses are often correlated with eating disorders in both males and females. Norris et al. (2012) found 12% of males with eating disorders reported histories of abuse, and Feldman and Meyer (2007) found that sexual abuse was significantly correlated with eating disorders in homosexual males. However, various types of negative life experiences can impact males and may be a factor in developing an eating disorder.

Neglectful parenting behavior, like low affection or physical neglect, can put a child at risk for later development of disordered eating (Johnson et al. 2002). Parent and peer comments, teasing about physical appearance, or talk about dieting can be associated with onset of eating disorders or body dysmorphic disorder (Tremblay and Lariviere 2009). Often, males with eating disorders report being teased during childhood or adolescence and attribute those experiences to body dissatisfaction (Anderson 1999). With these individual and environmental factors in mind, one of the biggest risks for onset and perpetuation of an eating disorder in males can be body image disturbances or disordered eating behavior going unnoticed. Early identification is crucial for all individuals suffering from any psychopathology. Clinicians need to have an understanding of presentations of eating disorders in males so that treatment is not delayed by lack of appropriate diagnosis and treatment.

SYMPTOM PRESENTATION AND ASSESSMENT IN MALES

On the whole, males and females experience many of the same eating disorder symptoms. Although the eating disorder field has much to still research, there are some differences that are already known in the male presentation. Nuances of the male body image concerns and behavioral presentations are described below. Table 9.1 provides some proposed diagnostic considerations for males.

TABLE 9.1

Considerations for Applying Eating Disorder Diagnoses in Males

Anorexia nervosa (Binge-eating/purging type or restricting type)	• More concern about muscle mass or percentage body fat than about weight gain • Use of steroids or muscle-building supplements
Bulimia nervosa	• Exercise as a more frequent compensatory behavior • Differences in experiencing a binge, such as no feeling of loss of control
Binge-eating disorder	• Differences in experiencing a binge, such as no feeling of loss of control • May be less likely to restrict intake prior to bingeing
Other specified feeding or eating disorder (OSFED)	• This category encompasses subthreshold disordered eating behavior as well as nondesignated criteria, such as night eating syndrome and purging disorder • For both men and women OSFED is likely the most common diagnosis

Body Image and Muscle Dysmorphia

Presenting somatic and psychological symptoms are mostly similar in males and females with a few key differences. Relative to women, some men may be more likely to focus on particular body parts, (e.g., arms, stomach), body fat percentage, and muscle mass rather than global overweight and shape concerns (Calzo et al. 2013; Pope et al. 2005; Robb and Dadson 2002; Weltzin et al. 2005).

Previously called "reverse anorexia," muscle dysmorphia is a specifier for body dysmorphic disorder. Muscle dysmorphia is characterized by preoccupations about increasing musculature and body mass as well as severe body image distortion (Grieve 2007; Ranzenhofer et al. 2012; Griffiths et al. 2014). Men experiencing muscle dysmorphia may obsessively exercise and lift weights, take weight gain supplements, restrict carbohydrates, and eat high-protein diets, yet no matter how fit, they never feel that they are adequately muscular. Frequent mirror-checking and social comparison to the "ideal" male body are often symptoms as well. However, a separate diagnosis of body dysmorphic disorder with muscle dysmorphia cannot be made if the muscle dysmorphia symptoms are primarily linked to the eating disorder symptoms (Mayo and George 2014). A study using vignettes about AN and muscle dysmorphia with male and female college students examined the perception and stigma around eating disorders (Griffiths et al. 2014). A large effect of character diagnosis on masculinity was observed, such that characters with AN were perceived as less masculine than characters with muscle dysmorphia, and this effect was more pronounced among male participants. A second study examined over 700 male and female university students using the Eating Attitudes Test (EAT) to asses risk for eating disorders and the Bodybuilder Image Grid (BIG) to assess body dissatisfaction and perceptual attractiveness (Mayo and George 2014). The study found 28% of the males were at risk based on their EAT scores which showed a positive correlation between the EAT scores and fat dissatisfaction and a negative correlation between the EAT scores and muscle dissatisfaction (muscle dissatisfaction indicated the person wanted smaller muscle mass). The males chose a significantly leaner and more muscular body as attractive compared to the female students' perception of an ideal male figure (Mayo and George 2014).

Binge Eating

Binge eating may functionally serve a different purpose in males than in females. Very little research has examined differential characteristics and predictors of binge eating in males. However, from our clinical experience, there are several ways in which the presentation of binge eating may differ for some males. First, males tend to have a difficult time identifying the sense of loss of control while binge eating. This challenges the diagnostic criterion for loss of control during a binge, in that some individuals may still experience other characteristics (e.g., eating more rapidly than normal, extreme guilt after-the-fact) that may indicate severity or impairment when loss of control is not present.

Second, some males may binge for different reasons than females. The subjective precipitants to a binge may rely more heavily on negative affect than an interaction of negative affect with dietary restraint in men compared to women. For example, males may binge as a coping mechanism for dealing with negative feelings, regardless of possible food intake restriction prior to the binge. This relationship may exist more frequently in males because of the societal pressure for males to not show emotion and be self-sufficient. Thus, emotion regulation capabilities may play a significant role in binge eating for males (Womble et al. 2001).

Finally, binge eating alone may not impact functioning in some males as much as in females; adolescent males who are obese and report binge eating have reported slightly higher quality of life than females (Mayo and George 2014). This may because it is more socially acceptable for males than females to indulge in large quantities of food.

COMPENSATORY AND PURGING BEHAVIORS

Behaviorally, men and women differ in compensatory actions, with exercising as a common compensatory behavior in men, while laxatives are not frequently utilized (Lewinsohn et al. 2002; Norris et al. 2012). Particular attention should be paid to the use of exercise as a compensatory behavior. However, overall, males may not utilize compensatory behaviors as often as females (Hudson et al. 2007).

ASSESSMENT

Health professionals should screen for eating disorder behavior in males and be cognizant of the possible nuances of male disordered eating characteristics. Although there is normative data for males (Lavender et al. 2010) on the "gold-standard" self-report questionnaire, the Eating Disorder Examination Questionnaire (Fairburn and Beglin 2008), the measure does not have the same sensitivity in males and females. Males in residential treatment for AN and BN scored lower than females across all Eating Disorder Examination Questionnaire scales, regardless of having the same diagnosis and severity level (Zayas et al. 2015). However, measures to better assess eating disorder symptoms in males are being developed. Forbush et al. (2013) created a 45-item self-report measure, called the Eating Pathology Symptom Inventory (EPSI). The EPSI is geared toward both men and women and includes questions particularly relevant for some males (e.g., "I thought my muscles were small;" "I used muscle building supplements"). Early identification is of utmost importance and effective, inclusive assessment tools are essential to filling the current gap in treatment access for men with disordered eating.

TREATMENT CONSIDERATIONS

Males may receive less intensive treatment than females, and services in general for eating disorders may not be meeting the population's needs (Striegel-Moore et al. 2000). Despite the lack of data available on male treatment outcomes specifically, males most likely do not have a poorer prognosis than females (Greenberg and Schoen 2008). Regardless, the main goals of treatment are the same for both sexes and, as always, it is crucial to treat the individual and his specific symptoms.

THERAPEUTIC RELATIONSHIP

An important consideration for males is that they are less likely than females to seek treatment. The stigma of eating disorders as "female disorders" combined with the societal pressure of masculine self-sufficiency could inhibit some men from asking for help. When entering treatment, some men may resist from fully engaging because of a fear of being dependent on another person for recovery. The therapeutic relationship can help break down such barriers.

Like females, males may want to fight for control over their eating and may take time to be able to let go of disordered eating behaviors (Greenberg and Schoen 2008). In therapy, a clinician may have to take engagement steps more slowly and possibly have the client first discuss relational examples that occurred outside of therapy. Men with eating disorders may hold personal rules regarding what their body "should" look like, what nutrition their body requires, and what their emotional allowance and needs are. By acknowledging a partnership between the clinician and the client, clinicians can emphasize to the client that treatment involves working on a problem together. In many cases, using a multidisciplinary approach with medical oversight, nutrition consultation, and psychotherapy can be helpful.

GOALS FOR TREATMENT

Currently, males are treated with various therapy modalities, including cognitive behavioral therapy. Family-based therapy has shown preliminary efficacy in adolescents and may be effective for some male clients Lock et al. (2010). In addition, because of the likelihood of symptom fluctuation, a full history of a client's symptoms can be helpful to prevent relapse.

SUMMARY AND CONCLUSIONS

Eating disorders in men have slowly become more recognized, discussed, and researched, but there is much that is still unknown for both males and females suffering from disordered eating. The next integral steps to take by researchers and clinicians for men with eating disorders are the following:

1. Increase awareness of male eating disorders and primary care physician screening
2. Introduce more higher level of care treatment facilities (e.g., residential) that are open to men with eating disorders
3. Investigate genetic, neuroendocrine, and neural correlates in males
4. Clarify the influence of risk factors and devise prevention strategies
5. Discover the potential moderating role of gender in treatment efficacy

CASE STUDIES

To help gain a better clinical understanding of eating disorders in males, two cases are described with relevant details for determining diagnoses and treatment. The information presented is a composite of cases and identifying information has been altered to protect privacy.

CASE STUDY 9.1

Steven

Steven is a 34-year-old male who is currently employed part-time and has been happily married for 5 years. He presents with sparse prior treatment history and no definitive diagnoses. Previously, he met with various therapists for only one to three sessions each and participated briefly in a support group. He is still trying to find a different treatment option. When asked about what he thinks he needs help with, he says that he is concerned about "the feelings I have around exercising."

Upon physical examination, he appears to be physically healthy with stable vital signs and normal laboratory findings. Body mass index (BMI) is in the slightly overweight category at 26.2, but percent body fat is 5%. Steven reports that he exercises daily for 2 hours each session and is currently taking 25 mg/day of creatine monohydrate, a controversial supplement typically used to increase muscle mass. While he does engage in cardiovascular activities, he mainly spends his time lifting weights. If he is not able to get to the gym on a particular day, he experiences increased worrying about his body and restricts his food intake. Steven reports that he has to build more strength and that he needs to exercise, because he wants to keep his muscularity stable. His goal is to have more muscle definition in the lateral and deltoid areas of his arms as well as a six-pack abdomen. When asked about body checking behaviors, he describes constantly checking for changes in the size of his upper half of his body, above his hips—on most mornings, he would spend over an hour checking his size in the bathroom mirror.

Further inquiry into his eating habits helps clarify his case. During the evaluation, he divulges impaired eating behaviors with minimal insight. He describes a typical day of no breakfast, a 300–400 cal lunch and occasional snacks of fruit or plain coffee. He has set rules for his daytime eating not to exceed 600 cal. When he misses a day of exercising, he restricts at night with a 300 cal frozen dinner. Over the past 6 months, he has engaged in objective binge episodes four times a week, when alone typically after dinner. Binges typically start off with "healthy" food such as a bag of baby carrots with hummus and then evolve into foods such as a large order of take-out Thai food or two medium pizzas. During all episodes, he experiences loss of control (i.e., feeling as though he cannot stop). He reports that he tries to not keep his "trigger" foods in the house. Describing conscious binges that occur throughout the night, he reports distress afterward and often exercising more intensely or longer the following day. He recalls approximately three unconscious nocturnal binges a week, when he finds empty food containers that he does not have any recollection of consuming. The unconscious binges seem to occur more frequently when he is under heightened stress, such as interviewing for a job or even worrying about missing a workout. He denied any history of laxative or diuretic use or self-induced vomiting but will increase the amount of his exercise the day after a binge to directly compensate for the food he consumed. When asked what most concerns him about his eating, he replies, "I hate when I wake up in

(Continued)

CASE STUDY 9.1 (CONTINUED)

the morning and there is food missing." He often consciously binges when he is unable to fall asleep.

His bingeing habits appear to have started in childhood, with a mother who struggles with late-night binge eating as well. At age 20, Steven had a highest weight of 220 lb. at 5'10" with a BMI of 31.6. In college, out of his home environment, he began to be more concerned about his appearance and started restricting minimally during the day but bingeing at night with a sense of loss of control. After marrying at age 29, he started to exercise and became obsessive about gaining muscle mass. He describes his relationship with food as a way to escape stress that is going on in his life.

Stephen was diagnosed with BN. A diagnosis of body dysmorphic disorder with muscle dysmorphia could not be made because his preoccupation with his muscles was better explained by his eating disorder.

CASE STUDY 9.2

Alex

Alex is a post-pubertal 16-year-old boy who had just entered the 11th grade. He and his parents emigrated to the United States from Eastern Europe, and both of his parents worked full-time. He presented to an adolescent inpatient unit with a 50-lb. weight loss over 3 months during his summer break. His BMI at admittance to an inpatient treatment facility is 14, though he is physically stable. Alex identified his sexual orientation as asexual, and his overall mood was anhedonic. In addition to obsessing about his weight and exercise, he would worry constantly about germs and contamination, engaging in hand washing more than 10 times a day and a ritualistic showering routine. He was diagnosed with AN, restricting type and obsessive–compulsive disorder. He had no prior psychiatric treatment history and no history of trauma.

Upon admission, Alex had no understanding of the gravity of his low weight or the effect of his eating and exercise behaviors. When Alex started swim team at the beginning of the summer, he began to compare himself to the other boys on the team and felt that his "belly was too fat" and wanted to lose weight. He had constant thoughts about his weight and size but had no target weight to meet. He wanted to fit into pants with a 22-inch waist and had no desire to increase muscle mass. On top of regular swim practice, he began a daily exercise routine of a 5-mile run and 200 abdominal crunches. While on the unit, he accepted that he was not able to exercise but feared he would get "fat" and was found trying to exercise with crunches and other isometric exercises whenever he was sitting down or alone in his room.

For an adolescent male in puberty, his meals were not sufficient to meet his body's functional needs and were not conducive to growth. On an inpatient unit with all non-eating disorder males, his peers in treatment talked

(Continued)

about their lunches consisting of a double cheeseburger, French fries, a bag of chips, and two chocolate milks. Although not nutritionally balanced, the other boys' lunch of 1000–1500 cal was starkly in contrast to Alex's 300-cal lunch. At the time of admittance, a typical day of eating included one cup of low-sugar cereal with one-half cup of skim milk for breakfast, one slice of turkey on white bread with an orange and a one-half cup of skim milk for lunch, and 4 oz. of protein with vegetables and occasional grains for dinner. His daily calorie intake typically totaled between 800 and 1000 cal. Alex was not aware of the amount of his calorie intake, and his parents did not realize that his intake was abnormal for his age. Based on his activity level, Alex's maintenance calorie intake would have been roughly 3200 cal.

While on the unit, Alex was fearful of eating fatty or sugary foods and any meat. He reported that he had to eat meat for dinner, because his parents were watching him. Feared foods were slowly introduced back into his diet, and he was mostly adherent to the meal plan. To induce weight restoration, he was started at 1200-cal oral intake and 800-cal nasogastric intake with increases over 2 weeks to a target 4000-cal oral intake and 1200-cal nasogastric intake, which was maintained over the remaining 6 weeks of hospitalization. At discharge, his BMI was 17.5, and he had some insight into his need to regain weight. He began an intensive outpatient program with a goal to return to a BMI of 19 and maintain a 5000-cal oral intake.

REFERENCES

American Psychiatric Association. *Diagnostic and Statistical Manual of Mental Disorders* (5th ed.). Washington, DC: Author, 2013.

Anderson, AE. Males with eating disorders: Medical considerations. In *Eating Disorders: A Guide to Medical Care and Complications*, edited by PS Mehler and AE Anderson, pp. 214–226. Baltimore, MD: Johns Hopkins University Press, 1999.

Barlett, CP, Vowels CL, and Saucier DA. Meta-analyses of the effects of media images on men's body-image concerns. *Journal of Social and Clinical Psychology* 27, no. 3 (2008): 279–310.

Brown, TA, and Keel PK. The impact of relationships, friendships, and work on the association between sexual orientation and disordered eating in men. *Eating Disorders* 21, no. 4 (2013): 342–359.

Bulik, CM. Exploring the gene—Environment nexus in eating disorders. *Journal of Psychiatry and Neuroscience* 30, no. 5 (2005): 335.

Calzo, JP, Corliss HL, Blood EA, Field AE, and Austin SB. Development of muscularity and weight concerns in heterosexual and sexual minority males. *Health Psychology* 32, no. 1 (2013): 42.

Calzo, JP, Sonneville KR, Haines J, Blood EA, Field AE, and Bryn Austin S. The development of associations among body mass index, body dissatisfaction, and weight and shape concern in adolescent boys and girls. *Journal of Adolescent Health* 51, no. 5 (2012): 517–523.

Carlat, DJ, Camargo CA, and Herzog DB. Eating disorders in males: A report on 135 patients. *American Journal of Psychiatry* 154, no. 8 (1997): 127–132.

Eddy, KT, Dorer DJ, Franko DL, Tahilani K, Thompson-Brenner H, and Herzog DB. Diagnostic crossover in anorexia nervosa and bulimia nervosa: Implications for DSM-V. *American Journal of Psychiatry* 165, no. 2 (2008): 245–250.

Fairburn, C. G., and Beglin, S. (2008). Eating Disorder Examination Questionnaire (EDE-Q 6.0). In C. G. Fairburn (Ed.), *Cognitive Behavior Therapy and Eating Disorders* (pp. 309–313). New York, NY: Guilford Press.

Feldman, MB, and Meyer IH. Eating disorders in diverse lesbian, gay, and bisexual populations. *International Journal of Eating Disorders* 40, no. 3 (2007): 218–226.

Fichter, M, and Krenn H. Eating disorders in males. In *Handbook of Eating Disorders*, edited by J Treasure, U Schmidt, and E van Furth, pp. 369–384. West Sussex, UK: Wiley, 2003.

Flahavan, C. Detection, assessment and management of eating disorders; How involved are GPs? *Journal of Psychological Medicine* 23, no. 3 (2006): 96–99.

Forbush, KT, Wildes JE, Pollack LO, Dunbar D, Luo J, Patterson K, Petruzzi L, Pollpeter M, Miller H, Stone A, Bright A, and Watson D. Development and validation of the Eating Pathology Symptoms Inventory (EPSI). *Psychological Assessment* 25, no. 3 (2013): 859.

Gottesman, II, and Gould TD. The endophenotype concept in psychiatry: Etymology and strategic intentions. *American Journal of Psychiatry* 160, no. 4 (2003): 636–645.

Greenberg, ST, and Schoen EG. Males and eating disorders: Gender-based therapy for eating disorder recovery. *Professional Psychology: Research and Practice* 39, no. 4 (2008): 464–471.

Grieve, FG. A conceptual model of factors contributing to the development of muscle dysmorphia. *Eating Disorders* 15, no. 1 (2007): 63–80.

Griffiths, S, Mond JM, Murray SB, and Touyz S. Young peoples' stigmatizing attitudes and beliefs about anorexia nervosa and muscle dysmorphia. *International Journal of Eating Disorders* 47, no. 2 (2014): 189–195.

Griffiths, S, Murray SB, and Touyzno S. Drive for muscularity and muscularity-oriented disordered eating in men: The role of set shifting difficulties and weak central coherence. *Body Image* 10, no. 4 (2013): 636–639.

Gueguen, J, Godart N, Chambry J, Brun-Eberentz A, Foulon C, Divac Phd SM, Guelfi JD, Rouillon F, Falissard B, and Huas C. Severe anorexia nervosa in men: Comparison with severe AN in women and analysis of mortality. *International Journal of Eating Disorders* 45, no. 4 (2012): 537–545.

Hart, LM, Granillo, M Teresa GM, Jorm AF, Paxton SJ. Unmet need for treatment in the eating disorders: A systematic review of eating disorder specific treatment seeking among community cases. *Clinical Psychology Review* 31, no. 5 (2011): 727–735.

Hoek, HW, and Van Hoeken D. Review of the prevalence and incidence of eating disorders. *International Journal of Eating Disorders* 34, no. 4 (2003): 383–396.

Hudson, JI, Hiripi E, Pope HG Jr, and Kessler RC. The prevalence and correlates of eating disorders in the national comorbidity survey replication. *Biological Psychiatry* 61, no. 3 (2007): 348–358.

Johnson, JG, Cohen P, Kasen S, and Brook JS. Eating disorders during adolescence and the risk for physical and mental disorders during early adulthood. *Archives of General Psychiatry* 59, no. 6 (2002): 545–552.

Lavender, JM, De Young KP, and Anderson DA. Eating Disorder Examination Questionnaire (EDE-Q): Norms in undergraduate men. *Eating Behaviors* 11, no. 2 (2010): 119–121.

Le Grange, D, et al. Eating disorder not otherwise specified presentation in the U.S. population. *International Journal of Eating Disorders* 45, no. 5 (2012): 711–718.

Leit, RA, Gray JJ, and Pope HG. The media's representation of the ideal male body: A cause for muscle dysmorphia? *International Journal of Eating Disorders* 31, no. 3 (2002): 334–338.

Lewinsohn, PM, Seeley JR, Moerk KC, and Striegel-Moore RH. Gender differences in eating disorder symptoms in young adults. *International Journal of Eating Disorders* 32, no. 4 (2002): 426–440.

Lock, J, Le Grange D, Agras WS, Moye A, Bryson SW, and Jo B. Randomized clinical trial comparing family-based treatment with adolescent-focused individual therapy for adolescents with anorexia nervosa. *Archives of General Psychiatry* 67, no. 10 (2010): 1025–1032.

Lopez, C, Roberts M, and Treasure J. Biomarkers and endophenotypes in eating disorders. In *The Handbook of Neuropsychiatric Biomarkers, Endophenotypes and Genes*, edited by MS Ritsner, pp. 227–237. New York, NY: Springer, 2009.

Lorenzen, LA, Grieve FG, and Thomas A. Brief report: Exposure to muscular male models decreases men's body satisfaction. *Sex Roles* 51, no. 11 (2004): 743–748.

Mayo, C and George V. Eating disorder risk and body dissatisfaction based on muscularity and body fat in Male University Students. *Journal of American College Health* 62, no. 6 (2014): 407–415.

Mickalide, AD. Sociocultural factors influencing weight among males. In *Males with Eating Disorders*, edited by A Anderson, Vol. 30, pp. 30–39, Philadelphia, PA: Brunner/Mazel, 1990.

Morton, R. *Phthisiologica-or Treatise of Consumption*. London: Smith and Walford, 1694.

Neumark-Sztainer, D, and Hannan PJ. Weight-related behaviors among adolescent girls and boys: Results from a national survey. *Archives of Pediatrics & Adolescent Medicine* 154, no. 6 (2000): 569–577.

Norris, M, Apsimon M, Harrison M, Obeid N, Buchholz A, Henderson KA, and Spettigue W. An examination of medical and psychological morbidity in adolescent males with eating disorders. *Eating Disorders* 20, no. 5 (2012): 405–415.

Peebles, R, Wilson JL, and Lock JD. Self-injury in adolescents with dating disorders: Correlates and provider bias. *Journal of Adolescent Health* 48, no. 3 (2011): 310–313.

Pollack, WS, and Levant RF. *New Psychotherapy for Men*. Hoboken, NJ: John Wiley & Sons, 1998.

Pope, HG, Olivardia R, Gruber A, and Borowiecki J. Evolving ideals of male body image as seen through action toys. *International Journal of Eating Disorders* 26, no. 1 (1999): 65–72.

Pope, CG, Pope HG, Menard W, Fay C, Olivardia R, and Phillips KA. Clinical features of muscle dysmorphia among males with body dysmorphic disorder. *Body Image* 2, no. 4 (2005): 395–400.

Pope, HG, et al. The growing commercial value of the male body: A longitudinal survey of advertising in women's magazines. *Psychotherapy and Psychomatics* 70, no. 4 (2001): 189–192.

Räisänen, U and Hunt K. The role of gendered constructions of eating disorders in delayed help-seeking in men: A qualitative interview study. *British Medical Journal* 4, no. 4 (2014): 1–9.

Ranzenhofer, LM, Columbo KM, Tanofsky-Kraff M, Shomaker LB, Cassidy O, Matheson BE, Kolotkin RL, Checchi JM, Keil M, McDuffie JR, and Yanovski JA. Binge eating and weight-related quality of life in obese adolescents. *Nutrients* 4, no. 3 (2012): 167–180.

Robb, AS. Eating disorders in children: Diagnosis and age-specific treatment. *Psychiatric Clinics of North America* 24, no. 2 (2001): 259–270.

Robb, AS and Dadson MJ. Eating disorders in males. *Child and Adolescent Psychiatric Clinics of North America* 11 (2002): 399–418.

Russell, CJ and Keel PK. Homosexuality as a specific risk factor for eating disorders in men. *International Journal of Eating Disorders* 31, no. 3 (2002): 300–306.

Støving, RK, Andries A, Brixen K, Bilenberg N, and Hørder K. Gender differences in outcome of eating disorders: A retrospective cohort study. *Psychiatry Research* 186, no. 2 (2011): 362–366.

Striegel-Moore, RH, Leslie D, Petrill SA, Garvin V, and Rosenheck RA. One-year use and cost of inpatient and outpatient services among female and male patients with an eating disorder: Evidence from a National Database of Health Insurance Claims. *International Journal of Eating Disorders* 27, no. 4 (2000): 381–389.

Swanson, SA, et al. Prevalence and correlates of eating disorders in adolescents: Results from the national comorbidity survey replication adolescent supplement. *Archives of General Psychiatry* 68, no. 7 (2011): 714–723.

Tremblay, L, and Lariviere M. The influence of puberty onset, body mass index, and pressure to be thin on disordered eating behaviors in children and adolescents. *Eating Behaviors* 10, no. 2 (2009): 75–83.

Ulfvebrand, S, et al. Psychiatric comorbidity in women and men with eating disorders results from a large clinical database. *Psychiatry Research* 230, no. 2 (2015): 294–299.

Weltzin, TE, Weisensel N, Franczyk D, Burnett K, Klitz C, and Bean P. Eating disorders in men: Update. *Journal of Men's Health and Gender* 2 (2005): 186–193.

Womble, LG, Williamson DA, Martin CK, Zucker NL, Thaw JM, Netemeyer R, Lovejoy JC, and Greenway FL. Psychosocial variables associated with binge eating in obese males and females. *International Journal of Eating Disorders* 30, no. 2 (2001): 217–221.

Yang, C-FJ, Gray P, and Pope HG Jr. Male body image in Taiwan versus the west: Yanggang zhiqi meets the adonis complex. *American Journal of Psychiatry* 162, no. 2 (2014): 263–269.

Zayas, L, et al. Sex differences in eating pathology of anorexia nervosa and bulimia nervosa across new DSM-5 severity categories. In *International Conference on Eating Disorders*. Boston, MA, 2015.

10 Eating Disorders and Type 1 Diabetes

Carolyn Costin, RD, CDE and Gail Prosser,
MA, MEd, LMFT, CEDS with special
thanks to Jacque Mular, MS, RD

CONTENTS

LEARNING OBJECTIVES

After reading this chapter, the reader should be able to do the following:

- Identify the prevalence and risk factors contributing to the comorbid presence of eating disorders and diabetes mellitus (DM)
- Recognize medical and mental health consequences of the comorbid presence of eating disorders and DM

CASE STUDY 10.1

Grace

Grace, a 24-year-old college student, presents for treatment at a residential eating disorder center, weighing 96 lb. at a height of 5'6". Grace's parents and providers state that she has anorexia nervosa (AN) but Grace claims that she does not have an eating disorder yet will attend the program to "gain some weight" and "satisfy my parents." Grace agrees she has lost too much weight, but explains that she gets distracted during school and just forgets to eat. She also admits she sometimes forgets to give herself the insulin injections she has required since the age of 12, when she was diagnosed with type 1 diabetes mellitus (DM1), but claims it has nothing to do with wanting to lose weight or be thin. In fact, she claims she wants to gain weight and says she will prove that to everyone. Grace reiterates often during the course of her stay that being in treatment is unnecessary.

Grace's eating behavior was so unusual for someone with AN that the other patients initially thought Grace might be right about not having an eating disorder. Grace readily put extra olive oil on her salads and ate hefty portions of avocado and cheese. She ate quickly and did not push food around on her plate or cut it into bits, as is commonly seen in someone with AN. However, Grace barely gained weight even after a few caloric increases in her meal plan. It was soon discovered that Grace was restricting her insulin.

Upon admission, Grace, her parents, and her physician all insisted that she be allowed to give herself her own insulin injections since she had been doing so for 12 years. The treatment team agreed to let Grace give herself the shots in front of an observing nurse. However, it turned out that Grace was reducing the amount of insulin she gave herself by leaking insulin out

(Continued)

of the syringe immediately before injecting herself, as well as pulling out the needle before all the insulin was injected. The nurses, while observing her, were not expecting someone who might try to underdose. They were unaware that Grace might try to reduce her insulin, a behavior similar to someone with AN who tries to reduce calories by hiding food in a napkin or under the table. It is important when monitoring patients to closely observe any self-administration of insulin. Clinicians need to understand that a person like Grace, with ED-DM1, may react to weight phobia by deliberately restricting insulin, even though insulin is a necessary, life-supporting medicine. Treatment providers should also be made aware that insulin has an odor that some people describe as petroleum jelly or pencils, and that, if this odor is present when a patient is injecting themselves, this may indicate leaking insulin. Even after being caught, Grace denied any responsibility for the leaking insulin claiming, "Why would I do that and risk my health?"

Grace had been dropping weight prior to being diagnosed with DM1 and was pleased with the weight loss. Upon learning she had diabetes, Grace was educated about her illness including how the lack of insulin causes an inability to obtain fuel from food thus resulting in nutrient deficiency and weight loss. She was taught how to control her blood sugar and how to give herself insulin injections. She not only regained the weight she lost, but also began overeating and gained even more weight. For the first time in her life, Grace started talking about being fat. She came to resent the insulin shots and began to think of them as "weight gain injections." Grace's family was very supportive and tried to help monitor her but once she left for college, she faced a tempting and dangerously easy way to shed unwanted pounds. She began skipping doses of insulin in order to lose weight. As time went on, restricting her insulin doses, lying about having taken insulin, and faking her blood-sugar results became the norm and Grace could not stop. Even though she had been taught the dangers of repeatedly letting her blood sugar get too high, including nerve damage, vision problems, and kidney failure, Grace thought she would be able to control her insulin restriction and not let it go too far. By the time she entered treatment, Grace had a full-blown eating disorder in addition to her DM and for a while was unable to tell the truth about what was really going on.

- Explain methods of manipulating insulin levels and reports of insulin levels
- Determine and appreciate appropriate safeguards in inpatient and outpatient settings for patients with eating disorders and DM

INTRODUCTION

Most people are familiar with the now widely known eating disorders, anorexia nervosa (AN), bulimia nervosa (BN), and binge-eating disorder (BED), but only recently has the co-occurrence of diabetes mellitus, type 1 (DM1) and insulin restriction been seen as a new variant of eating disorder manifestation. Some have referred to this condition as "diabulimia" because restricting insulin can be used as a way of purging or eliminating calories. Without the necessary insulin, the body's cells cannot utilize the energy from food. Diabulimia is not an official diagnostic term, and the combination of DM1 and an eating disorder is not yet recognized as a separate medical or psychiatric condition. The term diabulimia is also mislead-ing because not all patients with this condition binge, which is one of the main criteria for a diagnosis of bulimia. In order to avoid the shortcomings of the term *diabulimia* and escape the more lengthy and cumbersome *someone who has an eat-ing disorder and diabetes,* we have chosen to use the term *ED-DM1* for this chapter.

The combination of insulin-dependent diabetes and an eating disorder is becom-ing a more frequent presentation in clinicians' offices and treatment centers. It appears that insulin-dependent diabetes (DM1) may increase the risk of develop-ing an eating disorder in some individuals, yet there are few specialized programs and sparse literature on the subject. To help improve understanding of this complex condition, this chapter identifies risk factors, reviews basic medical information, and outlines steps to take when treating people who present with ED-DM1. We highlight difficulties that arise in diabetes management, both for individuals managing their own illness and for health professionals who treat them. It is important to understand that all the suggestions provided in this chapter should not be misconstrued as spe-cific recommendations for an individual case or used in lieu of professional advice.

EATING DISORDER-DIABETES MELLITUS 1

There are an increasing number of individuals like Grace, for whom insulin becomes a feared substance. In a culture obsessed with thinness, an easy weight loss method can be irresistible to people dissatisfied with their shape or size. Imagine a diet that allows you to eat all you want and not gain weight. Unlike AN, in which a person severely restricts calories or when calories are binged and purged as in bulimia nervosa, a person with DM1 who restricts insulin can eat whatever he or she wants without the calories being absorbed. The body's ability to convert glucose into energy is compro-mised when insulin is restricted. Insulin acts as a key to the door of our cells, thereby ushering the glucose into the cell to be converted into usable energy. When insulin is restricted, glucose is left outside the cell, rendering it ineffective. It is not surprising that we are increasingly seeing people with diabetes, particularly those with body image disturbance, weight phobia, and/or an obsession with calories, experiment with insulin restriction or manipulation and end up with an eating disorder.

People with ED-DM1 describe eating foods they routinely thought of as fattening such as cake, ice cream, or pizza and then essentially "getting rid" of the calories by omitting their insulin injections. This very serious, unhealthy practice of restricting insulin can lead to catastrophic consequences. The morbidity and mortality rates for individuals with a combination of disordered eating and diabetes are higher than that for those with diabetes alone (Rydall et al. 1997). In a 12-year study, research-ers followed 14 women, ages 25–42, who had ED-DM1. The results were grim. At the end of the 12 years, five of the women were dead, two were blind, and three were on dialysis or undergoing renal replacement therapy. All of the participants suf-fered some degree of irreversible medical problems (Walker et al. 2002). In another study comparing mortality rates over a 10-year period, individuals with DM1 alone had a mortality rate of 2.5%, individuals with AN and no history of diabetes had a mortality rate of 6.5%, and for those who had ED-DM1, the mortality rate jumped to 34.8% (Nielsen et al. 2002; Nielsen 2002).

BACKGROUND INFORMATION ON DIABETES

Simply put, diabetes, officially known as diabetes mellitus, is a metabolic disease in which a person has high blood sugar because either the pancreas does not produce enough insulin or cells do not respond to the insulin that is produced. Insulin, which is normally produced by the pancreas, is the hormone that allows our cells to absorb glucose to be used as fuel for the body.

TYPE 1 DIABETES MELLITUS

Type 1 diabetes mellitus is considered to be genetic and is usually diagnosed before the age of 40 with the peak age of diagnosis around 14 years of age. It is far less common than type 2. In DM1, the pancreas has lost its ability to produce insulin. Without insulin, the cells cannot absorb glucose for fuel and subsequently the glucose circulates in the bloodstream by raising blood-sugar levels. The terms *blood glucose* and *blood sugar* are used interchangeably and are symbolized using *BG*. When BG level rises above 200 mg/dL, the extra glucose is removed by the kidneys and flows into the urine, essentially eliminating calories. A high BG is harmful to the body in many ways that will be discussed in this chapter.

TYPE 2 DIABETES MELLITUS

The more common form of diabetes, type 2 diabetes mellitus (DM2), usually develops later in life and typically has a slower onset than type 1. These individuals can often control their blood-sugar level through diet, exercise, and oral medication. DM2 can result from insufficient insulin production by the pancreas or, more commonly, from an inability to efficiently use the insulin produced. Unlike type 1, DM2 is not an autoimmune disease, although genetic markers and a family history of diabetes are strong indicators that a person might develop diabetes in the future (Sargeant et al. 2000). DM2 is more likely to be a condition secondary to obesity and/or a sedentary lifestyle. DM2 was formerly referred to as adult onset diabetes because children and adolescents accounted for only 3% of all type 2 cases until relatively recently. However, in 2005, Pinhas-Hamiel and Zeitler found that adolescents account for 45% of new onset cases. This rise in type 2 prevalence rate in minors is attributed to a concurrent rise in childhood obesity worldwide (Pinhas-Hamiel and Zeitler 2005). Individuals with DM2 may manipulate insulin for weight loss but it is very rare, there is little or no data, and it is not the focus of this chapter.

FOOD, BLOOD SUGAR, AND INSULIN

Upon receiving a diagnosis of diabetes, people need to be educated on how to count carbohydrates, check blood sugars, and take medication, including how to dose and administer insulin appropriately. A registered dietician, physician, and diabetes educator can all be useful in developing an overall diabetes plan and nutrition program that provides balanced nutrition and helps to control BG in a desirable range.

The energy from our food comes in the form of protein, fat, or carbohydrate. Carbohydrates have the most substantial and immediate effect on BG and insulin use. Carbohydrates are more rapidly broken down into glucose, the sugar that fuels our cells, than protein or fat. A person's blood sugar rises and falls primarily based on the amount of carbohydrates consumed. Carbohydrates are the type of food that a person with diabetes needs to control and manage with insulin in order to regulate blood sugar.

Individuals with diabetes are taught the sources of carbohydrate in the diet, such as breads, grains, starchy vegetables, lentils, milk, fruit, desserts, and sugars. They are also taught how to limit carbohydrates in a meal plan, and how to *count carbs* either by grams or exchanges. An *exchange* or *carb serving* is generally equivalent to 15 g of carbohydrate. A one-ounce slice of bread, for example, or a small apple, or 1/2 cup cooked pasta equals 15 g of carbohydrate. A large banana, by contrast, contains about 30 g of carbohydrate, so it would be counted as 30 g or two exchanges. A sandwich (two slices of bread, lunch meat, cheese, mayo, and lettuce/tomato) would also have 30 g of carbohydrate, 15 g from each slice of bread. A lunch of sandwich and banana, thus, equals 60 g or four exchanges. Depending on the preference of the patient and clinician, some individuals with DM1 follow a *set meal plan* with three to four exchanges per meal (45–60 g of carbohydrate).

Another approach is to give the person with diabetes an insulin to carb ratio (ICR), so he or she can inject insulin based on the number of carbohydrates eaten. For example, an ICR of 1:15 means that 1 unit of rapid-acting insulin is injected for every 15 g of carbohydrates eaten. In the case of having a sandwich and banana for lunch, 60 g of carbohydrates would mean injecting 4 units of insulin. A sandwich, banana, and cup of milk would require 75 g or 5 units of insulin. The ICR allows for increased mealtime flexibility. A person can decide to eat a large carbohydrate meal such as a plate of pasta and garlic bread and take a large amount of insulin (the amount to replace what the pancreas would normally produce for a nondiabetic). Conversely, a person can decide to eat a very low carb meal, grilled chicken over salad, and thus have to take very little or even no insulin.

Individuals with DM1 are advised to check their blood-sugar levels at least four times a day and sometimes more often. This allows them to see if they need to adjust their insulin dosage and allows them to properly calculate the right amount of short-acting versus long-acting insulin needed.

Blood sugar can be checked by using a small medical device called a glucometer or BG meter. A drop of blood, typically taken from a needle prick by a lancet device, is placed onto a reactive test strip, the meter reads the test strip, and an estimated BG result can be read on the meter screen. Patients have to be taught to monitor low blood-sugar (hypoglycemia) as well as high blood-sugar (hyperglycemia) levels. Blood sugar needs to be kept in an optimum range, somewhere between 50 and 180 mg/dL. Having blood-sugar levels that are either too low or too high can cause a variety of symptoms and can potentially be very dangerous and even cause death (Table 10.1).

TABLE 10.1

SYMPTOMS OF HIGH OR LOW BLOOD SUGAR

SYMPTOMS OF HIGH BG CAN INCLUDE

Excessive thirst	Hunger	Stomach Ache
Excessive urination	Irritability	Deep breathing
Dehydration	Headache	Ketone body production (fruity breath odor)

PROLONGED OR SEVERE HIGH BG LEVELS CAN INCLUDE

Diabetic ketoacidosis (DKA), severe	Infections; most commonly urinary tract infections	Retinopathy (eye damage) leading to blindness
Neuropathy (nerve damage) leading to pain or lack of sensation in hands and feet	Kidney disease leading to kidney failure	Sexual dysfunction
Early death		

SYMPTOMS OF LOW BG CAN INCLUDE

Mood changes	Trembling	Sweating
Hunger	Fatigue	Weakness
Headache	Confusion	

SEVERE SYMPTOMS OF LOW BG CAN INCLUDE

Loss of consciousness	Seizure	Immediate death

INSULIN USE

Patients with diabetes are educated about the necessity of insulin and, if old enough, taught how to self-administer the required dose. They are often given a choice on how to administer insulin, either in multiple daily injections or the use of an insulin pump.

1. *Multiple daily injections* typically means the individual will give an injection or shot of insulin at meal and snack times using a short-acting type of insulin, such as Humalog, Novolog, or Apidra (three of the major brands used in the United States). Insulin must be given at every meal or snack that contains carbohydrate in order to keep BG levels in a desirable range. Another injection of a long-acting type of insulin, such as Lantus or Levemir, is given either once or twice a day. These long-acting types of insulin provide a background or base level of insulin, known as basal insulin, that keeps BG in check over 12–24 hours, similar to what a nondiabetic person's pancreas would do for them.

2. *Insulin pump therapy* is the use of a small device that is attached to the skin with a small plastic catheter called an infusion set. An insulin pump holds up to 300 units of rapid acting insulin programed to be continuously delivered in tiny amounts throughout the course of the day, providing the basal insulin. This replaces the need for long-acting insulin. There are several

advantages of using an insulin pump. People with diabetes who use a pump do not have to carry insulin vials and syringes and do not have to give themselves a shot every time they eat carbohydrates. Instead, the pump calculates how much insulin to deliver based on the BG level at the time and the amount of carbohydrates eaten. For the health-care practitioner, the pump records and stores valuable information on how much insulin was used, how many carbohydrates eaten, and the BG record.

THE PREVALENCE OF INSULIN RESTRICTION

Insulin restriction is the practice of manipulating how much insulin is taken in relationship to the carbohydrate content of the meal. When food or insulin is restricted, the end result is weight loss due to the inability of energy from the food to enter the cells of the body for use. Alarmingly, restricting insulin is not an uncommon practice among diabetics, with or without an eating disorder. Deliberate insulin omission is the most common method of purging calories in girls with DM2 and becomes progressively more common through the teen years (Colton et al. 2009). One study found that 2% of girls between 9 and 14 years old reported omitting their insulin in order to lose weight (Colton et al. 2004). Another study found that 14% of females between 12 and 18 years old were omitting or underdosing insulin, and at a 5-year follow-up the number had risen to 34% (Rydall et al. 1997). Similarly, a study by researchers at the University of Toronto found that one out of three women with DM1 reported skipping or underdosing their insulin to lose weight (Goebel-Fabbri et al. 2008).

Oslo University Hospital in Norway surveyed male and female DM1 teenagers using a tool called the Diabetes Eating Problem Survey-Revised (DEPS-R) to detect disturbed eating behavior. The study inquired specifically about insulin restriction as a behavior related to eating disorders. Nearly a third (31.6%) of the total group endorsed the DEPS-R item "When I overeat, I do not take enough insulin to cover the food" and 6.9% endorsed "After I overeat, I skip my next insulin dose." Among females, 36.8% reported restricting and 26.2% reported skipping insulin after overeating, while those proportions among males were 9.4% and 4.5%, respectively. Hemoglobin A1c (HbA1c) was also significantly higher among those who reported insulin restriction, 9.0% versus 8.3% ($p < .001$; Wisting et al. 2013).

METHODS USED TO RESTRICT, MANIPULATE, OR OTHERWISE AVOID INSULIN

Clinicians familiar with ED-DM1 have found that as the illness progresses, patients may go to increasingly extreme methods to avoid insulin. Anyone treating ED-DM1 will need to be aware of the various ways that patients can manipulate insulin in order to take in less insulin than they need, putting themselves at risk for serious medical complications.

As in the case of Grace, individuals who are giving themselves injections might lie or otherwise mislead health-care practitioners by, for example, not adequately reporting their sugars or "faking" their injections by leaking out insulin or not injecting appropriate tissue. An insulin pump might initially seem like a good alternative because the pump provides recordings on the amount of carbohydrate eaten and insulin received. However, the person with diabetes must routinely and accurately enter correct information. If trying to hide BG levels, carbohydrates consumed, or amount of insulin taken, the patient can enter incorrect data to manipulate the pump readings. Clinicians and parents have been fooled into thinking the information from the pump was accurate when it was actually recorded improperly by the patient. Furthermore, the meter only records that insulin has been delivered; it will not be able to detect if the insulin was actually delivered into the body.

Common pump manipulations:

1. Entering a reduced incorrect amount of carbohydrates at a meal. For example, eating 200 g of carbohydrates but recording 15–30 g so that the pump administers a smaller amount of insulin than what is needed.
2. Entering carbohydrates correctly but then overriding the pump calculations and delivering less insulin. This manipulation can easily be found in the pump discrepancy report.
3. Pump reports that consistently show a whole unit amount of insulin delivery, for example, 2 units or 10 units, instead of decimal units like 2.7 or 10.3, which are the type of numbers usually seen when using the pump calculations to deliver insulin.
4. Lack of information on carbohydrates, bolus (dose), or BG levels in the pump readings. This situation is commonly known as *riding the basal*. Since no information is entered into the pump, but the person is still eating meals, only the background, or basal, insulin is being received. Basal insulin provides enough insulin to prevent the patient from having acidosis and becoming very sick but still allows high BG levels to induce weight loss through glycosuria (glucose in the urine). Frequent urinary tract infections can result from glycosuria.
5. Frequent pump rewind. The amount of insulin put into the reservoir of the pump should last 2–3 days. If the pump has been rewound more frequently than this, the patient might be administering air rather than insulin. A supervising adult should watch pump refills to be sure that the insulin is filling the tubing and drops out of the end of the infusion set prior to placing the set under the skin. Depending on the length of the tubing used, 8–16 units of insulin can be underdosed using this technique.

Besides reducing, omitting, delaying, or manipulating the amount of insulin given through injections or by the pump, there are other ways of making insulin ineffective or manipulating BG readings. All health-care practitioners should be alerted to the various techniques that patients might use to avoid getting a proper insulin dose.

Techniques used to disable or impair insulin absorption:

- "Disabling insulin"
  - Heat exposure (putting insulin vial in hot water on the stove top, or leaving in a hot car intentionally)
  - Light exposure (letting insulin vial sit on the windowsill or on the car dashboard)

- Microwaving (denatures the protein molecule rendering it useless)

- Impairing absorption
  - Injecting into areas of atrophy (areas of poor absorption due to lack of subcutaneous fat tissue)
  - Injecting into areas of induration (areas of hardened skin and fat tissue)
  - Injecting into areas of hyperlipotrophy (areas of raised fatty lumps from frequent injections/overuse)
  - *Leaking the shots* (pulling the needle out from under the skin and letting insulin drip out of the syringe)

Manipulation of blood glucose in order to fool others regarding BG levels:

- Using a control solution for "perfect" readings. The control solution is red or blue in color. Unfortunately, the red color is often used to "fake" a BG check. The patient prepares a drop of the solution on the finger instead of their own blood and then tests BG in front of a parent or loved one to artificially prove normal BG range. However, it is important to note that having BG ranges within normal limits is difficult to achieve; therefore, perfect BG records should be suspect for having been manipulated or altered.
- Using a drop of alcohol on test strip.
- Diluting blood with water prior to testing.
- Using diluted orange juice instead of blood.
- Using ketchup instead of blood (reads 175 on glucometer and it is red).

RISKS OF ED-DM1

It is recommended that clinicians, physicians, educators, and parents continually assess for signs of disordered eating or a developing eating disorder in a person with diabetes. Likewise, people with eating disorders should be assessed for any problems with blood sugar or possible diabetes.

Although there is some debate about the rate of ED-DM1, most research identifies DM1 as a significant risk factor for disordered eating (Colton et al. 2004; Jones et al. 2000; Peveler et al. 1992; Rydall et al. 1997) and/or the development of a clinically diagnosable eating disorder (Jones 2000; Mannucci et al. 2005). One study reported young women with DM1 have 2.4 times more risk of developing an eating disorder than women of the same age without diabetes (Jones et al. 2000). Similarly, the University of Toronto researchers found that girls with DM1 are two to three times more likely to develop an eating disorder than their nondiabetic peers (Peveler et al. 1992). Another study found the rate of disordered eating and eating disorders in female teenagers with DM1 to be nearly double that of teens without diabetes (Jones 2000). Furthermore, children are developing eating disorders at younger and younger ages (Zhao and Encinosa 2011) and those with diabetes may be at an additional risk.

In a case-controlled study of young girls with DM1, girls as young as 9 years old were found to be at an increased risk for disordered eating when compared to non-diabetic children of the same age group (Colton et al. 2004).

CONTRIBUTIONS TO THE DEVELOPMENT OF ED-DM1

There is no specific research that can point to the exact etiology of what we are calling ED-DM1 but many factors can be considered as possible contributions to this complex disorder. We list a summary of these factors followed by a more detailed description.

Possible risk factors for developing ED-DM1:

1. Weight loss at onset of diabetes and weight gain with use of insulin
2. Dietary restraint due to management of blood sugar
3. Learning to base one's eating on external rather than internal cues
4. Exercise being promoted as a glucose control aid
5. Increased incidence of depression in diabetics (Anderson et al. 2001; Silverstein et al. 2005)
6. Availability of deliberate insulin omission as a weight-loss strategy

1. Weight loss at onset of diabetes and weight gain with use of insulin

People with diabetes quickly learn the connection between insulin use and weight gain. Individuals diagnosed with DM1 often notice weight loss prior to their diagnosis. Once diagnosed, these individuals are encouraged to engage in intensive insulin management. Since insulin is an anabolic hormone, it is often associated with weight gain due to the insulin causing the body to store glucose as fat if caloric needs are exceeded (DCCT Research Group 1988; The Diabetes Control and Complications Trial Research Group 1993). In our appearance-focused, thin-obsessed culture, weight gain is often difficult to accept and tolerate, even if a person is restoring to a healthy weight. The heightened attention to food along with any weight gain that occurs after starting insulin therapy can put diabetics at risk for developing an eating disorder.

2. Dietary restraint due to management of blood sugar

The necessary attention that has to be paid to meal planning, food portions (especially carbohydrates), blood sugars, weight, and exercise in the management of diabetes may promote or enhance the kind of rigid and obsessive thinking about food that is characteristic of women and men who develop eating disorders.

3. Learning to base one's eating on external rather than internal cues

With diabetes, food and meal times can become mechanical and unpleasant. Eating becomes ruled by external versus internal cues. Rather than providing pleasure and nourishment, eating can feel robotic and/or filled with conflict and distress. Having to count carbohydrates, test blood sugars, and inject insulin can create frustration, resentment, and resistance. All of the essential tasks for managing the diabetes can become "the enemy." Some individuals fight or rebel against the illness, and the necessary tasks of managing the diabetes, in an attempt to create a sense of autonomy or control or as a way of expressing their anger. People with eating disorders often share this dynamic of seeking a sense of control by controlling their food and weight.

4. **Exercise being promoted as a glucose control aid**
   People with diabetes are told they need to exercise as an additional tool to manage their BG. The emphasis on exercise for blood-sugar control may contribute to an obsession with exercise as a way to get rid of calories after eating, which is a cardinal feature of certain individuals with bulimia nervosa.

5. **Increased incidence of depression in diabetics**
   As cited above, there is an increased incidence of depression in individuals with diabetes. When added to other risk factors, the presence of depression or other disturbance in mood may increase the risk of developing an eating disorder in an already susceptible person with diabetes (DCCT Research Group 1988; The Diabetes Control and Complications Trial Research Group 1993).

6. **Availability of deliberate insulin omission as a weight-loss strategy**
   Insulin restriction is an easy way to limit caloric absorption and lose weight. The easy accessibility of insulin restriction to patients with diabetes provides what can seem like a relatively painless and simple way of getting rid of calories. One does not have to restrict food or purge via vomiting or laxatives. Like any eating disorder behavior, insulin restriction can become habitual and difficult to discontinue for susceptible individuals. Additionally, insulin restriction in people with diabetes seems to peak in late adolescence and early adulthood (Polonsky et al. 1994) which also coincides with the age range at the highest risk of developing an eating disorder (Hudson et al. 2007; Patton et al. 1999).

Many people with diabetes experiment with restricting insulin and engage in disordered eating behaviors (Goebel-Fabbri et al. 2008). Not all of these individuals develop an eating disorder but in certain susceptible individuals, a vicious cycle is quickly created as in the following example.

CASE STUDY

Shelly was obsessed with her weight and was being teased about being fat by her peers at school. Although she had been diagnosed with diabetes, Shelly so wanted to lose weight that she would intermittently restrict her food, which led to hypoglycemia (low BG), or she would eat but restrict her insulin, which led to hyperglycemia (high BG). Whether Shelly restricted food or insulin she would become intensely hungry, since in both cases the cells of her body were not getting the fuel she needed to support proper functioning. When Shelly felt the intense hunger she became anxious and depressed because she did not want to break down and eat. She always

(Continued)

worried that she would eat too much. Eventually, she would break down and eat, and usually end up bingeing, which caused even more anxiety and depression. Shelly felt bad about herself and her inability to control her urges for food. After overeating or bingeing, she knew she needed to take her insulin, but her disgust with herself for breaking down and eating, combined with her fear of weight gain, interfered with her doing so. Shelly would tell herself that she needed to "get rid" of excess food by restricting her insulin but would promise herself to get in better control of her eating. Unfortunately, restricting her insulin would cause her to become overwhelmed by hunger again and lose control of her eating, thus repeating the cycle over and over.

DETECTING ED-DM1

Individuals with ED-DM1, like others with disordered eating behaviors, usually keep their behaviors and their symptoms hidden and typically deny them when confronted with suspicions or even evidence. In order to avoid being recognized as someone who deliberately restricts insulin, people with ED-DM1 usually claim that they forgot their insulin or got too busy and took it late. They "forget" to bring their BG records to medical appointments and manipulate their BG meters or purposely leak their insulin.

Furthermore, what can make detection even harder is that people with ED-DM1 can appear to have normal eating behaviors and may even present as enthusiastic eaters. Unlike those with AN, these individuals usually do not delay eating by playing around with food, refusing to eat certain foods, or avoiding dietary fat. Unlike those with bulimia, they may not ever take laxatives or purge. People with ED-DM1 may eat normally, overeat, or binge with the plan to avoid absorbing the calories they consume if they restrict their insulin. When treating anyone with an eating disorder or diabetes, it is important to look for warning signs and to have the right knowledge and tools to do so.

The Diabetes Eating Problem Survey (DEPS-R; Markowitz et al. 2010) is an important tool to screen for eating problems and eating disorders specifically in the diabetic population. Other ED screenings ask questions about behaviors such as eating when not hungry or preoccupation with food. These may suggest disordered eating in the general population but are natural manifestations of DM1. Furthermore, the current generic eating disorder assessment tools do not assess for diabetes-specific problem behaviors such as insulin restriction. The DEPS-R is easy to administer and takes less than 10 minutes to complete. Since disordered eating can severely impair metabolic control, accelerate the development of diabetes complications, and is associated with increased mortality, this assessment tool should be added to standard diabetes care. Furthermore, since this screening tool indicated that nearly one in five children and adolescents with DM1 and one in four females has disturbed eating behavior, adolescents should be screened annually.

WARNING SIGNS OF ED-DM1

Clinicians, other health practitioners, educators, and parents should be aware of the following indicators which might be predictive of, or signal, an eating disorder in individuals with DM1:

- Changes in and preoccupation with food intake and/or eating habits
- Hoarding or hiding food
- Eating normally or even more than usual but still losing weight
- Preoccupation with body image and weight
- Rapid weight loss or weight gain
- Not wanting to eat around people
- Despite the appearance of compliance, poor metabolic control
- Unexplained elevations in HbA1c values
- Recurrent diabetic ketoacidosis
- Frequent urination, excessive thirst or drinking, high blood-sugar levels
- Frequent episodes of thrush/urine infections
- Low energy, fatigue, shakiness, irritability, confusion, anxiety, or even fainting
- Purging behaviors (such as vomiting, excessive exercise, or laxative use)
- Fear of injecting insulin, not injecting in front of other people
- Making excuses for forgetting insulin or frequently miscalculating amounts
- Unwillingness to follow through with medical appointments
- Frequent hospitalizations for poor blood-sugar control
- Delay in puberty or sexual maturation or irregular menses/amenorrhea
- Early onset of diabetic complications particularly neuropathy (peripheral nerve damage), retinopathy (damage to the retina of the eye), gastroparesis (impaired gastrointestinal [GI] motility), and nephropathy (kidney damage)
- Co-occurrence of depression, anxiety, or other psychological disturbance
- Overexaggerated fear of hypoglycemia
- Continually requesting new meters (for the control solution)
- Avoidance of diabetes-related health appointments
- Lack of blood-sugar testing/reluctance to test
- Over-or undert-reating hypoglycemic episodes
- A fundamental belief that insulin makes you fat
- Assigning moral qualities to food (i.e., good sugars/bad sugars)
- An encyclopedic knowledge of the carbohydrate content of foods
- Persistent requests for weight-loss medications
- If concurrent with hypothyroidism—abuse of levothyroxine
- Metformin abuse secondary to omission
- Nausea and stomach cramps
- Hair loss
- Delayed healing from infections/bruises
- Easy bruising
- Dehydration
- Dry skin

- Dental problems
- Blurred vision
- Osteopenia (low bone density) or recent history of fractures
- Iron deficiency anemia/other deficiencies

TREATMENT FOR ED-DM1

Treatment for someone with ED-DM1 calls for clinicians familiar with evidenced-based treatments for eating disorders as well as the management of diabetes. Both illnesses have to be considered when treating these individuals. Whether the patient can be treated on an outpatient basis or needs a more structured intensive program must be assessed by qualified professionals. Both the psychiatric condition of the patient and the medical condition need to be considered as does motivation and ability of the patient to care for himself or herself properly.

The patient needs to be assessed for the appropriate modality as well as level of care. For example, family-based treatment or the Maudsley approach has been shown to outperform other treatment modalities for young patients with AN (Lock et al. 2010). If the ED-DM1 patient is an adolescent with AN, a good assessment can indicate whether or not family-based treatment would be appropriate or whether the patient needs something more. Ongoing assessment of the treatment is necessary as well. The complication with diabetes makes it dangerous to continue treatment that is not working. It is very common that the complication of diabetes will warrant at least a residential level of care.

A multidisciplinary team approach is necessary at any level of care, including a physician specializing in diabetes, a psychiatrist for psychopharmacologic evaluation and treatment, psychotherapists to provide individual and family therapy, and a registered dietitian with experience and training in both the treatment of DM1 and eating disorders.

A medical exam including blood tests and other assessments also needs to be done to help determine the level of care needed. Routine lab tests include sodium, potassium, bicarbonate, blood urea nitrogen, creatinine, calcium, magnesium, phosphorus, liver enzymes, complete blood count with differential, and an erythrocyte sedimentation rate. Endocrine labs (luteinizing hormone, follicle stimulating hormone, and prolactin) to check for amenorrhea or lack of menstrual period should be ordered. An electrocardiogram (EKG) should be performed not only to check for a low heart rate (bradycardia) but also to rule out an irregular or prolonged QTc interval >0.44 seconds which would warrant hospitalization. The following is a list of other indications that hospitalization is necessary:

Criteria for Hospitalization

- Bradycardia: heart rate <45 beats per minute
- Prolonged QTc interval >0.44 seconds
- Orthostatic drop in systolic BP >10 mmHg or increase in pulse >35 bpm
- Hypothermia: temperature <96.6°F
- Hypokalemia: potassium <3.0 mEq/L
- Severe malnutrition: weight <75% ideal body weight (IBW)

OUTPATIENT TREATMENT

Outpatient treatment may involve seeing individual practitioners on a weekly basis or attending an intensive outpatient program (IOP) which could be a few hours a day or up to 8 hours a day. Patients with ED-DM1 may be seen on an outpatient basis but will require more medical monitoring than patients with either illness alone due to the complex issues involved when the two illnesses are combined. Laboratory tests (especially HbA1c and electrolytes) and weight checks should occur routinely and be shared with all the treating professionals. In order to provide the best quality treatment, open and frequent communication between team members is critical. As with any person with an eating disorder, a person with ED-DM1 may be an unreliable historian. Education about diabetes and the serious nature of restricting insulin or not managing it properly is an ethical responsibility for providers. Although the individual with ED-DM1 may dislike or resist being monitored, health and safety must come first. If the person is an adolescent, it is imperative to work with parents or guardians and welcome their involvement in the treatment team unless there is a serious reason to indicate otherwise. Until it can be established that the individual is getting the correct amount of insulin and keeping BG levels in the appropriate range, someone other than just the patient should monitor food, blood sugars, and insulin doses.

TESTING AND MONITORING BLOOD GLUCOSE AND INSULIN

Ketone Testing

All individuals with DM1 should have ketone test strips. When BG is elevated, the body is unable to use the glucose in the blood due to a lack of insulin. Muscle tissue breaks down, converting into a group of compounds collectively known as "ketone bodies." Before the advent of glucometer use, most diabetics could only tell when their BG was elevated by urinating on a ketone test strip. Generally, a high level is anything over 200 mg/dL (normal BG is 70–120 mg/dL). Some physicians will ask their patients to check for ketones at a BG of >250 mg/dL, and some may recommend testing when the BG is >350 or 400 mg/dL. This discrepancy happens when a person runs elevated BG levels often and has been noted to not develop ketones until a much higher number. This type of information is known by diabetes educators and practitioners but often members of the person's treatment team such as the psychologist, psychiatrist, nurse, dietitian, and even the physician, do not know this kind of information. For example, the most common form of ketone test strip abuse is using expired test strips. A parent may notice that BG seems to be elevated and ask the teen to check for ketones. By using expired test strips, the person can easily "prove" they are not in acidosis. When monitoring a patient, it is important to ensure the test strips are still good and not expired. Even better, there are more effective glucometers available that can use a blood sample rather than urine to check for ketone bodies.

Glucometers

Most diabetics and certainly all insulin-dependent diabetics will have a glucometer. This tiny device is palm sized and is used with test strips and a control solution.

There are many different brands of glucometers on the market. The small test strip is inserted into the glucometer and a tiny drop of blood is added to the end of the test strip. The BG result is displayed on a screen. The control solution is a liquid that is used to calibrate the glucometer, the result of the control solution is usually within a normal BG range 80–130 mg/dL (some meters vary).

Glucometers can be downloaded with a computer program or uploaded onto the Internet using a dongle, radio frequency, or flash drive that works with that particular glucometer brand. Patients should be asked to bring the printed reports for the health practitioner to see if the health-care center is unable to download. Practitioners should have a release form on file in order to legally share and review information between providers on the treatment team. If the patient does not have a computer, BG checks can be easily reviewed by using the history button or back button on the glucometer.

Blood Glucose Range

Patients usually check BG ranges four times a day: first thing in the morning prior to eating, before lunch, before dinner, and before bed. These are optimal times to check BG and give insulin, to adjust BG levels, and/or to cover for food eaten at the snack or meal. Frequent "forgetting" or omission of BG checks can be an indicator that the patient is trying to purposefully avoid documenting high BG.

HgbA1c Percentage

This test is used to give the patient and the health-care practitioner a good idea of the patient's general BG control for approximately 3 months prior to the test. *Hgb* is a symbol for *hemoglobin*. Hemoglobin is a protein in red blood cells that carries oxygen. *A1c* stands for the particle of the protein that is measured to indicate the degree of glucose exposure to the hemoglobin. If the BG has been elevated for a long duration, the HgbA1c level will be reflectively high. The most common finding for individuals with diabetes who also have an eating disorder is a high A1c. Typical goal A1c values depend on the age of patient and the type of diabetes. An A1c of <8.0% or <7.0% are typical goals. It is not uncommon to find A1c as high as >14% or >20%, and on rare occasions the levels are so dangerously elevated that the lab cannot detect a number. People with ED-DM1 have high A1c levels because they "purge" through insulin restriction. Simply omitting insulin while eating adequate food is an easy way of "purging" calories, much more comfortable and unnoticeable than other purging alternatives. An A1c that is normal or only slightly elevated can occur when BG levels are alternating between periods of high and low. BG may be elevated when a person binges on food and then "purges" with insulin omission. The BG level may also be low when insulin is given and food is restricted. When being monitored by others, patients with ED-DM1 often restrict food in order to drop their BG to a low, "but not too low" level, trying to find a "perfect time" to check their BG that makes the glucometer download look optimal and decreases the A1c%. This type of behavior causes a "roller coaster" of BG levels in the body and is very dangerous due to an increase in the frequency of severe hypoglycemia. After many events of severe hypoglycemia, people develop a condition called *hypoglycemia unawareness* where they become desensitized to and fail to perceive their blood sugar being low. Hypoglycemia unawareness is very dangerous and is a cause for sudden hypoglycemic death.

There is some benefit to testing HgbA1c more frequently than every 3 months. Because the test is more heavily weighted to the last month of BG control, healthcare practitioners can easily see an improvement if tested every month. Some patients may be unwilling to have their blood drawn this frequently, especially if they must pay for the expense outside of insurance reimbursement.

Insulin Pump

The insulin pump provides people with diabetes a convenient method for adjusting insulin needs more precisely. The pump can also store information that can be retrieved such as the amount of carbohydrates eaten at a snack or meal, the amount of insulin given to cover the food eaten, and BG information including any adjustments for high blood sugar that were needed. Keep in mind the precautions discussed earlier in the chapter regarding the manipulation of pump readings.

MEAL PLANS, EATING, AND EXERCISE

A structured meal plan provided by a dietitian in collaboration with the patient is important, especially in the beginning of treatment. Prescribing a meal plan is challenging because the person's eating disordered thoughts and behaviors may interfere with their ability to follow a diabetes meal plan, which can cause medical problems. If fear of weight gain trumps the need for insulin, people with ED-DM1 may put themselves at significant risk by restricting insulin. Individuals with a history of diabetes who develop an eating disorder have already spent time having to monitor and control their food and may express resentment about any imposed structure, lack of freedom, or monitoring, all of which are necessary to get ED-DM1 symptoms under control. Furthermore, dietitians (and other members of the treatment team) need to find a balance between asking someone with diabetes to count carbohydrates, insulin doses, and blood-sugar levels while at the same time trying to minimize the focus on calories and weight.

Initial meal plans for those with diabetes usually need to provide a different kind of structure than for those with eating disorders, especially depending on the type of eating disorder. For example, the dietitian is usually not concerned with someone with AN eating too many carbohydrates. Meal planning for those with ED-DM1 is more difficult and time consuming as many factors must be taken into account. Developing components like calorie ranges and the plan for eating and covering carbohydrates must be individualized for the ED-DM1 person. Much care is needed to explain things to the patient, get feedback, and check for understanding, willingness, motivation, and compliance. It is important not to let either diagnosis interfere with the other. For example, people with ED-DM1 might try to overly restrict carbohydrates using their diabetes as the reason. It is important to continually remind them about how to "cover," rather than restrict, their carbohydrates. On another note, it is easy for the treatment team to become overly concerned with variations in blood-sugar levels such that the food and BG monitoring becomes obsessive. During weight gain, BG levels will fluctuate more than normal and this must be allowed to happen without becoming overly alarmed.

If weight gain is indicated, resistance is to be expected as it is in any person with an eating disorder. Common justifications for not gaining weight or not finishing meals include statements such as "Portions are too large," "I'm not hungry," or "I don't like the food." If weight gain becomes problematic, guide the patient to consume protein and starch food items first and then finish with the lower calorie ones like green vegetables. Although green vegetables are healthy, it is common for someone with an eating disorder to gravitate toward this type of lower calorie food in lieu of other higher calorie foods. It might even be necessary to temporarily limit the amount of nonstarchy vegetable or salad items, if the patient is not able to consume the adequate amount of calories necessary.

The ED-DM1 sufferer will have an intense focus on weight. It is important to remember to help the individual place their focus on restoring health physically and emotionally. Discourage the consumption of any diet/fat free foods such as rice cakes, fat free milk, fat free salad dressing, and so on. These foods not only support a diet mentality but it is better for anyone with high blood-sugar problems to keep the added fat in their diet and even add fat to their meals to slow the rise in blood sugar after a meal. Reduce excessive consumption of diet soda, caffeinated drinks, or water, keeping in mind that excessive drinking is a way to create a false sense of being full without eating.

Exercise is important for everyone and is particularly good for helping control blood sugar but for those with ED-DM1, exercise can be another way to seek weight loss or avoid weight gain. Exercise improves the body's response to insulin and should be monitored closely in those who are taking insulin or hypoglycemic medication due to increased risk of hypoglycemia. Encourage consistency in the time of day a person exercises to promote greater consistency in BG. Note that a person with ED-DM1 may want to exercise right before or after meals to compensate for the calories eaten. This should be discouraged as it may strengthen disordered thinking around food, exercise, and BG. Additionally, if hypoglycemia is a concern, exercise should be avoided within 2 hours of a meal. Finally, insulin users may want to avoid exercise prior to bedtime as it may induce hypoglycemia during sleep, which can be a particularly dangerous situation. It may be advisable to check BG a few times in the middle of the sleep cycle to monitor the effect of exercise on BG. Limit exercise to 30–60 minutes per day, preferably low-impact exercise such as walking, biking, or swimming. Walking is the preferred type of exercise since it promotes well-being and improves strength and cardiovascular health.

Different types of exercise (aerobic vs. anaerobic) may have varying impacts on BG. Activities like CrossFit and interval training are largely anaerobic activities, which induce the production of glucagon, a hormone that triggers an increase in BG. This rise in BG may last for several hours after exercise, potentially necessitating the administration of additional insulin. Biking and/or swimming should only be allowed if the patient is willing to check BG prior to exercise. Low BG, or hypoglycemia, will increase risk of injury.

If the patient is on a weight gain plan but is unable to gain weight, or purging is suspected, ask the patient to use the bathroom prior to eating and then supervise bathroom use for 1 hour after eating. This helps control for purging and supports the digestion and metabolism of food and energy into the body. However, this should be a short-term intervention in outpatient treatment because if this kind of monitoring continues to be necessary then a referral for 24-hour care would be appropriate.

USE OF OTHER SUBSTANCES

Be sure to ask patients if they are taking any over-the-counter, illegal, or prescription drugs. If suspected, the treatment team might need to search for possession of these substances which should be banned from the treatment program. It might be appropriate for parents who have strong suspicions to look for appetite suppressants, herbal or caffeine containing stimulants, laxatives, sleep aids, amphetamines, glucose pills, marijuana, or other drugs. Parents have reported finding these items hidden in their child's room, and patients have been known to sneak all of these substances into treatment centers.

TREATMENT TIPS FOR THE CHILD/TEEN AT HOME

Have a parent or other adult (not a sibling) take responsibility for BG checks. Have the parent check the child or teen themselves, making a simple statement such as "It's time to check your blood sugar" or "We need to get a blood-sugar level." Often patients will resist this and try to check it themselves. If someone is trying to restrict insulin, this will typically be a time when the test strip is altered by a substance other than the patient's own blood. Other evasive behaviors include turning their back to the adult, "accidentally" dropping the meter, asking to do the check in the bathroom or bedroom, or stating that the meter needs "recalibration with control solution."

The treatment team should devise a plan to be carried out at school where the child or adolescent must go to the nurse's office or health technician for BG checks and observation of insulin administration by either pump or injection. A physician's signature may be necessary for the school to implement the plan. If the patient is on an insulin pump, the adult supervising will have to wait with the patient until the full amount of insulin is delivered. This can take several minutes and the patient might try to make excuses to run off before all the insulin is distributed. Patients who do this are often seeking to simply unplug the pump tubing from the infusion set that goes into the skin, thus leaking insulin out rather than having it go in the body. If this happens, checking the pump download will not show a missed dose or underdosing. For this reason, it is important while at school and at home that someone else is observing the full insulin delivery.

Clinicians need to spend time educating and preparing parents to be good monitors but do not assume the parent will be able to comply with treatment recommendations. Be sure to fully assess for how the monitoring is going and allow parents to be honest. Sometimes, it is too difficult for the parent, or the parent is not willing, to monitor the food, blood sugar, and insulin dosing. Parents might be too busy with work, have to travel away from home, or might not understand the seriousness of the disorder or the lengths their child may go to in order to restrict insulin. In any case where home monitoring is difficult or problematic, the treatment team, including a medical doctor, can write the school plan to include that long-acting insulin be administered at school, usually by a nurse. However, weekends will still be problematic if home monitoring and supervision is not taking place effectively. If problems persist or the home situation interferes with the person's ability to recover, then a higher level of care is likely needed.

OUTPATIENT TREATMENT TIPS FOR THE ADULT

Even with adults who have ED-DM1, it is important to have someone else help with monitoring BG and insulin use. With the patient's consent, ask a friend or other responsible adult to take responsibility for monitoring BG checks. Reassure both the patient and the significant other that this is not a long-term solution but a temporary step to help the patient get the blood sugar and other symptoms under control.

Meet with the significant other to help educate about ED-DM1 as well as how to monitor and provide support. Teach significant others about the psychological aspects of the illness and the fear that patients experience so that they can be understanding and compassionate. Educate significant others on the various ways in which patients try to manipulate insulin. Teach them to watch for any of these signs and discuss the importance of reporting this information to the treatment team. Furthermore, train significant others on strategies for how to best respond to various circumstances.

It is important to have joint sessions with the patient and the spouse or significant other. A variety of feelings and issues are bound to surface and should be discussed in these joint sessions. Eventually, as the patient's symptoms are under control, the monitoring can be reduced (although it must be restarted if the BG level again goes out of control or the patient is found restricting insulin).

TYPES OF THERAPY FOR A PERSON WITH ED-DM1

The ED-DM1 patient can likely benefit from a combination of individual, group, and family therapy. The goals of these three therapeutic modalities are the same as those described for use with patients who have eating disorders and are detailed in numerous other chapters in this book. However, there are a few nuances for the ED-DM1 patient listed below.

Individual Therapy

It is important for the ED-DM1 patient to have an individual therapist in order to work on aspects of the eating disorder unique to the concurrent diagnosis of diabetes. For example, resentments involving the paradoxical messages they encounter, such as "Count carbs appropriately, but don't get too obsessed with them," might be better dealt with in individual rather than group therapy. Additionally, these patients have many factors to deal with that other eating disorder patients do not have, such as BG monitoring and insulin dosing that may be understandable only to them and not relevant to other patients in a group setting. Unlike eating disorder patients who can fully recover, ED-DM1 patients will not ever be able to leave their DM diagnosis behind.

Group Therapy

Often the ED-DM1 individual feels different from other group members in an eating disorder treatment setting. These patients routinely make comments such as "I am different from all of you, I can't just eat dessert and not worry about it," "Unlike you all, I have to restrict my carbohydrates," "I don't have an eating disorder, I have complications from my diabetes," "I'm not like any of you, you don't see me pushing my food around on a plate," or "No one here can possibly understand me." It is important that ED-DM1 patients be able to express their feelings in group and other settings but learn how to do it in a way that does not turn others off or alienate them from their peers, parents, friends, and treatment providers. It is also important for group therapists to highlight what the ED-DM1 patient does have in common with other eating disorder patients (i.e., body image issues, fear of weight gain, the use of unhealthy behaviors to control food and weight). A good group therapist will be able to help bring out issues of comparison, competition, and resentment. Other group participants who do not have diabetes may feel the ED-DM1 patient is getting special treatment or they may be triggered by a discussion around counting carbs. Group therapy can help those with ED-DM1 find a way of incorporating their symptom management and communication about it into their social and everyday life.

Family Therapy

A person's family can be an integral part of successful treatment at any age. Having families involved by helping to support or monitor food and weight can be a critical aspect of successful recovery. Monitoring may be necessary due to the medical risks associated with diabetes alone and even more so with ED-DM1. Family members can either support or sabotage the patient's recovery, and it is immensely helpful if they can learn how best to do the former and avoid the latter. A family involved in treatment can learn how to best assist and encourage the patient and how best to monitor and set limits in age-appropriate ways. Family members need help too and may need to process their own feelings of frustration, anger, or fear.

OTHER OUTPATIENT THERAPY CONSIDERATIONS

During the course of outpatient treatment, it is important for clinicians, treatment team members, significant others, and patients to openly discuss the common issues we discuss in this chapter and the ones that are individual to each patient. Having good, supportive, and nonjudgmental role models is helpful. Empathy and understanding go a long way.

Patients and their families also need to be warned of possible consequences for continued behaviors or problems. For example, if a patient is out of control with blood sugars and/or has fainted, it might be appropriate to revoke driving privileges for a period of time. Any insulin-dependent person with diabetes is at risk for severe hypoglycemia and fainting. We have had many patients who reported having "dozed off" while driving. In fact, if frequent hypoglycemia or severe hypoglycemia is detected, it is the physician's obligation to report this information to the Department of Motor Vehicles (DMV). Reinstatement of driving can be achieved with demonstrated optimal BG control.

If the regulation of blood sugars continues to be problematic or eating disorder behaviors continue to be detected, a referral to a residential or inpatient eating disorder treatment program should be made where 24-hour care can be provided. This should be discussed ahead of time to prepare patients and families for this possibility.

CASE STUDY 10.2

Maria

Maria was diagnosed with DM1 when she was 11 years old, at a height of 5'5" and weight of 133 lb. Her body mass index (BMI) was above the 95% for her age. She presented with frequent thirst and urination, a 5 lb. weight loss, and fatigue. At the initial doctor's visit, Maria was negative for urine ketones and it was thought she might have DM2 but her lab tests indicated that she had markers for DM1 including pancreatic islet-cell antibodies. Maria and her family were educated on the use of insulin, both long-acting and short-acting, counting carbohydrates, and monitoring BG.

Maria did very well keeping her BG into a desirable target range until age 13, when she came to a diabetes clinic with a more than 20 lb. weight loss.

Maria insisted that she was not dieting to lose weight, but rather had changed her eating habits and cut out junk food in order to have a healthier diet for clear skin and silky hair. However, her HgbA1c was markedly elevated at 11% despite BG checks that were within normal limits. The treatment team questioned if somehow the BG checks belonged to someone else or if she had manipulated her BG reading in any way, which she adamantly denied.

A month later, while meeting with one of the diabetes educators, Maria broke down in tears, admitting that she had faked her BG reading by using the control solution because she wanted to lose weight as well as appease her parents, despite knowing she was hurting her body and did not feel well. She reported being desperate to lose weight, "to look good in her cheerleading uniform." Maria tearfully promised not to do this again and agreed to take her BG checks with real blood and take insulin as directed as long her parents allowed her to continue with cheerleading.

Over the next 6 months, Maria ate a high calorie, high carbohydrate diet and gained 25 lb. The weight gain upset Maria tremendously and triggered further eating disorder behaviors. Over the next 3 years, Maria's weight continued to cycle as she alternated between limiting her food intake, restricting her insulin, overeating, and bingeing. Once again she was unable to admit she had continued to tamper with her insulin. A recommendation to find a therapist was continually suggested by the diabetes educator. Both Maria and her mother felt that they could handle things without additional

(Continued)

CASE STUDY 10.2 (CONTINUED)

help. However, Maria was caught in a cycle which overwhelmed her. On one hand, she wanted to take her insulin and keep BG ranges in good control and please her family and her medical team. On the other hand, she felt envious of the other slender and fit girls on the cheer team and on campus felt compelled to restrict insulin in order to lose weight. She promised herself that once the weight was off, she would be able to control her carbohydrate cravings and keep it off.

Maria's behavior did not improve and eventually at age 16 she changed to a new diabetes clinic, where her team consisted of a pediatric endocrinologist, a registered nurse/diabetes educator, a dietitian/diabetes educator, and a mental health specialist. This team, familiar with ED-DM1, met with Maria and her family and educated them about the combination of insulin-dependent diabetes and an eating disorder and diagnosed Maria with this serious combination of illnesses. They recommended that Maria and her family attend an IOP.

The family was surprised to learn of the severity and insidious nature of Maria's condition. They had attributed her high BG ranges as a sign of being a lazy teenager. It was difficult for them to understand that she had continued to intentionally give herself less insulin, consciously making her BG high and damaging her health. However, Maria and her family agreed to attend the program.

Maria attended the group sessions and met weekly with a therapist for individual therapy; the entire family attended weekly family therapy sessions. Once a week, Maria also came to medical appointments, where her weight, vitals, and blood tests were taken. Sometimes, a urinary analysis would be performed to detect fasting or "water loading" (this result is seen in a low specific gravity of the urine, an indication of dilution of urine with excess water). These weekly tests were routine for everyone and Maria grew accustomed to meeting with the medical assistants, nurses, and dietitian.

Initially, Maria resented having to have so many appointments. She was unhappy that she had to miss some school and had less time to do homework and spend time with her friends. However, the program helped Maria learn about herself and her illness. She also learned how she dealt with her frustration and other feelings and improved greatly in her ability to relate to others. Maria and her family learned to communicate better and collaborate with each other with less conflict and fighting. Rather than being impatient about having to remind her to check her blood sugar and take her insulin shots, her parents learned how to listen to her, validate her feelings, and help her follow the treatment team's advice. Even her sister was included in being part of Maria's support system.

Maria was also able to share a common bond with the other teens in the program. She realized that although none of them had diabetes, they were all struggling with weight and distorted body image and had developed disordered eating habits in order to control their weight. This helped her admit and work on the eating disorder aspects of her illness. After 6 months

(Continued)

in the IOP program, Maria was able to graduate from the program having accomplished her goals. She was following her meal plan, taking insulin as directed, checking her BG with the appropriate frequency, maintaining her blood sugars correctly, and keeping her weight in the appropriate range. She also seemed happier and was able to verbalize her feelings in a more constructive way.

GUIDELINES FOR INPATIENT OR RESIDENTIAL TREATMENT

An inpatient or residential treatment eating disorder program may be needed for an individual with ED-DM1 to stabilize symptoms and ensure the patient is medically and psychologically stable enough to successfully engage in treatment without around-the-clock care. The staff of the treatment center should all be educated on the specialized treatment of ED-DM1. Many of the things described in the outpatient treatment section can apply in residential or inpatient treatment but with the patient under 24-hour care, there is a much more controlled environment and the patient can be prevented from engaging in certain behaviors, some of which could be dangerous. However, the treatment team needs to be knowledgeable on how best to treat, empathize with, supervise, and monitor patients in these settings.

SPECIAL CONSIDERATIONS FOR THE INPATIENT OR RESIDENTIAL ED-DM1 PATIENT (MAY BE USED AS GUIDELINES FOR STAFF)

1. Treat the person similar to a patient with bulimia; that is, just as you would ensure the patient is not purging by using observations after meals or locked bathrooms, make sure that insulin is not being misused or manipulated. Dietitians and nurses need to monitor carbohydrate counts and test blood sugars. Nurses should give the insulin injections. Patients with ED-DM1 have often been giving themselves shots for years and will do everything they can to convince the treatment team that taking away their ability to give themselves the shots is taking away their dignity. It is important to not let the patient be in control of the injections, at least in the beginning of treatment. A treatment goal could be for the patient to eventually take over their own injections but the health regulations and protocols of this must be checked in the individual treatment setting.

2. Patients with ED-DM1 will present differently than other eating disorder patients. Their eating behaviors seem more normal than other patients. Keep in mind that since individuals with ED-DM1 can restrict their insulin to lose weight, they may present as atypical around food compared to other patients with eating disorders.

3. The person with ED-DM1 will need to have labs, vitals, urine, et cetera tested periodically to evaluate how blood sugars are being managed, and how they are medically, and how they are progressing. If the person has to

gain weight it is probable that blood sugars will widely fluctuate and this needs to be tolerated. A knowledgeable physician who treats diabetes will be needed to help determine appropriate levels of BG fluctuation.

4. Be understanding but firm as you would with patients who have AN and who try to avoid weight gain in any way they can. Do not trust the ED-DM1 patient to tell you the truth about his or her blood sugars, insulin needs, or insulin injections. Be aware that using a BG meter or an insulin pump will not help ensure honesty and compliance as they can rig or otherwise manipulate their BG meters and pumps. To better understand and treat these patients, it is helpful to know that they often admit to having thoughts that their insulin injections are "shots of fat," "calorie injections," or "weigh gain serum." Knowing this should increase empathy and understanding for the patient.

5. Be prepared and prepare the client for the weight gain associated with reinstating the proper regimen and dosing of insulin. Patients need to be taught to identify insulin edema, which may make them feel fat, bloated, and uncomfortable, as temporary water retention that is different from the development of fatty tissue.

CASE STUDY 10.3

Carrie

Not every patient who has diabetes and an eating disorder restricts insulin. Carrie, a 25-year-old woman diagnosed with diabetes, became overly obsessed with food, began to binge, and became so frustrated with her lack of control over all of this she started purging. Carrie was admitted to residential treatment for BN as well as medical management and stabilization of her DM1. Carrie had been diagnosed with diabetes a few months earlier and reported no explanation from her doctors as to why she had become diabetic. She claimed she was not restricting her insulin but needed help because she was unable to manage her blood sugars due to her binge-purge episodes that started about 4 years earlier.

Carrie claims that prior to this, in high school, she briefly suffered from AN but gained weight and was better for 4 years after graduating.

On admission, Carrie's blood sugars were in the 300–400 range, and she reported this was customary for her postbingeing. Carrie said that her diabetes triggered her fear of carbohydrates and increased her obsession with food to the point that it reminded her of when she had suffered from AN. She said that in reality her negative thoughts about her weight and her body image had never completely gone away. She reported that dealing with her diabetes had quickly triggered her into "feeling fat" and wanting to lose weight. She reported being compliant with her insulin regimen but being unable to refrain from bingeing and purging.

(Continued)

The treatment team began to implement an aggressive sliding scale (Humalog insulin/short-acting and Lantus insulin/long-acting) and I:C ratio (carbohydrate count to insulin coverage). Her meal plan was devised with the registered dietician and included a moderate reduction in carbohydrates compared to the general patient's meal plan. Blood-sugar testing was done nine times daily including testing done in the middle of the night to manage nighttime lows. Glucose tablets were ordered to manage any blood-sugar dips that went too low. Carrie worked daily with the nurses and dietitian and gained confidence in choosing foods that were more appropriate for her diabetes while dealing with her hunger and fullness and achieving enough satisfactions to prevent cravings. Her sliding scale was modified frequently to accommodate shifts in her blood sugars, especially managing the lows. Carrie required much education about her condition. She was encouraged to join a diabetic support group to help her accept and incorporate her diabetes into her lifestyle. Carrie was open about her resentment toward her diagnosis and was able to process with the nursing staff and in her group and individual therapy sessions. Discussing her discomfort with her illness and the resentment she had for even having diabetes was a significant part of Carrie's treatment. A big part of her binge/purge episodes had to do with nonacceptance of, and even rebellion against, her situation. In therapy, Carrie learned the concept of acceptance versus resistance, which helped her to accept and respond to her illness rather than rebel and react. Once Carrie's eating was normalized and the binge/purge episodes stopped, Carrie's blood sugars stabilized. With increased freedom and responsibility for her blood sugars while still in residential treatment, Carrie demonstrated that she could manage her food and blood sugars on her own. With stable blood sugars, normalized eating, and remission of bingeing and purging, Carrie was able to discharge to a day treatment program.

SUMMARY OUTLINE FOR TREATMENT OF EDM1

- Medical assessment
  - Complications of DM
  - Complications of ED
- Psychiatric assessment
  - Psychiatric condition and stability
  - ED and other comorbidity diagnoses/treatment needs
  - Readiness for change
- Formalize diagnosis of ED-DM1 and appropriate level of care indicated
- Treatment (three phases): stabilize, manage, transition
  1. Stabilize = All care assumed by staff until patient is stable
  2. Manage = Collaborative/joint care by staff and patient
  3. Transition = Patient weans off supervision transitioning to self-care
- Initially aim for modest glucose control and gradually aim for "tighter control"

- Institute protocols for insulin management and testing for BG
- Consistency with protocols is imperative

PRINCIPLES FOR MANAGING THE ED-DM1 PATIENT

- Structure and monitoring (with the goal of returning self-care to the patient)
- Multidisciplinary expert team with experience in treating DM and ED
- Diabetic care retraining for patient and family with ED emphasis
- Educate and resolve diabetic exchanges versus actual grams of carbohydrates
- Help patient recognize "relative hypoglycemia"
- Address tendency to overcontrol, for example, obsessing on BG levels and overregulating
- Weight gain instituted with improved diabetic control
- No special foods provided
- Begin using treatment center's glucometers and insulin, later the patient's
- Discuss and determine benefits and risks of exercise and devise a plan
- Put in place a thorough discharge plan
- Advise patient and family about returning to the antirecovery environment that exists in the culture
- Identify red flags indicating relapse

FUTURE DIRECTIONS AND CONCLUSION

It is imperative that eating disorder and diabetes professionals inform each other and work together. Early detection and ongoing screening of all DM1 patients for ED will save lives and money and prevent suffering. Research into evidence-based approaches to modify diabetes education and management for individuals with increased risk for ED is an emerging area and will require attention from professionals working with this population. Some believe that research is needed to develop additional types of insulin that do not promote weight gain. However, many of the newer agents have the same potential for misuse as the older insulin agents so this may not be a feasible reality. There are also suggestions that ED-DM1 for possible inclusion in the next *Diagnostic and Statistical Manual of Mental Disorders (DSM)*.

An eating disorder coupled with diabetes represents a complex illness, difficult to treat both medically and psychologically. Many factors seem to influence the development of an eating disorder among patients with diabetes. Having to put extraordinary focus on what one is eating or not eating, counting carbohydrates, and having to take insulin are among the factors which increase risk. Since insulin affects the cells' ability to take in glucose for fuel, it greatly affects weight gain and loss, making it a powerful and tempting agent in one's ability to manipulate weight. An experienced team of health-care practitioners and support from friends and family members is essential in treating patients with ED-DM1. Outpatient, residential, and inpatient treatment providers who see patients with diabetes or eating disorders need to do a thorough assessment as well as continued monitoring of patients in order to ascertain who might have or be in danger of developing ED-DM1. They must also be prepared to properly treat patients who have this combined condition or be able to make appropriate referrals. Given the extent of the problem among individuals with diabetes, and the severe medical risks associated with it, further research aimed at understanding and preventing this combined illness as well as improving treatments is critical to the future health of this at-risk population.

REFERENCES

Anderson, RJ, Freedland KE, Clouse RE, and Lustman PJ. The prevalence of comorbid depression in adults with diabetes: A meta-analysis. *Diabetes Care* 24, no. 6 (2001): 1069–1078.

Colton, P, Olmsted M, Daneman D, Rydall A, and Rodin G. Disturbed eating behavior and eating disorders in preteen and early teenage girls with type 1 diabetes: A case-controlled study. *Diabetes Care* 27, no. 7 (2004): 1654–1659.

Colton, P, Rodin G, Bergenstal R, and Parkin C. Eating disorders and diabetes: Introduction and overview. *Diabetes Spectrum* 22, no. 3 (2009): 138–142.

DCCT Research Group. Weight gain associated with intensive therapy in the diabetes control and complications trial. *Diabetes Care* 11, no. 7 (1988): 567–573.

Goebel-Fabbri, AE, Fikkan J, Franko DL, Pearson K, Anderson BJ, and Weinger K. Insulin restriction and associated morbidity and mortality in women with type 1 diabetes. *Diabetes Care* 31, no. 3 (2008): 415–419.

Hudson, JI, Hiripi E, Pope HG Jr, and Kessler RC. The prevalence and comorbidity survey replication. *Biological Psychiatry* 61, no. 3 (2007): 348–358.

Jones, JM. *Eating Disorders in Adolescent Females with Type 1 Diabetes Mellitus: A Controlled Three-Site Study*. Canada: University of Toronto, 2000.

Jones, JM, Lawson ML, Daneman D, Olmsted MP, and Rodin G. Eating disorders in adolescent females with and without type 1 diabetes: Cross sectional study. *British Medical Journal* 320, no. 10 (2000): 1563–1566.

Lock, J, Le Grange D, Agras WS, Moye A, Bryson SW, and Jo B. Randomized clinical trial comparing family-based treatment with adolescent-focused individual therapy for adolescents with anorexia nervosa. *Archives of General Psychiatry* 67, no. 10 (2010): 1025–1032.

Mannucci, E, Rotella F, Ricca V, Moretti S, Placidi GF, and Rotella CM. Eating disorders in patients with type 1 diabetes: A meta-analysis. *Journal of Endocrinological Investigation* 28, no. 5 (2005): 417–419.

Markowitz, Jessica T, Butler DA, Volkening LK, Antisdel JE, Anderson BJ, and Laffel LMB. Brief screening tool for disordered eating in diabetes. *Diabetes Care* 33, no. 3 (2010): 495–500.

Nielsen, S. Eating disorders in females with type 1 diabetes: An update of a meta-analysis. *European Eating Disorders Review* 10, no. 4 (2002): 241–254.

Nielsen, S, Emborg C, and Mølbak AG. Mortality in concurrent type 1 diabetes and anorexia nervosa. *Diabetes Care* 25, no. 2 (2002): 302–312.

Patton, GC, Selzer R, Coffey C, Carlin JB, and Wolfe R. Onset of adolescent eating disorders: Population based cohort study over 3 years. *British Medical Journal* 318, no. 7186 (1999): 765–768.

Peveler, RC, Fairburn CG, Boller I, and Dunger D. Eating disorders in adolescents with IDDM: A controlled study. *Diabetes Care* 15, no. 10 (1992): 1356–1360.

Pinhas-Hamiel, O, and Zeitler P. The global spread of type 2 diabetes mellitus in children and adolescents. *Journal of Pediatrics* 146, no. 5 (2005): 693–700.

Polonsky, WH, Anderson BJ, Lohrer PA, Aponte JE, and Jacobson AM. Insulin omission in women with IDDM. *Diabetes Care* 17, no. 10 (1994): 178–185.

Rydall, AC, Rodin GM, Olmsted MP, Devenyl RG, and Daneman D. Disordered eating behavior and microvascular complications in young women with insulin-dependent diabetes mellitus. *New England Journal of Medicine* 336, no. 26 (1997): 1849–1854.

Sargeant, LA, Wareham NJ, and Khaw KT. Family history of diabetes identifies a group at increased risk for the metabolic consequences of obesity and physical inactivity in EPIC-Norfolk: A population-based study. *International Journal of Obesity and Related Metabolic Disorders* 24, no. 10 (2000): 1333–1339.

Silverstein, J, Klingensmith G, Copeland K, Plotnick L, Kaufman F, Laffel L, Debb L, Grey M, Anderson B, Holzmeister LA, and Clark N. Care of children and adolescents with type 1 diabetes. *Diabetes Care* 28, no. 1 (2005): 186–212.

The Diabetes Control and Complications Trial Research Group. The effect of intensive treatment of diabetes on the development and progression of long-term complications in insulin-dependent diabetes mellitus. *New England Journal of Medicine* 329, no. 14 (1993): 977–986.

Walker, JD, Young RJ, Little J, and Steel JM. Mortality in concurrent type 1 diabetes and anorexia nervosa. *Diabetes Care* 25, no. 9 (2002): 1664–1665.

Wisting, L, Frøisland DH, Skrivarhaug T, Dahl-Jørgensen K, and Rø Ø. Disturbed eating behavior and omission of insulin in adolescents receiving intensified insulin treatment. *Diabetes Care* 36, no. 11 (2013): 3382–3387.

Zhao, Y, and Encinosa W. *An Update on Hospitalizations for Eating Disorders, 1999 to 2009.* Vol. 120. Rockville, MD: Agency for Healthcare Research and Quality, September 2011.

11 Eating Disorders in Racial/Ethnic Minorities

Anna M. Bardone-Cone, PhD,
M. K. Higgins Neyland, PhD,
and Stacy L. Lin, MA

CONTENTS

LEARNING OBJECTIVES

After reading this chapter, the reader should be able to do the following:

- Summarize existing research on eating disorder prevalence rates in racial/ethnic minorities
- Recall cultural risk factors that may contribute to the development and maintenance of eating disorders in US racial/ethnic minority groups

- Recognize the challenges in assessment and treatment of eating disorders in racial/ethnic minority populations
- Illustrate how cultural factors such as ethnic identity and acculturation may inform treatment goals and approaches

BACKGROUND AND SIGNIFICANCE

Racial/ethnic minorities in the United States have historically been viewed as protected from eating disorders. To the degree that eating disorders are culture-bound disorders (Keel and Klump 2003), it has been argued that racial/ethnic minority groups that do not subscribe to the importance of thinness for females have immunity against disordered eating. However, it is now clear that racial/ethnic minorities do struggle with eating disorders, challenging "the myth of the golden girl" (Smolak and Striegel-Moore 2001), and research has begun to examine eating pathology in these populations using models with support in primarily Caucasian samples and, more recently, culturally specific models. While research in these populations is still in its infancy in terms of validating assessment tools, identifying risk factors, and proposing treatment approaches, progress has been made; this is important for the health and well-being of racial/ethnic minorities in their own right and because of the growing racial/ethnic minority presence in the United States.

In this chapter, we review some of the key findings related to eating disorders in African American/Black, Hispanic/American/Latino/a/x, Asian American, and Native American individuals. At the outset, we note that these different racial/ethnic minority groups are themselves heterogeneous; for example, Latinxs and Asian Americans in the United States have origins in a wide range of countries. We will sometimes be using terms interchangeably (e.g., African American and Black), understanding this is often an oversimplification, and will use the nomenclature used by the study authors when applicable. To date, little is known about within-group variability in relation to eating disorder prevalence and risk factors, with some exceptions (e.g., finding that partner violence was associated with binge eating in Caribbean Black women but not African American women; Lacey et al. 2015). We also note that most of the limited research has focused on females and, thus, most of the research cited comes from female (or primarily female) samples. Lastly, our focus is on diagnostically defined eating disorders, although disordered eating attitudes and behaviors will also be discussed, especially in relation to assessment and potential risk factors.

PREVALENCE

The best information about prevalence comes from epidemiological research, such as the National Survey of American Life (NSAL), which collected data on Black adults, and the National Latino and Asian American Study (NLAAS). Using pooled data from the National Institute of Mental Health (NIMH) Collaborative Psychiatric Epidemiological Studies, which combined data from the aforementioned NSAL, NLAAS, and the National Comorbidity Survey Replication (NCS-R), and applying statistical approaches that improve the accuracy of estimates in the context of

TABLE 11.1
Lifetime Prevalence Rates

National Survey of American Life: Lifetime Prevalence Rates (Taylor et al. 2007)		Pooled Data: NIMH Collaborative Psychiatric Epidemiological Studies Lifetime Prevalence Rates (Marques et al. 2011)	
	Black Females (%)	Black Males (%)	Black Females (%)	Non-Latina Caucasian Females (%)
BED	2.36	0.78	2.22	1.91
BN	1.90	0.97	1.74	0.97
AN	0.14	0.20	0.12	0.64

National Latino and Asian American Study: Lifetime Prevalence Rates (Alegria et al. 2007; Nicdao et al. 2007)			
	Latina Females (%)	Latino Males (%)	Latina Females (%)
BED	2.31	1.55	2.71
BN	1.91	1.34	2.34
AN	0.12	0.03	0.12
	Asian American Females (%)	Asian American Males (%)	Asian American Females (%)
BED	2.67	1.35	1.66
BN	1.42	0.71	1.87
AN	0.12	0.05	0.13

small sample sizes yielded estimated eating disorder prevalence rates across various racial/ethnic minority groups (see Table 11.1). It was found that binge-eating disorder (BED) was the most prevalent of the eating disorders and anorexia nervosa (AN) the least, with bulimia nervosa (BN) falling in between.

Extensive epidemiological data related to eating disorder diagnoses are not available for Native Americans. Preliminary evidence suggests that Native American women are as likely as Caucasian women to ever have been diagnosed with an eating disorder—4.3% of Native American women reported having received a diagnosis, compared with 4.6% of non-Latina Caucasian women (Striegel-Moore et al. 2011). For both Native American and non-Latino Caucasian men, 0.4% indicated that they had been previously diagnosed with an eating disorder (Striegel-Moore et al. 2011). In general, Native Americans report among the highest rates of disordered eating when examined across ethnicities (Lynch et al. 2004, 2007; Smith and Krejci 1991).

No significant group differences emerged between any of the racial/ethnic minority groups for lifetime rates of BED, BN, or AN for females. The prevalence rates for males were uniformly lower than those for females, highlighting that the gendered component of eating disorders exists in racial/ethnic minorities as it does for non-Latino Caucasians. Interestingly, Latino males had significantly higher rates of BN than their Caucasian peers. (See Table 11.1 for the prevalence estimates for males in the different racial/ethnic minority groups.)

In sum, epidemiological work finds that prevalence rates across racial/ethnic minority groups of African Americans, Latinxs, Asian Americans, and non-Latinx Caucasians are similar, with binge eating-related disorders (i.e., BN and BED) more common than AN. Gender differences in prevalence rates are comparable to those found in Caucasian samples; females are more likely than males to have eating disorders across racial/ethnic minority groups. While less is known about Native Americans in terms of diagnosed eating disorders, rates of disordered eating are high in this group.

ASSESSMENT AND EVALUATION

Research examining eating pathology and related factors (e.g., body dissatisfaction) has generally used assessment tools validated in primarily non-Latina Caucasian female samples. Without psychometric data for measures in racial/ethnic minority samples, it is not clear to what degree these assessments are appropriate for different races/ethnicities. It is also important to consider that components of an eating disorder may not manifest in the same way across all races/ethnicities. In considering evaluation, it is important to note that using Western criteria for eating disorders may be misleading; if components of an eating disorder do not manifest in the same way across all races/ethnicities, prevalence rates of eating disorders in minority populations may be distorted (Wildes et al. 2001).

To date, only a small number of studies explicitly test and report the psychometric properties of eating disorder instruments in racial/ethnic minority groups. Table 11.2

TABLE 11.2
Measures of Body Dissatisfaction and Disordered Eating with Some Psychometric Support among Racial/Ethnic Minorities

Measure	Citation	Comments
Bulimia Test-Revised (BULIT-R)	Thelen et al. (1991)	Reliability and validity demonstrated in African American females (Bardone-Cone and Boyd 2007)
		Similar factor structure for African American, Latina, Asian American, and non-Latina Caucasian samples (Fernandez et al. 2006)
		Similar factor structure for African American and non-Latina Caucasian samples (Kelly et al. 2012)
Binge-Eating Scale (BES)	Gormally et al. (1982)	Reliability demonstrated in African American females (Kelly et al. 2012)
		Different factor structure for African American and non-Latina Caucasian samples (Kelly et al. 2012)
Restraint subscale of the Three Factor Eating Questionnaire (TFEQ)	Stunkard and Messick (1985)	Reliability and validity demonstrated in African American females (Bardone-Cone and Boyd 2007)

(Continued)

TABLE 11.2 *(CONTINUED)*

Measures of Body Dissatisfaction and Disordered Eating with Some Psychometric Support among Racial/Ethnic Minorities

Measure	Citation	Comments
Eating Attitudes Test-26 (EAT-26)	Garner et al. (1982)	Reliability demonstrated in African American females (Kelly et al. 2012)
		Different factor structure for African American and non-Latina Caucasian samples (Kelly et al. 2012)
		Different factor structure for a Latina and female sample (Rutt and Coleman 2001)
Bulimia, Drive for Thinness, and Body Dissatisfaction subscales of the Eating Disorder Inventory (EDI)	Garner et al. (1983)	Reliability and validity of the Bulimic subscale demonstrated in African American females (Bardone-Cone and Boyd, 2007)
		Reliability of the Drive for Thinness and Body Dissatisfaction subscales demonstrated in African American females (Kelly et al. 2012)
		Different factor structure for the Drive for Thinness and Body Dissatisfaction subscales for African American and non-Latina Caucasian samples (Kelly et al. 2012)
		Reliability and similar factor structure to Caucasian, non-Latinos of the Bulimia, Drive for Thinness, and Body Dissatisfaction subscales for Latina undergraduate women (Cordero et al. 2013)
		Theoretical support for the three-factor model among Latina and Caucasian undergraduate females; measurement invariance was only observed in the Drive for Thinness subscale (Belon et al. 2015)
		Reliability and convergent and discriminant validity of the Body Dissatisfaction subscale demonstrated in African American college women, but two factors were a better fit to the data than the originally proposed single factor (Kashubeck-West et al. 2013)
Eating Disorder Diagnostic Scale (EDDS)	Stice et al. (2000)	Reliability demonstrated in African American females (Kelly et al. 2012)
		Different factor structure for African American and non-Latina Caucasian samples (Kelly et al. 2012)
Eating Disorder Examination Questionnaire (EDE-Q) (subscales: Restraint, Eating Concern, Weight Concern, Shape Concern)	Fairburn and Beglin (1994)	Reliability for all subscales and validity for the Restraint subscale demonstrated in African American females (Bardone-Cone et al. 2007)
		Reliability and validity demonstrated in Latina females (Franko et al. 2012)
		Factor structure supported in a Latina sample (Franko et al. 2012)
		Concordance between binge-eating frequencies and subscales across the self-report questionnaire (EDE-Q) and the interview format (Eating Disorder Examination [EDE]) in African American patients with BED, with scores higher on questionnaire vs. interview format (Lydecker et al. 2016)

(Continued)

TABLE 11.2 *(CONTINUED)*

Measures of Body Dissatisfaction and Disordered Eating with Some Psychometric Support among Racial/Ethnic Minorities

Measure	Citation	Comments
Spanish version of the EDE-Q	Grilo et al. (2005)	Reliability and validity demonstrated in monolingual Spanish-speaking Latina females (Elder and Grilo 2007)
Spanish version of the EDE	Grilo et al. (2005)	Reliability demonstrated in monolingual Spanish-speaking Latina females (Grilo et al. 2005)
		Different factor structure for monolingual Spanish-speaking Latino/as (Grilo et al. 2012)
Multidimensional Body-Self Relations Questionnaire- Appearance Scales (MBSRQ)	Cash (1994)	Reliability and convergent validity of the Appearance Evaluation subscale of the MBSRQ demonstrated in African American females (Kelly et al. 2012)
		Similar factor structure for African American and non-Latina Caucasian samples (Kelly et al. 2012)
		Reliability and convergent and discriminant validity supported in African American college women, but a single factor was a better fit to the data than the originally proposed two factors (Kashubeck-West et al. 2013)
Body Shape Questionnaire (BSQ)	Cooper et al. (1987)	Reliability and validity demonstrated in Latina females (Franko et al. 2012)
Body Esteem Scale for Adolescents and Adults	Mendelson et al. (2001)	Reliability and validity demonstrated in Latina females (Franko et al. 2012)
Objectified Body Consciousness Scale (OBCS)	McKinley and Hyde (1996)	Modest reliability demonstrated in African American females (Kelly et al. 2012)
		Similar factor structure for African American and non-Latina Caucasian samples (Kelly et al. 2012)
Sociocultural Attitudes Toward Appearance Questionnaire-3 (SATAQ-3)	Thompson et al. (2004)	Reliability and validity demonstrated in Latina females (Franko et al. 2012)
		Similar four-factor structure (but with fewer items) in African American college women. Reliability and convergent and discriminant validity supported in this sample (Kashubeck-West et al. 2013)

includes a sample of measures that have been psychometrically evaluated to some degree in racial/ethnic minorities. To provide some exemplars, Bardone-Cone and Boyd (2007) found support for the reliability and validity of several eating disorder measures in an African American female sample. While they found that measures of dieting had lower temporal stability than other eating disorder measures, this may validly represent the dieting experiences of African American females who are less embedded in a maintenance culture of dietary restriction than their non-Latina Caucasian counterparts (e.g., less likely to have friends they are dieting with). The Bulimia Test-Revised (BULIT-R; Thelen et al. 1991), in particular, stands out among eating disorder assessments as a measure that has demonstrated factorial invariance across African Americans, Latinas, Asian Americans, and non-Latina Caucasians (Fernandez et al. 2006). Some other measures, however, appear to yield different factor structures in racial/ethnic minority samples. For example, a study of several measures of body image in African American college women yielded factors different from the subscales identified in initial research (on primarily Caucasian samples) (Kashubeck-West et al. 2013). An investigation of the Drive for Muscularity Scale (McCreary and Sasse 2000), a measure of an individual's desire to become more muscular (a risk factor for body dissatisfaction and other negative outcomes that may be particularly salient for men), found that in a group of Asian men living in the United States and Canada, the two-factor structure proposed by McCreary and Sasse was a poor fit for the data (Keum et al. 2015). However, after the removal of three items, the two-factor model emerged in the Asian sample, suggesting that a modified version of the Drive for Muscularity Scale may be used with Asian American men.

Psychometric research on the Eating Disorder Examination (EDE) interview (Fairburn and Cooper 1993) and the Eating Disorder Examination Questionnaire (EDE-Q; Fairburn and Beglin 1994), the self-report questionnaire version of the interview, is highlighted at this point given the widespread use of these measures in clinical and research settings. Patterns of concordance have been found for the two measures for both binge-eating frequencies and eating pathology subscales (restraint, eating concern, shape concern, weight concern) in a sample of Black patients (primarily female) with BED; while scores were significantly positively correlated across the two measures, scores tended to be higher on the self-report questionnaire compared to the interview (Lydecker et al. 2016). This pattern was similar to the pattern found in the White patients with BED. Within a Latina undergraduate sample, support has been found for the factor structure of the EDE-Q (Franko et al. 2012).

When considering the assessment of eating disorders in racial/ethnic minorities, well-validated translations of instruments may be particularly important for specific minority groups. Individuals of ethnic groups with higher percentages of immigrants (e.g., Asian Americans and Latinxs) may be more likely not to speak English fluently, raising the concern of whether their symptoms are being adequately captured by English versions of these instruments, and complicating the process of assessing these populations (Tsong and Smart 2014). Research on Spanish translations of the EDE (interview) and the EDE-Q (questionnaire) has garnered some support in monolingual Spanish-speaking Latinx samples (Elder and Grilo 2007; Grilo et al. 2005). Although the more commonly used instruments have been translated into some Asian languages (Lee et al. 1997; Tseng et al. 2014), to our knowledge, in many cases there has not been rigorous and comprehensive evaluation of their psychometric properties in the target populations.

Additional factor analyses of eating disorder assessments could establish ways in which symptom patterns might differ between ethnic groups (Cummins et al. 2005); establishing these patterns will help researchers and clinicians study prevalence and develop assessments and treatment protocols. Being more culturally sensitive to the assessment of body dissatisfaction among racial/ethnic minorities and examining its validity as a predictor of eating disorders will be important. For example, Asian Americans express particular dissatisfaction with racially defined aspects of their bodies (e.g., eyelids, height, and leg shape) that cannot be altered by weight loss (Mintz and Kashubeck 1999). More recent research has identified variability in dissatisfaction of other facial and body features across a female sample of African Americans, non-Latina Caucasians, and Caucasians, with Latinas in particular reporting more areas of dissatisfaction (Warren 2014). More research is needed on the assessment of racially/ethnically specific sources of body dissatisfaction and the examination of possible linkages between those body concerns and disordered eating.

One reason assessments may not be equivalent across races/ethnicities is if eating disorders manifest differently in different groups. The need to consider this has been made most salient for the fear of fat criterion for AN (under-endorsed by Asian American women otherwise meeting AN criteria) and time-related concepts, such as frequency and duration for bulimic behaviors (Franko 2007). These issues may have been somewhat resolved with the more inclusive criteria for AN and BN in the fifth edition of the *Diagnostic and Statistical Manual of Mental Disorders* (*DSM-5*; American Psychiatric Association 2013), which allows persistent behavior interfering with weight gain as an alternative to the fear of fat criterion and includes a lower frequency threshold of bulimic behaviors of once per week on average rather than twice a week as in the previous edition. As other examples of potentially different manifestations of eating disorder symptoms, it was reported that Asian Americans found vomiting to be the most distressing eating disorder symptom, whereas the other ethnicities studied all found binge eating to be the most distressing (Franko et al. 2007), and that binge eating and purging were not significantly correlated in Native American girls, while they were significantly positively correlated in Caucasian girls (Lynch et al. 2007).

Of note, the psychometric support reported in Table 11.2 was most often established in undergraduate female samples, meaning that reliability and validity in other demographics of racial/ethnic minority groups (e.g., males, community samples representing a greater diversity of ages, etc.) is not yet known. Also, most of the psychometric work of measure has used African American or Latinx samples. In an overview of the assessment of eating pathology in Asian Americans, there was an emphasis on the lack of data on the reliability and validity of measures for Asian Americans (Tsong and Smart 2014). To our knowledge, no published work focuses on the psychometrics of eating disorder instruments in Native Americans.

Regarding the intersection of race/ethnicity and evaluation, there is evidence that eating disorders in minority groups are less likely to be detected, probably due to the common (erroneous) belief that they are much less likely to suffer from them than non-Latinx Caucasians. Analogue studies have demonstrated that when undergraduate student participants were given the same vignette of eating disorder symptoms, differentiated only by the race/ethnicity assigned the subject of the vignette, eating disorder symptoms were more often recognized when the subject was Caucasian (93%) than when she was either Latina or African American (both 79%; Gordon et al. 2002). When this study was replicated with clinicians as participants, the clinicians identified disturbed eating patterns in the vignettes of Latina and non-Latina Caucasian subjects at equivalent rates (40.5% and 44.4%, respectively), but under-identified symptoms in African Americans (16.7%; Gordon et al. 2006). Though it appears this has not yet been studied, identification of eating disorders among Asian

Americans may be hampered if clinician bias leads to assumptions that lower body mass indices (BMIs) are expected; the presence of this potential stereotype may result in fewer concerns being raised by what may in actuality be tendencies toward AN. Evaluation for Native Americans tends to focus on obesity and little research has explored eating disorders in these populations, despite the fact that being overweight means individuals are more likely to try unhealthy weight loss strategies (which may include eating disorder symptoms) than normal weight individuals (Neumark-Sztainer et al. 1997).

Other research further supports differences regarding evaluation and the expected consequences of referral. A study involving ethnic minority college students showed that they were less likely to be assessed for eating disorders than Caucasian students, and also less likely to be referred for further evaluation if they endorsed concerns about disordered eating (Becker et al. 2003). This effect was found even after controlling for severity of eating disorder symptoms and BMI, pointing to an ethnic disparity in evaluation and subsequent treatment referral among eating-disordered individuals. Asian Americans were significantly less likely to be referred for further evaluation than other ethnicities despite engaging in eating disorder behaviors at comparable levels (Franko et al. 2007). The bias of overlooking or downplaying symptoms of an eating disorder in racial/ethnic minority populations is not trivial. When eating disorders are recognized in racial/ethnic minorities, they are often diagnosed only when symptoms have become relatively serious and arguably more difficult to treat (Cummins et al. 2012; Gordon et al. 2002; Root 1990).

In sum, although some of the more well-known measures of eating pathology have exhibited psychometric support in African American and Latinx samples, the same cannot be said for Asian American and Native American samples. Most psychometric work has used undergraduate female student samples, which may limit generalizability of findings. Accurate evaluation of eating disorders, which is closely tied to assessment, is constrained among racial/ethnic minorities, which has serious implications for the early detection important for best outcomes.

GENERAL RISK FACTORS IN RACIAL/ETHNIC MINORITY GROUPS

Longitudinal or experimental research is necessary to posit true risk factors, and minimal such research has been done in racial/ethnic minority samples. We primarily discuss here correlates of eating pathology although we use the heading "risk factors" to suggest possible (although not always tested) causal relations. Here, we review findings in racial/ethnic minorities as they relate to established risk factors from primarily Caucasian samples (e.g., those identified in meta-analytic work) (Stice 2002), as well as findings examining more culturally specific potential risk factors.

BODY DISSATISFACTION

Body dissatisfaction is considered "one of the most consistent and robust risk and maintenance factors for eating pathology" (Stice 2002), but this comes from primarily Caucasian samples. Given different cultural expectations and messages regarding physical attractiveness across different racial/ethnic groups, it is not clear if body dissatisfaction confers the same risk. Meta-analytic work indicates that levels of body dissatisfaction are not generally significantly different across most racial/ethnic minority groups of females (Grabe and Hyde 2006). In particular, pairwise comparisons among African American, Latina, Asian American, and non-Latina Caucasian women yielded only two small effect sizes, with non-Latina Caucasians reporting greater body dissatisfaction than African Americans (mean effect size of 0.29), even though African American girls/women tend to weigh more than Caucasians (Boyd et al. 2011), and Latina women reporting greater body dissatisfaction than African Americans (mean effect size of –0.18).

Greater body satisfaction among African American females is likely due to a variety of reasons; in African American samples, research finds that the ideal body size is larger (Freedman et al. 2004); ideas of what is attractive are more flexible (Parker et al. 1995; Webb et al. 2013); males prefer larger female body sizes (Greenberg and LaPorte 1996; Root 1990); investment in the importance of thinness is lower (Boyd et al. 2011); "fat talk" is less prevalent (Nichter 2009); and weight-based stigmatization and bias is less prominent (Barnes et al. 2014; Gray et al. 2011). For Latinas, some work suggests that their largest body discrepancy may be between their perceived body shape and their perceived ethnic group ideal, and less so between perceived body shape and perceived mainstream ideal (Gordon et al. 2010). In a study of female undergraduates, Asian Americans had lower BMIs than Caucasian and African American students, but the body discrepancy reported by Asian Americans was still higher than African Americans' even after controlling for BMI, indicating a larger difference between their current and ideal bodies (Gluck and Geliebter 2002). In a sample of African American, Asian American, and Caucasian men—in one of the small number of studies focused on racial/ethnic minority males—Asian American men reported significantly higher levels of body image concerns than the other two groups (Kelly et al. 2015), suggesting that Asian American men may experience increased risk for disordered eating and attitudes.

For all racial/ethnic minority groups, there is evidence that body dissatisfaction is associated with eating pathology (e.g., in African Americans—Rogers Wood and Petrie [2010], Latinas—Kroon Van Diest et al. [2014], Asian Americans—Franko and Striegel-Moore [2002], and Native Americans—Stevens et al. [1999]). However, the strength of association between body dissatisfaction and eating pathology may differ across groups. For example, correlations between body dissatisfaction measures and binge eating were found to be stronger for Caucasian females than African American females (Kelly et al. 2012). Another study found the correlation between body dissatisfaction and unhealthy weight control behavior was weaker for African American boys than for all other groups (girls and boys; African American, Asians, Latinos, and non-Latino Caucasians; Bucchianeri et al. 2015). In a study comparing Caucasian to Asian American females, body discrepancy accounted for significant variance in bulimic symptoms in the Caucasian sample, but not the Asian sample (Chang et al. 2014b). Some research has investigated body dissatisfaction in more complex models including mediational models where, for example, body dissatisfaction mediates the relationship between BMI and eating disorder risk in Native Americans (Lynch et al. 2008; Neumark-Sztainer et al. 1997) as well as the relationship between ethnic identity and disordered eating attitudes/behaviors in Asian Americans (Tsai et al. 2003).

SOCIOCULTURAL MODEL

Sociocultural pressure to be thin and thin-ideal internalization are risk factors for eating pathology in Caucasian samples that may not be as relevant in racial/ethnic minorities. However, among racial/ethnic minorities who do experience these socio-cultural pressures and internalization, models of eating pathology may be similar to non-Latina Caucasians. For example, a sociocultural model provided a good fit to the data of African American female undergraduates, with sociocultural pressures regarding thinness contributing to thin-ideal internalization and body concerns which, in turn, were related to disordered eating (Rogers Wood and Petrie 2010). Of note, lower levels of ethnic identity were associated with greater internalization of the thin ideal. A sociocultural model centered around objectification theory, including thin-ideal internalization and body monitoring in relation to body dissatisfaction and disordered eating, was found to apply to African American women (Mitchell and Mazzeo 2009). That is, the structural model of these constructs was invariant across African American and non-Latina Caucasian samples, suggesting that the relationships between these constructs are similar. African American college women showed an increase in dietary restraint across their first semester, with this increase predicted by thinness expectancies, even after controlling for baseline restraint. Interestingly, this effect was not moderated by level of ethnic identity (Stojek and Fischer 2013).

Support for the sociocultural model has also been evidenced among samples of Latinx youth. Social comparison to models in the media, thin-ideal internalization, perceived appearance pressure, and eating pathology were all positively correlated for both male and female adolescents; however, females exhibited significantly higher mean levels on all of these factors. Additionally, when taking into account generational status, higher generational status was associated with more social comparison to models in the media, thin-ideal internalization, perceived appearance pressure, and eating pathology for females only (Warren et al. 2010). Support was found for two sociocultural mediational models in a sample of Latino undergraduate men: (1) awareness of Western values of appearance was associated with perceived pressure to attain the ideal promoted in the media which in turn was associated with athletic-ideal internalization and (2) perceived pressure to attain the ideal was associated with athletic-ideal internalization which in turn was associated with muscle dissatisfaction/body image problems (Warren and Rios 2013). Additionally, in this sample of Latino males, social comparison to models was associated with perceived pressure to attain the ideal as well as athletic-ideal internalization. In a sample of preadolescent Latina and African American girls, weight-related teasing from a parent (but not such teasing from a peer) was associated with binge eating (Olvera et al. 2013). Support for additional sociocultural models exists, including studies involving objectification theory among Latinas (Velez et al. 2015) and media-influenced sociocultural values and ideals about appearance, where Latina girls showed a stronger relationship between these values/ideals and disordered eating and body image concerns than did their male peers (Lopez et al. 2013).

Sociocultural pressures regarding thinness and thin-ideal internalization are also concepts relevant to Asian Americans. For example, for Asian American women, perceived pressure for thinness was associated with body preoccupation directly as well as indirectly through internalization of the thin ideal, and body preoccupation predicted eating disorder symptoms (Phan and Tylka 2006). Asian Americans and non-Latino Caucasians showed significantly more thin-ideal internalization than African Americans and Latinas (Shaw et al. 2004). The sociocultural pressures of thin-ideal internalization, media influence, and peer influence have been found to be associated with body dissatisfaction in Asian American women, but note that, surprisingly, family influence was not associated with body dissatisfaction in this sample (Javier and Belgrave 2015).

Little work has examined the applicability of sociocultural models in Native American samples, but existing research provides opportunities for speculation. For Native Americans, the finding that youth with higher BMIs also tended to report higher levels of body dissatisfaction implies some internalization of the value of thinness (Davis and Lambert 1999). Further, in this sample of Native American children, 61% reported trying to lose weight, a rate similar to same-aged non-Hispanic white children, which also suggests a valuing of weight loss (Davis and Lambert 1999).

NEGATIVE AFFECT

Negative affect is a potentially culturally neutral risk factor for eating pathology that may be applicable across racial/ethnic minority groups; indeed, support has been found for a negative affect/eating pathology linkage in samples of combined racial/ethnic minorities. For example, in a community sample of African American and Latina women, stress impact scores and clinically significant levels of depression were associated with binge-eating severity (Adamus-Leach et al. 2013). In a sample of African American, Latinx, and Caucasian children and adolescent males and females, depressive symptoms were associated with binge-eating and disordered eating attitudes (Elliott et al. 2013). Fear of negative evaluation by peers, which reflects social anxiety, was positively associated with body image discrepancy among a sample of African American, Latina, and Caucasian fifth-grade girls (Michael et al. 2014).

Additional support for links to negative affect comes from research focused on single, rather than combined, racial/ethnic groups. Among African Americans, some evidence supports a relationship between negative affect such as anxiety and depressive symptoms and disordered eating (Blue and Berkel 2010; Mitchell and Mazzeo 2004). Other support for a linkage between negative affect and eating disorders comes from the comorbidity of major depressive disorder and social phobia with BED in African American women (Pike et al. 2001). Among Latinas, depressive symptomatology has been associated with eating pathology (Granillo et al. 2005; Sánchez-Johnsen et al. 2008). Additionally, in a sample of middle school students, Latinas experienced the most comorbidity when assessing depression, anxiety, aggression, and eating pathology, pointing to a possible relationship between negative affect and disordered eating (McLaughlin et al. 2007). Anxiety has been additionally associated with binge eating among Latina psychiatric inpatients (White and

Grilo 2005). In South Asian female American college students, negative affect was significantly and positively associated with drive for thinness, bulimic symptoms, and body dissatisfaction; these relations were not found in the male sample (Chang et al. 2014a). Emotional distress appears to be strongly related to binge eating among Native American women (Clark and Winterowd 2012). Of note, all of the studies described above reflect correlational research; to date, only cross-sectional designs examine the topic of negative affect and eating pathology, with prospective work needed to confirm negative affect as a causal or maintenance factor for eating pathology in racial/ethnic minorities.

PERSONALITY FACTORS: PERFECTIONISM AND IMPULSIVITY

Personality factors such as perfectionism and impulsivity have been linked to AN and BN in primarily Caucasian samples, with perfectionism being associated with both eating disorders and impulsivity to BN and to the binge/purge subtype of AN (Bardone-Cone et al. 2007; Hoffman et al. 2012; Stice 2002; Wonderlich et al. 2005). Very limited work exists regarding personality features and eating disorders in minority populations.

Perfectionism has been associated with eating pathology in African American samples. For example, African American women who exhibited high levels of socially prescribed perfectionism (a maladaptive type of perfectionism involving the perception that others expect too much of you) and perceived themselves to be overweight (regardless of actual weight status) exhibited the highest levels of bulimic symptoms (Bardone-Cone et al. 2009).

The negative effects of high expectations from important others may be buffered, however, in groups who are disadvantaged in a dominant culture. Among African American college women who perceived high expectations from their parents (i.e., a type of socially prescribed perfection), those who interpreted those expectations positively as demonstrating confidence and support were protected from bulimic symptoms compared to those who interpreted the expectations negatively as being too demanding (Bardone-Cone et al. 2012). While striving for perfection is relevant in many ethnicities including Asian American samples, for example, feeling pressure to represent "perfect" examples of Asian femininity and to be perfect in order to combat negative stereotypes (Hall 1995), connections between perfectionism and eating pathology have not been extensively assessed. One study found that perfectionism did not account for significant variance in drive for thinness in their Asian American sample (Chang et al. 2014c). To our knowledge, there is no research examining the relation between perfectionism and eating pathology in Latinx or Native American populations.

Regarding impulsivity, parental report of daughters' impulsivity in first grade was associated with bulimic symptoms in late adolescence among African American females (Bodell et al. 2012). Impulsivity was also significantly positively associated with bulimic symptoms in an African American female undergraduate sample; further, the combination of high body shame and high impulsivity was associated with the highest levels of bulimic symptoms, thus identifying a moderator model involving impulsivity (Higgins et al. 2015). Among psychiatric inpatient adolescent Latinas, impulsivity and body image dissatisfaction accounted for the most variance in dietary restraint (White and Grilo 2005). We did not find studies specifically investigating the link between impulsivity and bulimic symptomatology in Asian Americans or Native Americans.

In sum, there is great variability in terms of how extensively eating pathology risk factors found in primarily non-Latino Caucasian samples have been examined in racial/ethnic minorities. Body dissatisfaction and sociocultural models have been investigated more so than negative affect and personality, but for all constructs more research is needed across racial/ethnic groups, in more complex moderator and mediation models involving these empirically supported risk factors from Caucasian samples, and using longitudinal and experimental designs.

RISK FACTORS SPECIFIC TO RACIAL/ETHNIC MINORITY GROUPS

It is critical that an examination of risk factors in racial/ethnic minorities extend beyond those typically examined in the dominant culture in the United States. Here, we review some of the promising contenders for models of risk for eating pathology among minorities.

ACCULTURATION

The process of aligning with a new culture is known as acculturation and includes both "the extent to which the individual maintains cultural beliefs and practices of his/her country of origin, and the extent to which the individual adopts similar aspects of the new dominant culture" (Ayala et al. 2007). Seminal work by Becker et al. (2002) found support for an acculturation effect on disordered eating in a naturalistic experiment in Fiji. They examined the impact of the introduction of television on eating pathology in a sample of Fijian adolescent girls, a media-naïve population, finding consequences of more prevalent disordered eating and reports of interest in weight loss prompted by comparisons with television characters. To the degree that eating disorders can be thought of as "culture-bound" within the United States, it makes sense that the more a person aligns and identifies with mainstream US culture which centers on the thin ideal for women, the more a woman may be at risk for developing body dissatisfaction and eating disorders (Ayala et al. 2007).

In a sample of Latina and Asian American females, women who were more acculturated (e.g., less likely to be bilingual, more likely to have parents born in the United States) were more likely to experience disordered eating (Cachelin et al. 2000). Level of acculturation was also found to be associated with partial syndrome eating disorders among Latinas; among a sample of 9th–12th-grade Latinas, 13.6% of the more acculturated participants were diagnosed with partial syndrome eating disorders versus 0% of those participants who were less acculturated (Gowen et al. 1999). The few studies isolating Asian American women to address this issue seem to indicate that thus far, acculturation has not been related to symptoms of eating disorders in most studies (Akan and Grilo 1995; Nicdao et al. 2007; Yoshimura 1995). It should be noted, though, that these studies were limited in the sense that they failed to differentiate between specific cultural groups contained within the Asian American category and in most cases had relatively small sample sizes that might have lacked the power to detect differences (Cummins et al. 2005).

ACCULTURATIVE STRESS

It is also theorized that discrepancy between the ideals and attitudes of two cultures, reflecting acculturative stress, might affect racial/ethnic minority individuals' assessment of themselves and development of disordered eating (Yoshimura 1995). Acculturative stress can be considered the stress and reduction in health status that one experiences while undergoing the process of acculturation/adaptation to a new culture (Berry 1970, 1997; Berry et al. 1987) and has been linked to a number of unhealthy psychological outcomes, including broad eating pathology among Latina and Asian American women (Claudat et al. 2016) and bulimic symptoms among African American and Latina women (Gordon et al. 2010; Perez et al. 2002). Native Americans may experience unique cultural influences of feelings of historical loss, related to the systematic oppression of Native Americans throughout history, via genocide, forced assimilation, and other tragedies, which may be experienced as acculturative stress. Feelings of historical loss were related to binge eating in a sample of Native American women (Clark and Winterowd 2012). Conceptually, acculturative stress could influence eating pathology in two ways: (1) individuals may restrict in order to achieve some sense of control or (2) they may binge eat as an escape from the overwhelming stress of acculturation.

Some of the research involving acculturative stress has examined this construct in the context of moderator/interactive, mediator/pathway, or unique variance models. Among a sample of African Americans and Latinas, body dissatisfaction interacted with acculturative stress to identify women with the highest levels of bulimic symptomatology (Perez et al. 2002). Thus, it appears that African American and Latina women with body dissatisfaction may engage in bulimic behaviors if they are also experiencing acculturative stress. In terms of a pathway, among a sample of undergraduate male and female Latinxs, acculturative stress was related to body image disturbance in part through its association with thin-ideal internalization (Menon and Harter 2012). When investigating acculturative stress among African Americans, Asian Americans, and Latinas, acculturative stress was significantly associated with bulimic symptoms when controlling for general life stress, highlighting the impact of acculturative stress in the manifestation of bulimic symptoms over and above general stress (Kroon Van Diest et al. 2014).

Some researchers postulate that acculturative stress serves as a more potent risk factor for eating disorders than acculturation (Gordon et al. 2010; Reddy and Crowther 2007). To support this point, higher levels of acculturative stress were associated with a higher drive for thinness among Latinas; however, level of acculturation was not similarly associated with this construct (Gordon et al. 2010). Among a sample of Latino males, acculturation was not associated with social comparison, perceived pressure from media to attain the ideal appearance, awareness of Western media ideals of appearance, athletic-ideal internalization, or body image, whereas acculturative stress was positively associated with all of these constructs (Warren and Rios 2013). These findings support the contention that it is the *stress* of acculturating which may be detrimental, rather than acculturation itself. Thus, racial/ethnic minorities who experience a high degree of acculturative stress may be coping with this stress in maladaptive ways (e.g., eating pathology).

ETHNIC IDENTITY

A construct related to acculturation, but often more broadly applied across racial/ethnic minority groups, is ethnic identity. Several studies have shown that ethnic identity can serve as a risk factor for eating disorders among racial/ethnic minorities. Among African American females, low levels of ethnic identity are associated with higher levels of binge eating and eating pathology (Henrickson et al. 2010; Shuttlesworth and Zotter 2011). African American women with low ethnic identity are more likely to buy into the importance of thinness which increases their risk for engaging in weight-control behaviors that may be problematic (Rogers Wood and Petrie 2010). Flowers et al. (2012) parsed apart aspects of ethnic identity to find that self-hatred of African American group membership was related to eating pathology directly, as well as indirectly related via body dissatisfaction. Lower ethnic identity is also associated with eating disorder symptoms among Latinas (Ayala et al. 2007). For example, among Mexican American women, lower levels of Mexican ethnic identity were associated with binge-eating behavior (Stein et al. 2010) and female Latinas who were less identified with Latin culture made more negative comments about their own bodies after viewing sexualized, thin-ideal media images of Caucasian women when compared to those who identified more with Latin culture (Schooler and Daniels 2014). In contrast, a relation was not found between ethnic identification and disordered eating among South Asian Americans (Iyer and Haslam 2003). However, in a study involving African American, Latina, and Asian American undergraduate women, ethnic identity was negatively associated with eating and weight concerns (Rakhkovskaya and Warren 2014). Furthermore, ethnic identity moderated the relationship between thin-ideal internalization and eating concerns, such that the relationship was stronger for those with lower ethnic identity. In a study that examined ethnic identity among Native Americans, the levels of Native American cultural identity were not associated with binge eating or purging although, surprisingly, higher levels of ethnic identity were associated with greater weight control behaviors (Lynch et al. 2007).

The majority of these findings suggest that ethnic identity may serve a protective function against body dissatisfaction and disordered eating, at least for African American and Latina women. Perhaps those high in ethnic identity are less attuned to majority culture and less exposed to majority messages about the body (Striegel-Moore and Cachelin 2001). Additionally, for some racial/ethnic groups, embracing an ethnic identity that may include a larger body size and receiving messages about their bodies and self-worth from "culturally consistent sources" (e.g., family, ethnic media sources) that are more supportive of their natural body sizes/shapes may be ways that ethnic identity buffers against eating pathology (Rogers Wood and Petrie 2010). An interesting aspect of ethnic identity that may increase risk for bulimic pathology among African American women is the "strong Black woman" ideology, which refers to the inherent resilience and strength of Black women, self-reliance, and the ability to handle all challenges (Harrington et al. 2010). While generally perceived as a positive quality among African American female trauma survivors, trauma exposure and distress influenced the internalization of the strong Black woman ideology which facilitated turning to binge eating as an acceptable means of emotional regulation since it does not undercut the self-reliance important to this ideology.

DISCRIMINATION

Lastly, although not much work has examined discrimination as a risk factor for eating disorders, to the degree that it represents an ego-threatening stressor it may function as part of an escape theory of binge eating (Heatherton and Baumeister 1991). According to this theory, ego threats are distal factors in a chain of contributory causes that lead to the aversive self-awareness and negative affect, which are proximal motivators of binge eating; discrimination experiences may be minority-relevant, ego-threatening stressors in this model. Eating problems may arise in economically disadvantaged racial/ethnic minorities as a way to cope with racism and poverty (Thompson 1992). Greater acculturative stress has been associated with more experiences of discrimination, which in turn have been linked to binge eating symptoms among African American women (Harrington et al. 2006). Among Latina women, discrimination was positively associated with body shame and eating disorder symptoms, and discrimination was indirectly associated with eating disorder symptoms through its relationship with body shame, such that more discrimination led to more body shame, which led to more eating disorder symptoms (Velez et al. 2015). Among South Asian Americans, discrimination in the form of racial teasing has been associated with disordered eating (Iyer and Haslam 2003). Furthermore, perceived racial discrimination was associated with disordered eating both directly and indirectly in a sample of Asian American women (Cheng 2014). Among Native Americans, experiences of racism have been related to binge eating (Clark and Winterowd 2012).

In sum, preliminary evidence supports the value of continuing to investigate acculturation, acculturative stress, ethnic identity, and discrimination among racial/ethnic minorities for their roles in contributing to or protecting against eating pathology.

HEALTH CONSEQUENCES

Health consequences for those suffering from eating disorders are similar across different racial/ethnic minority groups. Since obesity is a health consequence of BED, health problems related to obesity are relevant. Obesity is an especially prevalent health concern among African Americans and Hispanic Americans, afflicting those in these racial/ethnic minority groups across the life span at a higher rate than other races and ethnicities (National Heart Lung and Blood Institute and National Institutes of Health 2009; Ogden et al. 2008). Rates of obesity in Native Americans are also high and significantly greater than in Caucasians; in fact, the incidence of obesity in Native American youth is around three times higher than that of the general population (Story et al. 1999; Zephier et al. 1999). Health consequences of obesity are numerous and include concerns such as high blood pressure, high cholesterol, cardiovascular disease, hypertension, difficulty sleeping, and diabete (Burroughs et al. 2008; Field et al. 2001).

Since eating disorders may be overlooked or diagnosed later in minority groups, there is a greater likelihood that the disorder may be more severe by the time it is diagnosed, and this could lead to worse health consequences (e.g., osteoporosis, bradycardia, liver, and kidney damage). In the case of AN, a later age of presentation is associated with greater risk for mortality (Arcelus et al. 2011), suggesting that if AN is identified and treated later because of incorrect evaluation, lack of referral, or lack of resources related to being an ethnic/racial minority, than rates of death from AN may be elevated among these groups.

Nutrition/Food Management

Food choices and nutrition are obvious topics in treating individuals with eating disorders. For racial/ethnic minorities struggling with eating pathology, eating that is influenced by residing in obesogenic environments should be part of any treatment discussion. Obesogenic food environments, sometimes called "food deserts," refer to living in areas where calorie-dense foods high in fat and sugar are readily available through fast food restaurants and convenience stores, while access to fresh fruits and vegetables is limited (Larson et al. 2009; U.S. Department of Agriculture n.d.). For example, many reservations do not have large supermarkets, requiring residents to travel great distances to obtain affordable, healthy food, which may be prohibitively expensive (McKinnon et al. 2009). Indeed, a survey of Native American children in fifth grade found that one of the major perceived barriers to following a set of guidelines for healthy dietary choices was environmental barriers including lack of affordable, accessible food (Jahns et al. 2015). Individuals who are economically disadvantaged, regardless of their race or ethnicity, often reside in obesogenic environments; further, their economic status means that healthy foods may be less feasible cost-wise. All of these circumstances can contribute to unhealthy eating and potentially binge eating and obesity.

Interventions to improve food environments must function at multiple levels, both environmental and individual, with changes in one domain ideally complemented by reinforcement for changes in other domains (Gittelsohn and Rowan 2011). As an illustration of the multiple levels of influence, qualitative analysis of interviews with African American adolescents from low-income families highlighted four environmental contexts that influenced food-related habits: neighborhood (e.g., accessibility of food), school food environment, family (e.g., modeling, monitoring), and peer behaviors (Christiansen et al. 2013). Thus, one important avenue to healthier outcomes involves improving access to healthy foods through strategies such as limiting unhealthy food accessibility, improving food transportation networks, constructing supermarkets, increasing the range of healthy food options and promoting these options in local food stores, and facilitating farmers' markets. Another avenue might involve a school focus, such as the Pathways intervention that trained school food-service workers in best practices food ordering and preparation and encouraged teachers to use nonfood rewards in Native American communities (Gittelsohn and Rowan 2011). Yet another avenue may focus on the family, such as the web-based program "Family Eats" that provided nutritional education and guidance to families in setting food-related change goals, resulting in better outcomes for African American families in terms of a healthy home food environment, for example, more fruit available at home, healthier food preparation practices, and healthier dining out practices (Cullen et al. 2013). Of note, in the ideal scenario, these multiple spheres of influence would be targeted concurrently.

Another way to think about nutrition/food management in racial/ethnic minorities is to assess whether they have culturally influenced diets or cultural values/traditions that may contribute to healthy or unhealthy eating. For example, Mexican Americans appear to consume low amounts of leafy green vegetables and fruits and reduced-fat dairy products (Carrera et al. 2007), although there is also evidence that Latinxs may have higher quality diets than African Americans and Caucasians based on the 2003–2004 National Health and Nutrition Examination Survey (Hiza et al. 2013). There is also research suggesting that Native Americans' diets are often poor in fresh produce and micronutrients but heavy in refined carbohydrates, fat, and sodium (Harnack et al. 1999; Sharma et al. 2008). With a careful assessment of diet and a culturally informed and culturally sensitive approach to recommended changes, additions or modifications (e.g., in food preparation, such as not using lard) are feasible. One study of Latinx families that relied on parental input found that parents were receptive to integrating healthy substitutes in their traditional meals: "We have to keep our traditional foods, but realize that we can make them more nutritious" (Flores et al. 2012).

It is important that nutrition- and food-related interventions reflect an understanding of culture, such as the importance of eating traditional foods and the possible conflicts between cultural norms and healthy eating. For example, to the degree that parents may equate making food with showing love, there may be conflict when a child does not want to eat as much as is expected, which could turn meals into a power struggle. Focus groups of adolescent African American females and their mothers noted the centrality of food in social and family gatherings in African American culture, with adolescents reporting feeling pressure to eat large amounts and certain kinds of traditional foods when with family or at community functions (Palmberg et al. 2014). As another example of the need for cultural understanding, many Native Americans may view being overweight or obese as healthy due to historical lack of food availability, suggesting that nutritional education might be beneficial for encouraging healthier food choices (Berg et al. 2012). Modifications of existing nutrition education programs should consider factors such as bilingual–bicultural educators and the use of community health workers as well as the acknowledgement and incorporation of cultural values and cultural practices around mealtime in order to increase acceptance and adherence (Broyles et al. 2011; Mier et al. 2009).

TREATMENT

Regarding treatment goals, the first goal is connecting racial/ethnic minorities with eating pathology to treatment providers. We already addressed possible public and clinician bias that limits identification and referral rates, a common first step to seeking treatment, as well as commented on intervention related to nutrition. Here, we focus on psychological treatment and its access. Minority women are less likely than Caucasian women to seek care for eating disorders and once they do seek care for eating disorders, ethnic minorities are less likely to receive treatment (Becker et al. 2003). Once identified and referred, financial aspects may play a role in treatment received for some minorities. One study found that among youth hospitalized with an eating disorder (AN, BN, or what was formerly called eating disorder not otherwise specified [EDNOS]), Latinxs and African Americans were less likely to have private insurance (Calderon et al. 2007). Thus, issues related to insurance or financial status may have an impact on whether or not clients are able to seek and/or receive treatment.

Ethnic identity and degree of acculturation may also play a role in whether or not minorities seek treatment for an eating disorder. As aforementioned, the strong Black woman ideology, while a positive aspect of African American female identity (Harrington et al. 2010), may also hinder treatment seeking for an eating disorder because of the belief that one should solve one's problems without help. For cases where ethnic identity includes the concept that problems are taken care of within the family, this aspect of identity may dissuade racial/ethnic minorities from seeking treatment. An examination of acculturation among Latinas in a community sample found that of those who were diagnosed with eating disorders, those who were less acculturated (e.g., bilingual, foreign born, had parents who were foreign born) were less likely to seek and receive treatment for their eating disorder symptoms in the past year, when compared with those who were more acculturated (Cachelin et al. 2000). For Asian Americans, the stigma attached to psychological disorders and the loss of "face" they cause in many Asian cultures could serve to keep these problems from coming to light and discourage Asian Americans with eating disorders from drawing attention to themselves by seeking treatment or participating in research (Cachelin et al. 2000). There are concerning implications for delayed referrals and treatment seeking in that when racial/ethnic minorities do present for treatment, eating disorder symptoms (e.g., binge eating in a sample of African Americans seeking treatment for BED; Lydecker and Grilo 2016) and psychiatric comorbidities are often more severe (e.g., mood and anxiety disorders in a sample of African Americans and Latinxs seeking treatment for BED; Grilo et al. 2013).

The most efficacious and recommended treatment for eating disorders is cognitive-behavioral therapy (CBT), but many treatment studies do not include racial/ethnic minorities in their trials (Cummins and Lehman 2007) and fewer have examined culturally specific adaptations. Franko (2007) argues for a two-step approach in intervention work with racial/ethnic minorities, first examining if existing empirically supported treatments are effective in these groups and, if this is not the case, developing and assessing culturally specific modifications of existing treatments or entirely new treatment programs.

Using a randomized, controlled multisite study design, CBT and interpersonal therapy (IPT) were examined in Caucasian and ethnic minority women with BN (Chui et al. 2007). At the end of treatment in this exploratory research, all racial/ethnic groups in the study (Caucasian, African American, Hispanic, and Asian) displayed higher abstinence rates of binge eating and purging for CBT than IPT, supporting CBT as the treatment of choice in these groups.

The efficacy of a variety of psychosocial treatments for BED was assessed by aggregating data across multiple randomized, controlled trials to examine the relative influence of race/ethnicity on the outcome of treatment. In a sample of African American, Latinx, and non-Latino Caucasian patients, it was found that race/ethnicity generally did not influence treatment outcome. More specifically, race/ethnicity did not moderate the effect of format of treatment (individual vs. group) or treatment length on posttreatment BED symptom levels (Thompson-Brenner et al. 2013). In a study of a cognitive-behaviorally based nutrition and physical activity treatment in a sample of African American and Caucasian obese women, differential effects of race/ethnicity on treatment outcome (body satisfaction change) were not found (Annesi et al. 2014). However, there is some evidence that African Americans are more likely to drop out of treatment for BED than Caucasians, suggesting a greater need for attention to the retention of African Americans in treatment for BED (Thompson-Brenner et al. 2013). Researchers seeking an intervention that may be more feasible and sustainable among racial/ethnic minority women, who may less likely seek treatment in clinics, tested a "lifestyle intervention" promoting healthy dietary habits and physical activity (Mama et al. 2015). They found that this behavior intervention, with its focus on physical activity, contributed to decreased binge-eating symptoms among African American and Latina women.

Research in other psychological disorders suggests that thoughtful, data-driven modifications to existing treatments may yield better outcomes for racial/ethnic minorities (e.g., treatment adaptations for the treatment of depression; Miranda et al. 2003). Preliminary research is being done to adapt CBT for bulimia nervosa (CBT-BN; Fairburn and Wilson 1993) for Latinxs living in the United States. The adaptations attend to the following specific values of Latinxs: familismo (familism), personalismo (personalism), and fatalism (Reyes-Rodriguez et al. 2014); for example, attention to familism can be seen in the cultural adaptation of family member involvement. Incorporating the factors of familism and personalism in particular serve to reduce patient drop out, a problem commonly seen among Latinxs seeking mental health care (Añez et al. 2008). In terms of fatalism, which is the belief that certain events are bound or destined to happen due to external factors and is represented in the statement "No matter what I do, if I am going to get sick, I will get sick" (Wallston and Strudler Wallston 1981), therapeutic interventions focus on the patient's self-efficacy for change, with specific focus on bringing the influence of fatalism on therapy and disordered eating into the patient's awareness and challenging distorted cognitions. This culturally adapted treatment of CBT-BN led to decreased binge eating and purging, depression, and acculturative stress, suggesting promise for use among Latinxs (Reyes-Rodriguez et al. 2014). To our knowledge, there are no widespread culturally sensitive treatments that have been specifically tailored to African American, Asian American, or Native American clients.

Treatment goals and approaches with racial/ethnic minorities should consider cultural factors. For example, collectivism, which is emphasized in many minority groups more so than the individualistic values in the dominant US culture (Gaines et al. 1997), may be a lens therapists should look through to better understand their clients' worldviews. Another example of a culturally emphasized concept that should potentially be considered is that of "saving face." It has been suggested that face-saving be accommodated as a normative component of treatment for individuals from Chinese cultures, instead of being treated as avoidance (Lester and Ma 2013). In the case of Native Americans, researchers stress that clinicians must strive to understand the collective Native American experience. Native Americans have been systematically subjected to a number of traumatic experiences throughout their history, including genocide, forced assimilation, and culture loss; these collective experiences should be considered with culturally competent clinicians assessing risk factors unique to this population and being sensitive to their significance in shaping individuals' identities and psychopathology (Clark and Winterowd 2012).

Treatment for eating disorders in ethnic minorities should also recognize the significance of racially defined features and how internalized racism, in the form of aspirations toward the Caucasian physical ideal, can negatively impact body esteem and produce unhealthy weight control behaviors. There is some evidence that Asian Americans in particular may be more likely to desire Caucasian features than other racial/ethnic minorities (Evans and McConnell 2003). Given that low levels of ethnic identity appear to confer risk for body dissatisfaction and eating pathology among racial/ethnic minorities (and that the converse is also true: high levels of ethnic identity may be protective), treatment may want to incorporate an examination of ethnic identity and the benefits of embracing one's culture. Relatedly, level of acculturation should be examined to help understand what factors may be in place that increase risk for or maintain the eating disorder. For example, Asian Americans who are very highly acculturated to White culture may face unique stresses in terms of conflicts with less acculturated parents that may prompt dietary restriction as an attempt to gain control or binge eating as a means of escape; they may also experience maintenance factors shared by Caucasian peers, such as dieting frequently. Lastly, while a goal of a strong therapeutic alliance is always advised in therapy, this may be especially important in treating eating disorders in racial/ethnic minorities, since these groups may feel out-of-step with their cultural group (even though prevalence rates of eating disorders generally do not differ across racial/ethnic group), may be more inexperienced with therapy, may be more interested in seeing a counselor of the same ethnicity, and may be more distrustful of health-care professionals (López et al. 1991; Pomales and Williams 1989).

In sum, racial/ethnic minorities are less likely to receive treatment for an eating disorder than non-Hispanic Caucasians and little intervention research has examined the efficacy of treatment specifically in different racial/ethnic groups. Preliminary evidence suggests that CBT may be efficacious in African American, Latina, and Asian American individuals with BN, and that a modification of CBT incorporating values important to Latinxs has shown promise in reducing bulimic symptoms and acculturative stress among Latinas. Health-care professionals working with racial/ethnic minorities with eating disorders may want to keep in mind aspects specific to these groups (e.g., collectivism, ethnic identity, and level of acculturation) as a way to foster a strong therapeutic alliance, to better understand their clients' world views, and to possibly bolster protective factors related to culture.

PREVENTION

Testing and improving upon eating disorder interventions for racial/ethnic minorities are clearly important. Although less work has been done on testing and improving prevention efforts for racial/ethnic minorities, this work is equally critical. As referred to earlier, some race/ethnicity constructs seem to provide a buffering effect against body dissatisfaction and disordered eating, namely ethnic identity. Here, we review examples of more systematic prevention efforts focused on racial/ethnic minorities. A cognitive dissonance-based prevention program with substantial support in non-Latina Caucasian samples, the Body Project, was found to be equally effective in reducing body dissatisfaction and disordered eating for Latinas and non-Latina Caucasians (Stice et al. 2014). Similarly, a dissonance-based prevention program was found to be equally effective in reducing thin-ideal internalization, body dissatisfaction, and disordered eating symptoms among Latina, Asian American, and non-Latina Caucasian adolescent and young adult women aged 13–20 (Rodriguez et al. 2008). Based on these findings, it may be that tailoring prevention programs to participants' ethnicities is not necessary, but more work is needed to conclusively determine this across a range of racial/ethnic minority groups of both genders.

There is also evidence supporting the use of the online prevention program, StayingFit, with racially/ethnically diverse high school students (Jones et al. 2014). This program has two tracks: weight management (for those who are overweight) and healthy habits (for those who are normal weight). Researchers found that in their sample of primarily Latinx, African American, and multiracial adolescents, those in the weight management track reduced their BMIs and those in the normal weight track maintained their BMIs. Furthermore, weight/shape concerns significantly decreased among participants in both tracks who had elevated concerns at baseline. Fruit and vegetable intake increased among participants in both tracks, while physical activity increased and soda and television consumption decreased among participants in the weight management track. This prevention program appears to be effective at reducing weight for those who are overweight, while encouraging healthy eating habits and reducing weight/shape concerns for both groups. The use of an online format for this and other prevention efforts may be especially important for reaching racial/ethnic minorities who for financial, stigma, or other reasons may be less likely to participate in in-person prevention programs.

The following are two case studies of racial/ethnic minority females with eating disorders that include some of the topics addressed above, followed by questions one might consider in approaching treatment with these individuals.

CASE STUDY 11.1

CT

CT is a 19-year-old African American female college student. Her high school years were spent at a predominantly Caucasian school where she had mainly Caucasian friends and did not identify strongly with African

(Continued)

CASE STUDY 11.1 (*CONTINUED*)

American culture. Now attending a predominantly Caucasian university, her friend group continues to be mainly Caucasian, but she feels more pressure from her peers to look a certain way. In particular, her friends talk a lot about their bodies (often making negative comments about how they look) and engage in dieting to lose weight. When CT compares her body to theirs, she easily finds unwanted discrepancies: she is heavier than her friends and has bigger hips. As part of trying to fit in to the new environment of college, she has been skipping lunch to lose weight, but finds that later in the day she usually loses control of her eating and ends up binge eating on food from the cafeteria or snacks she has in her dorm. While the binge eating actually provides some escape from her negative feelings about her body, she is also worried that she will gain weight. Thus, after a month of recurrent binge eating, CT starts self-inducing vomiting as an attempt to counteract the binges.

QUESTIONS

1. It is unclear how strong CT's racial/ethnic identity is given the peer culture she grew up in—how might racial/ethnic identity be approached in treatment and what are the ways to help engage her with this part of her identity?
2. In the context of CBT, how might overvaluation of weight/shape be broached, recognizing her sociocultural milieu (where thinness is clearly highly valued), her desire to fit in, and her body size (heavier, larger hips)?
3. How might an exploration of discrimination experiences inform treatment and provide greater understanding of CT's disordered eating behaviors?

CASE STUDY 11.2

AK

AK is a 30-year-old, first-generation Chinese American female. Her immigrant parents expected her to be married by this age or to at least have gotten further in a prestigious career. AK feels stress from living in a bicultural world where she feels her parents have one set of expectations that differ from those she sees for herself or that she sees amid her peers. She wants to make her parents proud and has perfectionistic personality traits that make her want to excel to the extreme. As a result of her perceiving that she does not meet up to her parents' standards or her own, she begins to feel both anxious and depressed and not in control of her life. AK finds that she is

(Continued)

able to exert control over eating by limiting her calorie intake and excluding high-fat foods from her diet. This eating pattern provides some comfort to her as she feels that she has agency over food whereas she does not have full agency over parental expectations, her romantic relationship, and her career. This eating pattern has resulted in her losing a great deal of weight to the point that her friends and family are concerned; however, given her feelings of shame associated with possibly having an eating disorder, AK is not willing to seek help.

QUESTIONS

1. What role might perfectionism play in terms of the disordered eating behaviors and potential comorbidities, and how might a nuanced discussion of perfectionism, including a focus on maladaptive, socially prescribed perfectionism, help diminish negative effects of perfectionism?
2. Acculturative stress appears relevant to AK's presentation—in a CBT context, how might exploration of these tensions help both with understanding her lived experience and with identifying areas she can adaptively have agency over?
3. It is important that therapists understand the cultural motivation to "save face," while also recognizing that this could act as an impediment to treatment. Should this individual come in for therapy, how can this be addressed in a way so that what motivates her may shift and she more likely stays in treatment?

SUMMARY AND CONCLUSIONS

In conclusion, burgeoning research contradicts long-held assumptions by health-care professionals and public opinion that racial/ethnic minorities do not experience eating disorders. Research demonstrates that racial/ethnic minorities may experience these disorders at equivalent or elevated rates to their Caucasian, non-Latinx counterparts, although minorities tend to be diagnosed later and referred less than majority clients. Although we have new knowledge regarding prevalence, there is much more to be learned about the experience of eating disorders by racial/ethnic minorities. Psychometrics of eating disorder instruments are beginning to be tested among minority samples, although the status of validated measures varies dramatically between racial/ethnic groups. Preliminary research has found that many of the risk factors identified in Caucasian, non-Latinx majority samples generalize to minorities as well. However, there are also culturally specific risk factors that must be considered when working with racial/ethnic minorities. Regarding treatment, there is some support for CBT for racial/ethnic minorities struggling with BN, but much more intervention research is needed to test existing treatments and consider culturally adapted treatments, including possible modifications of treatment goals and approaches. The field of prevention of eating disorders in racial/ethnic minorities is quite young, with more research needed to test the effectiveness of such prevention efforts and whether improvements would result from culturally adapted modifications.

The eating disorder field is at an exciting point in regard to expanding our knowledge about eating pathology among diverse populations. In addition to further identifying psychometrically strong assessments, examining risk factors (both those established in primarily Caucasian samples and those relevant to racial/ethnic minorities), and developing optimal intervention and prevention strategies, future research should explore an array of other topics. For example, research is needed examining Other Specified Feeding or Eating Disorders (OSFED; formerly known as EDNOS) in minorities, including atypical but distressing eating patterns (e.g., purging disorder). Future work should broaden the demographics of the samples investigated to include males, community samples, and clinical samples. Given the challenges inherent in getting large enough sample sizes of racial/ethnic minorities, multisite research may be needed to attain the power necessary to test hypotheses. Research is also needed considering nuances of race/ethnicity; for example, minimal research has examined multiracial/ multiethnic individuals or within-group heterogeneity (e.g., Asian Americans of different Asian origins). Lastly, research should be theory-driven and test complex models that would help identify conditions under which racial/ethnic minorities are at greater risk for eating disorders (i.e., moderator models) and pathways through which racial/ethnic minorities develop eating disorders (i.e., mediation models).

REFERENCES

Adamus-Leach, HJ, Wilson PL, O'Connor DP, Rhode PC, Mama SK, and Lee RE. Depression, stress and body fat are associated with binge eating in a community sample of African American and Hispanic Women. *Eating and Weight Disorders-Studies on Anorexia, Bulimia and Obesity* 18, no. 2 (2013): 221–227.

Akan, GE, and Grilo CM. Sociocultural influences on eating attitudes and behaviors, body image, and psychological functioning: A comparison of African-American, Asian-American, and Caucasian College Women. *International Journal of Eating Disorders* 18, no. 2 (1995): 181–187.

Alegria, M, Woo M, Cao Z, Torres M, Meng XL, and Striegel-Moore RH. Prevalence and correlates of eating disorders in Latinos in the United States. *International Journal of Eating Disorders* 40, no. 3 (2007): S15–S21.

American Psychiatric Association. *Diagnostic and Statistical Manual of Mental Disorders* (5th ed.). Washington, DC: Author, 2013.

Añez, LM, Silva MA, Paris M, and Bedregal LE. Engaging Latinos through the integration of cultural values and motivational interviewing principles. *Professional Psychology: Research and Practice* 39, no. 2 (2008): 153–159.

Annesi, JJ, Tennant GA, and Mareno N. Treatment-associated changes in body composition, health behaviors, and mood as predictors of change in body satisfaction in obese women effects of age and race/ethnicity. *Health Education and Behavior* 41, no. 6 (2014): 1–9.

Arcelus, J, Mitchell AJ, Wales J, and Nielsen S. Mortality rates in patients with anorexia nervosa and other eating disorders: A meta-analysis of 36 studies. *Archives of General Psychiatry* 68, no. 7 (2011): 724–731.

Ayala, GX, Mickens L, Galindo P, and Elder JP. Acculturation and body image perception among Latino youth. *Ethnicity and Health* 12, no. 1 (2007): 21–41.

Bardone-Cone, AM, and Boyd CA. Psychometric properties of eating disorder instruments in black and white young women: Internal consistency, temporal stability, and validity. *Psychological Assessment* 19, no. 3 (2007): 356–362.

Bardone-Cone, AM, Harney MB, and Boyd CA. What if high expectations feel good? Perceived parental expectations, their meanings, and bulimic symptoms in black and white college women. *Eating Behaviors* 13, no. 2 (2012): 170–173.

Bardone-Cone, AM, Weishuhn AS, and Boyd CA. Perfectionism and bulimic symptoms in African American college women: Dimensions of perfectionism and their interactions with perceived weight status. *Journal of Counseling Psychology* 56, no. 2 (2009): 266–275.

Bardone-Cone, AM, Wonderlich SA, Frost RO, Bulik CM, Mitchell JE, Uppala S, and Simonich H. Perfectionism and eating disorders: Current status and future directions. *Clinical Psychology Review* 27, no. 3 (2007): 384–405.

Barnes, RD, Ivezaj V, and Grilo CM. An examination of weight bias among treatment-seeking obese patients with and without binge eating disorder. *General Hospital Psychiatry* 36, no. 2 (2014): 177–180.

Becker, AE, Burwell RA, Gilman SE, Herzog DB, and Hamburg P. Eating behaviours and attitudes following prolonged exposure to television among ethnic Fijian adolescent girls. *British Journal of Psychiatry* 180, no. 6 (2002): 509–514.

Becker, AE, Franko DL, Speck A, and Herzog DB. Ethnicity and differential access to care for eating disorder symptoms. *International Journal of Eating Disorders* 33, no. 2 (2003): 205–212.

Belon, KE, McLaughlin EA, Smith JE, Bryan AD, Witkiewitz K, Lash DN, and Winn JL. Testing the measurement invariance of the eating disorder inventory in nonclinical samples of Hispanic and Caucasian women. *International Journal of Eating Disorders* 48, no. 3 (2015): 262–270.

Berg, CJ, Daley CM, Nazir N, Kinlacheeny JB, Ashley A, Ahluwalia JS, Greiner KA, and Choi WS. Physical activity and fruit and vegetable intake among American Indians. *Journal of Community Health* 37, no. 1 (2012): 65–71.

Berry, JW. Immigration, acculturation, and adaptation. *Applied Psychology* 46, no. 1 (1997): 5–34.

Berry, JW. Marginality, stress and ethnic identification in an acculturated aboriginal community. *Journal of Cross-Cultural Psychology* 1, no. 3 (1970): 239–252.

Berry, JW, Kim U, Minde T, and Mok D. Comparative studies of acculturative stress. *International Migration Review* 21, (1987): 491–511.

Blue, EL, and Berkel LA. Feminist identity attitudes, negative affect, and eating pathology in African American College Women. *Journal of Black Psychology* 36, no. 4 (2010): 426–445.

Bodell, LP, Joiner TE, and Ialongo NS. Longitudinal association between childhood impulsivity and bulimic symptoms in African American adolescent girls. *Journal of Consulting and Clinical Psychology* 80, no. 2 (2012): 313–316.

Boyd, EM, Reynolds JR, Tillman KH, and Martin PY. Adolescent girls' race/ethnic status, identities, and drive for thinness. *Social Science Research* 40, no. 2 (2011): 667–684.

Broyles, SL, Brennan JJ, Burke KH, Kozo J, and Taras HL. Cultural adaptation of a nutrition education curriculum for Latino families to promote acceptance. *Journal of Nutrition Education and Behavior* 43, no. 4 (2011): S158–S161.

Bucchianeri, MM, Fernandes N, Loth K, Hannan PJ, Eisenberg ME, and Neumark-Sztainer D. Body dissatisfaction: Do associations with disordered eating and psychological well-being differ across race/ethnicity in adolescent girls and boys? *Cultural Diversity and Ethnic Minority* 22, no. 1 (2015): 137–146.

Burroughs, VJ, Nonas C, Sweeney CT, Rohay JM, Harkins AM, Kyle TK, and Burton SL. Self-reported comorbidities among self-described overweight African-American and Hispanic adults in the United States: Results of a national survey. *Obesity* 16, no. 6 (2008): 1400–1406.

Cachelin, FM, Veisel C, Barzegarnazari E, and Striegel-Moore RH. Disordered eating, acculturation, and treatment-seeking in a community sample of Hispanic, Asian, Black, and White women. *Psychology of Women Quarterly* 24, no. 3 (2000): 244–253.

Calderon, R, Vander Stoep A, Collett B, Garrison MM, and Toth K. Inpatients with eating disorders: Demographic, diagnostic, and service characteristics from a nationwide pediatric sample. *International Journal of Eating Disorders* 40, no. 7 (2007): 622–628.

Carrera, PM, Gao X, and Tucker KL. A study of dietary patterns in the Mexican-American population and their association with obesity. *Journal of the American Dietetic Association* 107, no. 10 (2007): 1735–1742.

Cash, TF. *The Multidimensional Body-Self Relations Questionnaire.* Norfolk, VA: Old Dominion University, 1994.

Chang, EC, Perera MJ, and Kupfermann Y. Predictors of eating disturbances in South Asian American females and males: A look at negative affectivity and contingencies of self-worth. *Asian American Journal of Psychology* 5, no. 3 (2014a): 172–180.

Chang, EC, Yu EA, and Kahle ER. BMI, body discrepancy, and self-construal as predictors of eating disturbances in European and Asian American females. *Eating Behaviors* 15, no. 2 (2014b): 328–330.

Chang, EC, Yu EA, and Lin EY. An examination of ethnic variations in perfectionism and interpersonal influences as predictors of eating disturbances: A look at Asian and European American females. *Asian American Journal of Psychology* 5, no. 3 (2014c): 243–251.

Cheng, HL. Disordered eating among Asian/Asian American women racial and cultural factors as correlates. *Counseling Psychologist* 42, no. 6 (2014): 821–851.

Christiansen, KM, Qureshi F, Schaible A, Park S, and Gittelsohn J. Environmental factors that impact the eating behaviors of low-income African American adolescents in Baltimore city. *Journal of Nutrition Education and Behavior* 45, no. 6 (2013): 652–660.

Chui, W, Safer DL, Bryson SW, Agras WS, and Wilson GT. A comparison of ethnic groups in the treatment of bulimia nervosa. *Eating Behaviors* 8, no. 4 (2007): 485–491.

Clark, JD, and Winterowd C. Correlates and predictors of binge eating among Native American women. *Journal of Multicultural Counseling and Development* 40, no. 2 (2012): 117–127.

Claudat, K, White EK, and Warren CS. Acculturative stress, self-esteem, and eating pathology in Latina and Asian American female college students. *Journal of Clinical Psychology* 72, no. 1 (2016): 88–100.

Cooper, PJ, Taylor MJ, Cooper Z, and Fairburn GC. The development and validation of the body shape questionnaire. *International Journal of Eating Disorders* 6, no. 4 (1987): 485–494.

Cordero, ED, Julian AK, and Murray KE. Measurement of disordered eating in Latina college women. *Eating Behaviors* 14, no. 2 (2013): 220–223.

Cullen, KW, Thompson DI, and Chen A. The impact of goal attainment on the outcomes of family eats, a web-based program on healthy home food environments for African-American families. *Journal of the Academy of Nutrition and Dietetics* 9, no. 113 (2013): A46.

Cummins, LH, and Lehman J. Eating disorders and body image concerns in Asian American women: Assessment and treatment from a multicultural and feminist perspective. *Eating Disorders* 15, no. 3 (2007): 217–230.

Cummins, LH, Lehman JD, and Liu RC. Eating disorders in Asians. In *Handbook of Adult Psychopathology in Asians: Theory, Diagnosis, and Treatment,* edited by LH Cummins and EC Chang, pp. 249–289. New York, NY: Oxford University Press, 2012.

Cummins, LH, Simmons AM, and Zane NW. Eating disorders in Asian populations: A critique of current approaches to the study of culture, ethnicity, and eating disorders. *American Journal of Orthopsychiatry* 75, no. 4 (2005): 553–574.

Davis, SM, and Lambert LC. Body image and weight concerns among Southwestern American Indian preadolescent schoolchildren. *Ethnicity and Disease* 10, no. 2 (1999): 184–194.

Elder, KA, and Grilo CM. The Spanish language version of the Eating Disorder Examination Questionnaire: Comparison with the Spanish language version of the eating disorder examination and test–retest reliability. *Behaviour Research and Therapy* 45, no. 6 (2007): 1369–1377.

Elliott, CA, Tanofsky-Kraff M, and Mirza NM. Parent report of binge eating in Hispanic, African American and Caucasian youth. *Eating Behaviors* 14, no. 1 (2013): 1–6.

Evans, PC, and McConnell AR. Do racial minorities respond in the same way to mainstream beauty standards? Social comparison processes in Asian, Black, and White women. *Self and Identity* 2, no. 2 (2003): 153–167.

Fairburn, CG, and Beglin SJ. Assessment of eating disorders: Interview or self-report questionnaire? *International Journal of Eating Disorders* 16, no. 4 (1994): 363–370.

Fairburn, CG, and Cooper Z. The eating disorder examination. In *Binge Eating: Nature, Assessment and Treatment* (12th ed.), edited by CG Fairburn and GT Wilson, pp. 317–360. New York, NY: Guilford Press, 1993.

Fairburn, CG, and Wilson GT. *Binge Eating: Nature, Assessment, and Treatment.* New York, NY: Guilford Press, 1993.

Fernandez, S, Malcarne VL, Wilfley DE, and McQuaid J. Factor structure of the Bulimia Test-Revised in college women from four ethnic groups. *Cultural Diversity and Ethnic Minority Psychology* 12, no. 3 (2006): 403–419.

Field, AE, Coakley EH, Must A, Spadano JL, Laird N, Dietz WH, Rimm E, and Colditz GA. Impact of overweight on the risk of developing common chronic diseases during a 10-year period. *Archives of Internal Medicine* 161, no. 13 (2001): 1581–1586.

Flores, G, Maldonado J, and Durán P. Making tortillas without lard: Latino parents' perspectives on healthy eating, physical activity, and weight-management strategies for overweight Latino children. *Journal of the Academy of Nutrition and Dietetics* 112, no. 1 (2012): 81–89.

Flowers, KC, Levesque MJ, and Fischer S. The relationship between maladaptive eating behaviors and racial identity among African American women in college. *Journal of Black Psychology* 38, no. 3 (2012): 290–312.

Franko, DL. Race, ethnicity, and eating disorders: Considerations for DSM-V. *International Journal of Eating Disorders* 40, Suppl. (2007): S31–S34.

Franko, DL, Becker AE, Thomas JJ, and Herzog DB. Cross-ethnic differences in eating disorder symptoms and related distress. *International Journal of Eating Disorders* 40, no. 2 (2007): 156–164.

Franko, DL, Jenkins A, Roehrig JP, Luce KH, Crowther JH, and Rodgers RF. Psychometric properties of measures of eating disorder risk in Latina college women. *International Journal of Eating Disorders* 45, no. 4 (2012): 592–596.

Franko, DL, and Striegel-Moore RH. The role of body dissatisfaction as a risk factor for depression in adolescent girls: Are the differences Black and White? *Journal of Psychosomatic Research* 53, no. 5 (2002): 975–983.

Freedman, RE, Carter MM, Sbrocco T, and Gray JJ. Ethnic differences in preferences for female weight and waist-to-hip ratio: A comparison of African–American and White American college and community samples. *Eating Behaviors* 5, no. 3 (2004): 191–198.

Gaines, SO, Marelich WD, Bledsoe KL, Steers WN, Henderson MC, Granrose CS, Barájas L, Hicks D, Lyde M, Takahashi Y, Yum N, Ríos DI, García BF, Farris KR, and Page MS. Links between race/ethnicity and cultural values as mediated by racial/ethnic identity and moderated by gender. *Journal of Personality and Social Psychology* 72, no. 6 (1997): 1460–1476.

Garner, DM, Olmsted MP, Bohr Y, and Garfinkel PE. The eating attitudes test: Psychometric features and clinical correlates. *Psychological Medicine* 12, no. 4 (1982): 871–878.

Garner, DM, Olmstead MP, and Polivy J. Development and validation of a multidimensional eating disorder inventory for anorexia nervosa and bulimia. *International Journal of Eating Disorders* 2, no. 2 (1983): 15–34.

Gittelsohn, J, and Rowan M. Preventing diabetes and obesity in American Indian communities: The potential of environmental interventions. *American Journal of Clinical Nutrition* 93, no. 5 (2011): 1179S–1183S.

Gluck, ME, and Geliebter A. Racial/ethnic differences in body image and eating behaviors. *Eating Behaviors* 3, no. 2 (2002): 143–151.

Gordon, KH, Brattole MM, Wingate LR, and Joiner TE. The impact of client race on clinician detection of eating disorders. *Behavior Therapy* 37, no. 4 (2006): 319–325.

Gordon, KH, Castro Y, Sitnikov L, and Holm-Denoma JM. Cultural body shape ideals and eating disorder symptoms among White, Latina, and Black college women. *Cultural Diversity and Ethnic Minority Psychology* 16, no. 2 (2010): 135–143.

Gordon, KH, Perez M, and Joiner TE. The impact of racial stereotypes on eating disorder recognition. *International Journal of Eating Disorders* 32, no. 2 (2002): 219–224.

Gormally, J, Black S, Daston S, and Rardin D. The assessment of binge eating severity among obese persons. *Addictive Behaviors* 7, no. 1 (1982): 47–55.

Gowen, LK, Hayward C, Killen JD, Robinson TN, and Barr Taylor C. Acculturation and eating disorder symptoms in adolescent girls. *Journal of Research on Adolescence* 9, no. 1 (1999): 67–83.

Grabe, S, and Hyde JS. Ethnicity and body dissatisfaction among women in the United States: A meta-analysis. *Psychological Bulletin* 132, no. 4 (2006): 622–640.

Granillo, T, Jones-Rodriguez G, and Carvajal SC. Prevalence of eating disorders in Latina adolescents: Associations with substance use and other correlates. *Journal of Adolescent Health* 36, no. 3 (2005): 214–220.

Gray, WN, Simon SL, Janicke DM, and Dumont-Driscoll M. Moderators of weight-based stigmatization among youth who are overweight and non-overweight: The role of gender, race, and body dissatisfaction. *Journal of Developmental and Behavioral Pediatrics* 32, no. 2 (2011): 110–116.

Greenberg, DR, and LaPorte DJ. Racial differences in body type preferences of men for women. *International Journal of Eating Disorders* 19, no. 3 (1996): 275–278.

Grilo, CM, Crosby RD, and White MA. Spanish-language Eating Disorder Examination interview: Factor structure in Latino/as. *Eating Behaviors* 13, no. 4 (2012): 410–413.

Grilo, CM, Lozano C, Elder KA. Inter-rater and test-retest reliability of the Spanish language version of the Eating Disorder Examination interview: Clinical and research implications. *Journal of Psychiatric Practice* 11, no. 4 (2005): 231–240.

Grilo, CM, White MA, Barnes RD, and Masheb RM. Psychiatric disorder co-morbidity and correlates in an ethnically diverse sample of obese patients with binge eating disorder in primary care settings. *Comprehensive Psychiatry* 54, no. 3 (2013): 209–216.

Hall, CCI. Asian eyes: Body image and eating disorders of Asian and Asian American women. *Eating Disorders* 3, no. 1 (1995): 8–19.

Harnack, L, Sherwood N, and Story M. Diet and physical activity patterns of urban American Indian women. *American Journal of Health Promotion* 13, no. 4 (1999): 233–236.

Harrington, EF, Crowther JH, Payne Henrickson HC, and Mickelson KD. The relationships among trauma, stress, ethnicity, and binge eating. *Cultural Diversity and Ethnic Minority Psychology* 12, no. 2 (2006): 212–229.

Harrington, EF, Crowther, JH and Shipherd JC. Trauma, binge eating, and the "strong Black woman." *Journal of Consulting and Clinical Psychology* 78, no. 4 (2010): 469–479.

Heatherton, TF, and Baumeister RF. Binge eating as escape from self-awareness. *Psychological Bulletin* 110, no. 1 (1991): 86–108.

Henrickson, HC, Crowther JH, and Harrington EF. Ethnic identity and maladaptive eating: Expectancies about eating and thinness in African American Women. *Cultural Diversity and Ethnic Minority Psychology* 16, no. 1 (2010): 87–93.

Higgins, MK, Lin SL, Alvarez A, and Bardone-Cone AM. Examining impulsivity as a moderator of the relationship between body shame and bulimic symptoms in Black and White young women. *Body Image* 14 (2015): 39–46.

Hiza, HA, Casavale KO, Guenther PM, and Davis CA. Diet quality of Americans differs by age, sex, race/ethnicity, income, and education level. *Journal of the Academy of Nutrition and Dietetics* 113, no. 2 (2013): 297–306.

Hoffman, ER, Gagne DA, Thornton LM, Klump KL, Brandt H, Crawford S, Fichter MM, Halmi KA, Johnson C, Jones I, Kaplan AS, Mitchell JE, Strober M, Treasure J, Woodside DB, Berrettini WH, Kaye WH, and Bulik CM. Understanding the association of impulsivity, obsessions, and compulsions with binge eating and purging behaviours in anorexia nervosa. *European Eating Disorders Review* 20, no. 3 (2012): e129–e136.

Iyer, DS, and Haslam N. Body image and eating disturbance among south Asian-American women: The role of racial teasing. *International Journal of Eating Disorders* 34, no. 1 (2003): 142–147.

Jahns, L, McDonald L, Wadsworth A, Morin C, Liu Y, and Nicklas T. Barriers and facilitators to following the Dietary Guidelines for Americans reported by rural, Northern Plains American-Indian Children. *Public Health Nutrition* 18, no. 3 (2015): 482–489.

Javier, SJ, and Belgrave FZ. An examination of influences on body dissatisfaction among Asian American College Females: Do family, media, or peers play a role? *Journal of American College Health* 63, no. 8 (2015): 579–583.

Jones, M, Taylor Lynch K, Kass AE, Burrows A, Williams J, Wilfley DE, and Taylor CB. Healthy weight regulation and eating disorder prevention in high school students: A universal and targeted Web-based intervention. *Journal of Medical Internet Research* 16, no. 2 (2014): 28–39.

Kashubeck-West, S, Coker AD, Awad GH, Stinson RD, Bledman R, and Mintz L. Do measures commonly used in body image research perform adequately with African American college women? *Cultural Diversity and Ethnic Minority Psychology* 19, no. 3 (2013): 357–368.

Keel, PK, and Klump, KL. Are eating disorders culture-bound syndromes? Implications for conceptualizing their etiology. *Psychological Bulletin* 129, no. 5 (2003): 747–769.

Kelly, NR, Cotter EW, Tanofsky-Kraff M, and Mazzeo SE. Racial variations in binge eating, body image concerns, and compulsive exercise among men. *Psychology of Men and Masculinity* 16, no. 3 (2015): 326–336.

Kelly, NR, Mitchell KS, Gow RW, Trace SE, Lydecker JA, Bair CE, and Mazzeo S. An evaluation of the reliability and construct validity of eating disorder measures in white and black women. *Psychological Assessment* 24, no. 3 (2012): 608–617.

Keum, TB, Wong SN, DeBlaere C, and Brewster ME. Body image and Asian American men: Examination of the drive for muscularity scale. *Psychology of Men and Masculinity* 16, no. 3 (2015): 284–293.

Kroon Van Diest, AM, Tartakovsky M, Stachon C, Pettit JW, and Perez M. The relationship between acculturative stress and eating disorder symptoms: Is it unique from general life stress? *Journal of Behavioral Medicine* 37, no. 3 (2014): 445–457.

Lacey, KK, Sears KP, Matusko N, and Jackson JS. Severe physical violence and black women's health and well-being. *American Journal of Public Health* 105, no. 4 (2015): 719–724.

Larson, NI, Story MT, and Nelson MC. Neighborhood environments: Disparities in access to healthy foods in the US. *American Journal of Preventive Medicine* 36, no. 1 (2009): 74–81.

Lee, S, Lee AM, Leung T, and Yu H. Psychometric properties of the Eating Disorders Inventory (EDI-1) in a nonclinical Chinese population in Hong Kong. *International Journal of Eating Disorders* 21, no. 2 (1997): 187–194.

Lester, RJ, and Ma JL. Anorexia nervosa and family therapy in a Chinese context. *Culture, Medicine, and Psychiatry* 37, (2013): 565–568.

Lopez, V, Corona R, and Halfond R. Effects of gender, media influences, and traditional gender role orientation on disordered eating and appearance concerns among Latino adolescents. *Journal of Adolescence* 36, no. 4 (2013): 727–736.

López, SR, López AA, and Fong KT. Mexican Americans' initial preferences for counselors: The role of ethnic factors. *Journal of Counseling Psychology* 38, no. 4 (1991): 487–496.

Lydecker, JA, White MA, and Grilo CM. Black patients with binge-eating disorder: Comparison of different assessment methods. *Psychological Assessment* 28, no. 10 (2016): 1319–1324.

Lydecker, JA, and Grilo CM. Different yet similar: Examining race and ethnicity in treatment-seeking adults with binge eating disorder. *Journal of Consulting and Clinical Psychology* 84, no. 1 (2016): 88–94.

Lynch, W, Eppers K, and Sherrodd J. Eating attitudes of Native American and white female adolescents: A comparison of BMI- and age-matched groups. *Ethnicity and Health* 9, no. 3 (2004): 253–266.

Lynch, WC, Heil DP, Wagner E, and Havens MD. Body dissatisfaction mediates the association between body mass index and risky weight control behaviors among White and Native American adolescent girls. *Appetite* 51, no. 1 (2008): 210–213.

Lynch, WC, Heil DP, Wagner E, and Havens MD. Ethnic differences in BMI, weight concerns, and eating behaviors: Comparison of Native American, White, and Hispanic adolescents. *Body Image* 4, no. 2 (2007): 179–190.

Mama, SK, Schembre SM, O'Connor DP, Kaplan CD, Bode S, and Lee RE. Effectiveness of lifestyle interventions to reduce binge eating symptoms in African American and Hispanic women. *Appetite* 93 (2015): 269–274.

Marques, L, Alegria M, Becker AE, Chen CN, Fang A, Chosak A, and Diniz JB. Comparative prevalence, correlates of impairment, and service utilization for eating disorders across US ethnic groups: Implications for reducing ethnic disparities in health care access for eating disorders. *International Journal of Eating Disorders* 44, no. 5 (2011): 412–420.

McCreary, DR, and Sasse DK. An exploration of the drive for muscularity in adolescent boys and girls. *Journal of American College Health* 48, no. 6 (2000): 297–304.

McKinley, NM, and Hyde JS. The Objectified Body Consciousness Scale: Development and validation. *Psychology of Women Quarterly* 20, no. 2 (1996): 181–215.

McKinnon, RA, Reedy J, Handy SL, and Rodgers AB. Measuring the food and physical activity environments: Shaping the research agenda. *American Journal of Preventive Medicine* 36, no. 4 (2009): S81–S85.

McLaughlin, KA, Hilt LM, and Nolen-Hoeksema S. Racial/ethnic differences in internalizing and externalizing symptoms in adolescents. *Journal of Abnormal Child Psychology* 35, no. 5 (2007): 801–816.

Mendelson, BK, Mendelson MJ, and White DR. Body-esteem scale for adolescents and adults. *Journal of Personality Assessment* 76, no. 1 (2001): 90–106.

Menon, CV, and Harter SL. Examining the impact of acculturative stress on body image disturbance among Hispanic college students. *Cultural Diversity and Ethnic Minority Psychology* 18, no. 3 (2012): 239–246.

Michael, SL, Wentzel K, Elliott MN, Dittus PJ, Kanouse DE, Wallander JL, Pasch KE, Franzini L, Taylor WC, Qureshi T, Franklin FA, and Schuster MA. Parental and peer factors associated with body image discrepancy among fifth-grade boys and girls. *Journal of Youth and Adolescence* 43, no. 1 (2014): 15–29.

Mier, N, Ory MG, and Medina AA. Anatomy of culturally sensitive interventions promoting nutrition and exercise in Hispanics: A critical examination of existing literature. *Health Promotion Practice* 11, no. 4 (2009): 541–554.

Mintz, LB, and Kashubeck S. Body image and disordered eating among Asian American and Caucasian college students an examination of race and gender differences. *Psychology of Women Quarterly* 23, no. 4 (1999): 781–796.

Miranda, J, Azocar F, Organista KC, Dwyer E, and Areane P. Treatment of depression among impoverished primary care patients from ethnic minority groups. *Psychiatric Services* 54, no. 2 (2003): 219–225.

Mitchell, KS, and Mazzeo SE. Binge eating and psychological distress in ethnically diverse undergraduate men and women. *Eating Behaviors* 5, no. 2 (2004): 157–169.

Mitchell, KS, and Mazzeo SE. Evaluation of a structural model of objectification theory and eating disorder symptomatology among European American and African American undergraduate women. *Psychology of Women Quarterly* 33, no. 4 (2009): 384–395.

National Heart Lung and Blood Institute and National Institutes of Health. Who is at risk for overweight and obesity? 2009. Available at http://www.nhlbi.nih.gov.libproxy.lib.unc.edu/health/health-topics/topics/obe/atrisk.html.

Neumark-Sztainer, D, Story M, French SA, Hannan PJ, Resnick MD, and Blum RW. Psychosocial concerns and health-compromising behaviors among overweight and non-over weight adolescents. *Obesity Research* 5, no. 3 (1997): 237–249.

Nicdao, EG, Hong S, and Takeuchi DT. Prevalence and correlates of eating disorders among Asian Americans: Results from the National Latino and Asian American study. *International Journal of Eating Disorders* 40, no. S3 (2007): S22–S26.

Nichter, M. *Fat Talk: What Girls and Their Parents Say about Dieting.* Cambridge, MA: Harvard University Press, 2009.

Ogden, CL, Carroll MD, and Flegal KM. High body mass index for age among US children and adolescents, 2003–2006. *Journal of the American Medical Association* 299, no. 20 (2008): 2401–2405.

Olvera, N, Dempsey A, Gonzalez E, and Abrahamson C. Weight-related teasing, emotional eating, and weight control behaviors in Hispanic and African American girls. *Eating Behaviors* 14, no. 4 (2013): 513–517.

Palmberg, AA, Stern M, Kelly NR, Bulik C, Belgrave FZ, Trapp SK, Hofmeier SM, and Mazzeo SE. Adolescent girls and their mothers talk about experiences of binge and loss of control eating. *Journal of Child and Family Studies* 23, no. 8 (2014): 1403–1416.

Parker, S, Nichter M, Nichter M, Vuckovic N, Sims C, and Ritenbaugh C. Body image and weight concerns among African American and White adolescent females: Differences that make a difference. *Human Organization* 54, no. 2 (1995): 103–114.

Perez, M, Voelz ZR, Pettit JW, and Joiner TE. The role of acculturative stress and body dissatisfaction in predicting bulimic symptomatology across ethnic groups. *International Journal of Eating Disorders* 31, no. 4 (2002): 442–454.

Phan, T, and Tylka. TL. Exploring a model and moderators of disordered eating with Asian American college women. *Journal of Counseling Psychology* 53, no. 1 (2006): 36–47.

Pike, KM, Dohm FA, Striegel-Moore RH, Wilfley DE, and Fairburn CG. A comparison of black and white women with binge eating disorder. *American Journal of Psychiatry* 158, no. 9 (2001): 1455–1460.

Pomales, J, and Williams V. Effects of level of acculturation and counseling style on Hispanic students' perceptions of counselor. *Journal of Counseling Psychology* 36, no. 1 (1989): 79–83.

Rakhkovskaya, LM, and Warren CS. Ethnic identity, thin-ideal internalization, and eating pathology in ethnically diverse college women. *Body Image* 11, no. 4 (2014): 438–445.

Reddy, SD, and Crowther JH. Teasing, acculturation, and cultural conflict: Psychosocial correlates of body image and eating attitudes among South Asian women. *Cultural Diversity and Ethnic Minority Psychology* 13, no. 1 (2007): 45–53.

Reyes-Rodriguez, ML, Baucom DH, and Bulik CM. Culturally sensitive intervention for Latina women with eating disorders: A case study. *Revista Mexicana de Trastornos Alimentarios* 5, no. 2 (2014): 136–146.

Rodriguez, R, Marchand E, Ng J, and Stice E. Effects of a cognitive dissonance-based eating disorder prevention program are similar for Asian American, Hispanic, and White participants. *International Journal of Eating Disorders* 41, no. 7 (2008): 618–625.

Rogers Wood, NA, and Petrie TA. Body dissatisfaction, ethnic identity, and disordered eating among African American women. *Journal of Counseling Psychology* 57, no. 2 (2010): 141–153.

Root, MPP. Disordered eating in women of color. *Sex Roles* 22, no. 7–8 (1990): 525–536.

Rutt, CD, and Coleman, KJ. The evaluation of a measurement model for the Body Image Questionnaire and the Eating Attitudes Test in a Hispanic population. *Hispanic Journal of Behavioral Sciences* 23, no. 2 (2001): 153–170.

Sánchez-Johnsen, LA, Hogan K, Wilkens LR, and Fitzgibbon ML. Correlates of problematic eating behaviors in less acculturated Latinas. *Eating Behaviors* 9, no. 2 (2008): 181–189.

Schooler, D, and Daniels EA. "I am not a skinny toothpick and proud of it": Latina adolescents' ethnic identity and responses to mainstream media images. *Body Image* 11, no. 1 (2014): 11–18.

Sharma, S, Cao X, Gittelsohn J, Ethelbah B, and Anliker J. Nutritional composition of commonly consumed traditional Apache foods in Arizona. *International Journal of Food Sciences and Nutrition* 59, no. 1 (2008): 1–10.

Shaw, H, Ramirez L, Trost A, Randall P, and Stice E. Body image and eating disturbances across ethnic groups: More similarities than differences. *Psychology of Addictive Behaviors* 18, no. 1 (2004): 12–18.

Shuttlesworth, ME, and Zotter D. Disordered eating in African American and Caucasian women: The role of ethnic identity. *Journal of Black Studies* 42, no. 6 (2011): 906–922.

Smith, JE, and Krejci J. Minorities join the majority: Eating disturbances among Hispanic and Native American youth. *International Journal of Eating Disorders* 10, no. 2 (1991): 179–186.

Smolak, L, and Striegel-Moore, RH. Challenging the myth of the golden girl: Ethnicity and eating disorders. In *Eating Disorders: Innovative Directions in Research and Practice*, edited by RH Striegel-Moore and L Smolak, pp. 111–132. Washington, DC: American Psychological Association, 2001.

Stein, KF, Corte C, and Ronis DL. Personal identities and disordered eating behaviors in Mexican American women. *Eating Behaviors* 11, no. 3 (2010): 197–200.

Stevens, J, Story M, Becenti A, French SA, Gittelsohn J, Going SB, Juhaeri, Levin S, and Murray DM. Weight-related attitudes and behaviors in fourth grade American Indian children. *Obesity Research* 7, no. 1 (1999): 34–42.

Stice, E. Risk and maintenance factors for eating pathology: A meta-analytic review. *Psychological Bulletin* 128, no. 5 (2002): 825–848.

Stice, E, Marti CN, and Cheng ZH. Effectiveness of a dissonance-based eating disorder prevention program for ethnic groups in two randomized controlled trials. *Behaviour Research and Therapy* 55 (2014): 54–64.

Stice, E, Telch CF, and Rizvi SL. Development and validation of the eating disorder diagnostic scale: A brief self-report measure of anorexia, bulimia, and binge eating disorder. *Psychological Assessment* 12, no. 2 (2000): 123–131.

Stojek, MM, and Fischer S. Thinness expectancies and restraint in Black and White college women: A prospective study. *Eating Behaviors* 14, no. 3 (2013): 269–273.

Story, M, Evans M, Fabsitz RR, Clay TE, Holy Rock B, and Broussard B. The epidemic of obesity in American Indian communities and the need for childhood obesity-prevention programs. *American Journal of Clinical Nutrition* 69, no. 4 (1999): 747S–754S.

Striegel-Moore, RH, and Cachelin, FM. Etiology of eating disorders in women. *Counseling Psychologist* 29, no. 5 (2001): 635–661.

Striegel-Moore, RH, Rosselli F, Holtzman N, Dierker L, Becker AE, and Swaney G. Behavioral symptoms of eating disorders in Native Americans: Results from the ADD Health Survey Wave III. *International Journal of Eating Disorders* 44, no. 6 (2011): 561–566.

Stunkard, AJ, and Messick S. The three-factor eating questionnaire to measure dietary restraint, disinhibition and hunger. *Journal of Psychosomatic Research* 29, no. 1 (1985): 71–83.

Taylor, JY, Caldwell CH, Baser RE, Faison N, and Jackson JS. Prevalence of eating disorders among Blacks in the National Survey of American Life. *International Journal of Eating Disorders* 40, no. S3 (2007): S10–S14.

Thelen, MH, Farmer J, Wonderlich S, and Smith M. A revision of the bulimia test: The BULIT-R. *Psychological Assessment: A Journal of Consulting and Clinical Psychology* 3, no. 1 (1991): 119–124.

Thompson, BW. "A way outa no way": Eating problems among African-American, Latina, and White women. *Gender and Society* 6, no. 4 (1992): 546–561.

Thompson, JK, van den Berg P, Roehrig M, Guarda AS, and Heinberg LJ. The Sociocultural Attitudes Towards Appearance Scale-3 (SATAQ-3): Development and validation. International Journal of Eating Disorders 35, no. 3 (2004): 293–304.

Thompson-Brenner, H, Franko DL, Thompson DR, Grilo CM, Boisseau CL, Roehrig JP, Richards LK, Bryson SW, Bulik CM, Crow SJ, Devlin MJ, Gorin AA, Kristeller JL, Masheb R, Mitchell JE, Peterson CB, Safer DL, Striegel RH, Wilfley DE, and Wilson GT. Race/ethnicity, education, and treatment parameters as moderators and predictors of outcome in binge eating disorder. *Journal of Consulting and Clinical Psychology* 81, no. 4 (2013): 710–721.

Tsai, G, Curbow B, and Heinberg L. Sociocultural and developmental influences on body dissatisfaction and disordered eating attitudes and behaviors of Asian women. *Journal of Nervous and Mental Disease* 191, no. 5 (2003): 309–318.

Tseng, MC, Fang D, and Lee MB. Comparative validity of the Chinese versions of the Bulimic Inventory Test Edinburgh and Eating Attitudes Test for DSM-IV eating disorders among high school dance and nondance students in Taiwan. *International Journal of Eating Disorders* 47, no. 1 (2014): 105–111.

Tsong, Y, and Smart R. Assessing eating pathology in Asian Americans. In *Guide to Psychological Assessment with Asians*, edited by LT Benuto and BT Leany, pp. 243–260. New York, NY: Springer, 2014.

U.S. Department of Agriculture. Definition of a Food Desert. (n.d.). Available at http://www.ers.usda.gov/dataFiles/Food_Access_Research_Atlas/Download_the_Data/Archived_Version/archived_documentation.pdf

Velez, BL, Campos ID, and Moradi B. Relations of sexual objectification and racist discrimination with Latina women's body image and mental health. *Counseling Psychologist* 43, no. 6 (2015): 906–935.

Wallston, KA, and Strudler Wallston, B. Health locus of control scales. In *Research with the Locus of Control Construct*, edited by HM Lefcourt, pp. 189–243. New York, NY: Academic Press, 1981.

Warren, CS, and Rios, RM. The relationships among acculturation, acculturative stress, endorsement of Western media, social comparison, and body image in Hispanic male college students. *Psychology of Men and Masculinity* 14, no. 2 (2013): 192–201.

Warren, CS, Schoen A, and Schafer KJ. Media internalization and social comparison as predictors of eating pathology among Latino adolescents: The moderating effect of gender and generational status. *Sex Roles* 63, no. 9–10 (2010): 712–724.

Warren, CS. Body area dissatisfaction in White, Black and Latina female college students in the USA: An examination of racially salient appearance areas and ethnic identity. *Ethnic and Racial Studies* 37, no. 3 (2014): 537–556.

Webb, JB, Warren-Findlow J, Chou YY, and Adams L. Do you see what I see? An exploration of inter-ethnic ideal body size comparisons among college women. *Body Image* 10, no. 3 (2013): 369–379.

White, MA, and Grilo CM. Ethnic differences in the prediction of eating and body image disturbances among female adolescent psychiatric inpatients. *International Journal of Eating Disorders* 38, no. 1 (2005): 78–84.

Wildes, JE, Emery RE, and Simons AD. The roles of ethnicity and culture in the development of eating disturbance and body dissatisfaction: A meta-analytic review. *Clinical Psychology Review* 21, no. 4 (2001): 521–551.

Wonderlich, SA, Crosby RD, Joiner T, Peterson CB, Bardone-Cone A, Klein M, Crow S, Mitchell JE, Le Grange D, Steiger H, Kolden G, Johnson F, and Vrshek S. Personality subtyping and bulimia nervosa: Psychopathological and genetic correlates. *Psychological Medicine* 35, no. 5 (2005): 649–657.

Yoshimura, K. Acculturative and sociocultural influences on the development of eating disorders in Asian-American females. *Eating Disorders* 3, no. 3 (1995): 216–228.

Zephier, E, Himes, JH, and Story, M. Prevalence of overweight and obesity in American Indian school children and adolescents in the Aberdeen area: A population study. *International Journal of Obesity and Related Metabolic Disorders* 23, no. S2 (1999): S28–S30.

12 Eating Disorders in Women at Midlife and Beyond

A Biopsychosocial-Relational Perspective

*Margo Maine, PhD, FAED, CEDS
and Karen Samuels, PhD*

CONTENTS

LEARNING OBJECTIVES

After reading this chapter, the reader should be able to do the following:

- Illustrate the biopsychosocial and relational nature of eating disorders in adult women
- Describe the range and pattern of eating disorders and body image despair currently seen in adult women
- Understand the unique female bodily experiences at and beyond midlife that create risk for eating disorders
- Discriminate the differences between eating disorders at midlife and earlier onset
- Apply *relational cultural theory* (RCT) to understand and address clinical issues with adult eating disorders and related problems

INTRODUCTION

More adult women are seeking treatment for eating disorders than ever before. Adult female development has a rich and complex trajectory from young adulthood, through the midlife transition of the 30s and 40s, middle age, retirement, and later years. In the midst of the youth-obsessed attitude that "60 is the new 40," exact age parameters for these stages are difficult to define. The 40s may bring a first pregnancy or menopause; an empty nest or a growing family; a long and satisfying marriage or a return to the dating game; early retirement or becoming a grandparent; or the beginning of graduate school or a new career. Clearly the lives of contemporary women are nonlinear, with distinctly diverse life events and milestones now occurring in each decade or life stage (Maine et al. 2015). Thus, women are now at risk for eating disorders throughout adult development.

Over the past three decades, the "face" of eating disorders has changed significantly. Initially seen primarily in young Caucasian women in technologically advanced nations, they now appear across age, gender, race, ethnicity, class, culture, and place. In fact, between 1999 and 2009, inpatient admissions for eating disorders showed the greatest increase among older patients, with women over age 45 accounting for a full 25% of admissions (Zhao and Encinosa 2011). Outpatient practices have witnessed similar trends. In 2003, an urban community-based program served 43 patients age 38 or older, accounting for 9% of their patients. Only 4 years later, during the first 6 months of 2007, the program had treated nearly 500 patients in that same age category, approximately 35% of its clientele (Forliti 2007).

Some of these women have suffered for their entire lives and are coming forward for the first time. Others have recovered from an eating disorder earlier in their lives and relapsed as they encounter the challenges of midlife. Many have been preoccupied with food, weight, and body image for years, but at a subclinical level until midlife, while a small percentage develop clinical eating disorders for the first time as adults (Maine 2010).

Increased attention to eating disorder research and clinical presentations has raised difficult questions: Is the onset or return of disordered eating on the rise in adult women? Or, is this population presenting for treatment due to increased attention? Are they coming because we finally are providing an adequate environment for these women to seek professional guidance for their struggles? As the healthcare community becomes better educated, will primary care providers, psychotherapists, psychiatric professionals, and others better assess and refer their older women patients for appropriate care? How does the continuum of eating disorders manifest in women postmenopause as they navigate the aging process?

This increase in adult women seeking professional treatment for their disordered eating and body image distress requires that we find the best treatment modalities for women approaching menopause, as well as those who are postmenopausal. More questions arise. What are their special needs and medical concomitants? And where and how do we refer these patients for optimal care? Are there any specialized programs for postmenopausal women seeking residential eating disorder treatment? As an 85-year-old woman asked recently: "Who would think my eating disorder struggles are worthy of attention, at my age?"

Despite these compelling trends and unanswered questions, the research, treatment, and prevention in the field of eating disorders continue to focus primarily on early onset with young children, adolescents, and early adulthood targeted as the population for intervention. Many acute care and residential treatment programs provide some specialized groups to address the developmental needs of adults, but these tend to be an accessory to the programming instead of the core ingredient. Generally, women in their 40s, 50s, 60s, and beyond in need of a higher level of care find themselves in groups with much younger women. They often feel out of place and blame themselves for struggling with what they see as "a teenager's problem." If they do attend treatment, they will likely assume the familiar maternal role as caregiver within that milieu and, once more, they may not get what they need from the experience (Maine and Kelly 2016).

The authors have been working specifically with women at midlife and older with eating disorders, devoting special attention to postmenopause for over a decade. Practicing in different parts of the country, meeting at the annual Renfrew Foundation Conference, Feminist and Relational Perspectives on Eating Disorders, we have found much common ground in our experiences and are committed to help the field of eating disorders as well as the broader mental health and medical professions understand and treat adult women more effectively. This chapter describes the bodily experience of women at midlife and beyond, the developmental challenges they meet, and how a biopsychosocial-relational perspective best frames our thinking and treatment.

THE FEMALE BODILY EXPERIENCE AT MIDLIFE AND LATER

In the past, women's satisfaction with their bodies appeared to increase during midlife with a shift in focus from its appearance to its function. This is no longer the case—age certainly does not immunize women from body image preoccupation, weight and shape concerns, restrictive dieting, and disordered eating. The dramatic increase in eating disorders in the past 30 years and the ongoing gender disparity suggests that a sociocultural perspective will best explain this phenomenon (Maine and Bunnell 2010).

According to women's health expert Dr. Christiane Northrup: "The state of a woman's health is indeed completely tied up with the culture in which she lives and her position within it" (Northrup 2006). Indeed, contemporary women are navigating a fast-changing world. Our economic and social structures have rapidly become a globalized consumer culture, resulting in a major transformation of women's role in just this past generation. Women are now expected to pursue education and careers and to compete with men at the same time they maintain their families and feminine identity. While this new era offers women unprecedented opportunities, it also brings unprecedented stress. The media, fashion, cosmetic, and dieting industries constantly convey that women must do more, buy more, and be more to be successful, and that self-worth is based on how they look, what they weigh, and what they eat. The relentless pressure to do everything and to do it perfectly leads many women to feel that they do not measure up and to seek comfort in the rituals of disordered eating, rigid dieting, exercise, and other body rituals (Maine and Kelly 2016).

These pressures on women have truly transformed the experience of their bodies. A consumer economy thrives by making women feel they need to buy something or be something other than their natural selves—that they are not good enough as is. While the dieting industry has soared to a $60 billion gross annual income in the United States (Overweight and Weight Loss Statistics n.d.), the number of adult women with disordered eating and eating disorders has also soared. In a large-scale study of American women between ages 25 and 45, 75% reported disordered eating and body image dissatisfaction, and 6% were trying to lose weight, although over half of these dieters were already at a normal weight. Nearly 40% reported that concerns about weight or eating interfere with their happiness and skip meals regularly to lose weight. More than a quarter cut out whole food groups and 13% reported smoking to lose weight (Bulik and Reba-Harrelson 2008).

In a survey of Austrian women aged 40–60, 4.6% met full criteria for a clinical eating disorder and another 4.8% met subthreshold standards for an eating disorder. However, both groups reported the same degree of psychopathology, distress, and impairment, demonstrating that even a subclinical eating disorder seriously compromises the quality of a woman's life (Mangweth-Matzek et al. 2014).

Research on American women over the age of 50 is equally disturbing. About 60% reported that their concerns about weight and shape negatively affected their lives. As many as 79% described that weight and shape impacted their self-image and 41% weighed themselves daily. Another 36% spent at least half of the last 5 years dieting and as many as 8% reported purging. Over 13% have current eating disorder symptoms (Gagne et al. 2012) surpassing the 12.4% of American women who have breast cancer (National Cancer Institute 2015). Yet, we have consistently ignored eating disorders and the suffering they cause women in later life.

As women age past midlife into later years, they continue to be at risk for eating disorders. Today, disordered eating and the fear of aging seem to go hand-in-hand for many women (Lewis and and Cachelin 2001). When researchers asked a group of women aged 61–92 what bothered them most about their bodies, they identified weight as their greatest concern (Clarke 2002). Another study of a random nonclinical sample of women between the ages of 60 and 70, all at average weight and body mass index (BMI), found that 4% met the diagnostic criteria for an eating disorder, 4% were subclinical, 80% were actively controlling their weight, and 60% reported body dissatisfaction. Again, these occurred regardless of being at a normal weight (Mangweth-Matzek et al. 2006).

The Western culture's fixation on young, highly sexualized, and sculpted images of women rarely place an older woman in a position of power or influence. Media—be it Internet, social media, film, fashion, advertising, print, or television—systematically exclude older women's faces and bodies. Consequently, the natural process of aging disempowers women more and more quickly than it does men. Added to this is ongoing economic disparity, with women in the United States earning approximately 79% of what men earn (Institute for Women's Policy Research 2015). The body has become a form of currency for women who assume that a thin, sculpted, and beautiful appearance will give them legitimacy, power, and more income (Wolf 1990). In the current cultural climate, the natural impact of an aging body, along with sociopolitical-economic factors, may activate or reactivate eating disorders.

Regardless of age, eating disorders come in different shapes, sizes, and severities, from anorexia nervosa (AN), bulimia nervosa (BN), other specified feeding and eating disorders (OSFED), binge eating disorders (BED), and subclinical or partial syndrome eating disorders, including orthorexia. Orthorexia nervosa is marked by a fixation on "optimal health," via a natural or restrictive diet with self-imposed rules that exclude most food choices (Dunn and Bratman 2016). Dietary restrictions may escalate over time including the elimination of micro- and macronutrients that do not meet their standards for health or purity. Orthorexia often leads to great emotional distress in relation to food choices, as well as malnutrition, emaciation, depression, anxiety, and social isolation, much like clinical eating disorders. Recent reports indicated BED and OSFED were more common among midlife eating disorder treatment-seeking individuals relative to their younger counterparts (Elran-Barak et al. 2015).

In our clinical experience, adult eating disordered women often fall into the OSFED or partial syndrome categories. Their symptoms may have changed over time, having initially been more purely restricting AN or more prominently BN via self-induced vomiting. Gradually, they may have eaten more, stopped vomiting, and reached a stable, "normal" weight, but their relationship with food is still disordered and distressing. Because they engage in eating disorder behaviors less severely or less frequently, they feel that they no longer "have it," yet their behaviors and thoughts about food, weight, and their bodies are still distracting, obsessive, critical, and unhealthy. A woman might say "but I eat now," while eating far less than normal metabolic needs require and living in a chronic state of hypometabolism. She might believe she is no longer purging but has only traded vomiting for grueling hours of obsessive exercise or laxative abuse. Medical journals, magazine articles, and the popular self-help literature tend to focus on restricting AN or BN via self-induced vomiting. They neglect symptoms such as exercise abuse, laxatives, binge eating, or chronic restricting without significant weight loss. This creates a barrier to both self-diagnosis and to professional identification of eating disorders in adult women.

These startling statistics pose some difficult questions. What contributes to increased body image distress and disordered eating in adult women as they age? Is there a perfect storm of biopsychosocial-relational conditions? Are the hormonal changes that produce the sensation that one's "body is out of control" with age-specific symptoms a factor? What about the psychosocial factors associated with the transition to a new stage of women's development and to new personal meanings and identities? Does menopause resemble puberty with these major hormonal, psychological, and physical changes? As one's sexuality is changing, does this also influence the meaning of the body and its capacity to appeal to others, to respond, and to provide pleasure? Are these times critical to the onset or reactivation of disordered eating presentation? Are the "entrance" at menarche and the "exit" at menopause from our reproductive life both windows of vulnerability for eating disorders? (Mangweth-Matzek et al. 2013) These questions beg answers and yet few are taking the time to examine them. Unfortunately, eating disorders at midlife and beyond are still nearly invisible in our health-care system.

UNIQUE ISSUES AT AND BEYOND MIDLIFE

Adult women struggling with eating disorders present with many issues unique to their life stage. Certainly they share common ground with younger women, including personality characteristics of perfectionism, low self-esteem, a chronic sense of inadequacy, and a tendency to focus on others rather than on their own needs and desires. This perfectionism, keen desire to please, and difficulty identifying their own needs make them easy prey, whatever their age, to the unrealistic media images of beauty, the marketing of body-change technology (e.g., pills, surgeries, exercise equipment, cosmeceuticals), and the "war on obesity" fed by misinformation from the diet industry. Many who develop eating disorders grew up amid intergenerational patterns of body distress and preoccupation, dieting, and various attempts to sculpt the body to meet an unattainable ideal. In fact, one of the unique motivations for adult women entering treatment is a deep desire to stop this cycle and to protect their children from the pain of an eating disorder and a negative body image. Often the experience of parenting is what brings midlife women into treatment (Maine and Kelly 2016).

A striking observation when we first meet women suffering at midlife or later is their severe shame and embarrassment for having a "teenager's problem." They apologize for needing our time and attention, repeatedly blaming themselves because they "should know better." Having spent more years in the throes of the eating disorder, they may have some budding awareness of what it has cost them. Some can see the havoc it wreaked on relationships, marriages, jobs, and on their bodies as they age. The natural aging process increases anxiety about appearance and health, which can lead them to consider the impact of their eating disorder but also can reinforce some of the eating disorder thoughts and behaviors. They may have developed osteopenia or osteoporosis, or have significant dental issues, hair may have thinned, and skin wrinkled prematurely. Fatigue and muscle weakness may be keeping them from enjoying life, and they begin to recognize what they are missing, while also being unsure they deserve anything better than the compromised life of an eating disorder. The aging process can unfortunately intensify or legitimize an eating disorder, with the misguided belief that control of their food intake will ameliorate any problems associated with getting older.

Loss is a major theme as women navigate midlife. Parents may be aging or ill, and inevitably, loved ones begin to die off. They may also be facing their own loss of power and status as aging women. The rituals of an eating disorder can numb these feelings but cannot forestall the natural rhythm of life. The multiple stressors and losses that accompany adult development are major contributing factors to eating disorders at and beyond midlife (Maine and Kelly 2016; Maine 2010).

The life transitions at midlife are multifold including alterations in significant relationships such as empty nest or divorce, aging parents requiring more care, and the boomerang generation of young adult children returning home. For many, this period is marked by change. Menopause may be one physical contributing factor, but the multitude of threads contributing to personal and relational health and well-being are often shifting simultaneously. Numerous age- and life stage-related physical conditions coalesce at midlife.

The "deadline decade," the years between 35 and 45, can be particularly disruptive (Sheehy 2006). This culmination of the biopsychosocial developmental process supposedly indicates the prime of life, the halfway point, marking a time to assess, take stock, and set intentions for the future (Maine et al. 2015). Deciding to have children, then facing fertility and infertility trials, possible pregnancy, child-birth, and parenting are all factors that can trigger or reactivate eating disorders. Realization that parenting will not be part of a woman's life also ushers in a process of loss, acceptance, and change. With the biological clock ticking, and the window of fertility and reproduction closing, some women experience the loss of their fecundity as another factor in body despair. The paradox of being at their sexual prime (Easton et al. 2010) can be the tipping point, as increased interest in sexuality, role confusion, unsettling guilt, and perimenopausal changes shifting the body shape and size away from the cultural ideal occur simultaneously.

Many women describe the fear of becoming invisible, ghosts of their younger counterparts who represent youthful vitality and attractiveness. Preparing for their adult children's marriages and becoming a grandparent adds to anxiety and appre-hension. Moving from a demanding work environment, seeking the elusive "work–family balance," heading toward retirement, and shifting to caretaking grandchildren and elderly parents all compete with attention to self-care, self-empathy, and identity. The natural aging process may bring emotional upheaval rather than the peaceful perspective women anticipate.

Infidelity and divorce are also transitional triggers that can reactivate disordered eating in adult women. Women describe lifelong marriages suddenly torn apart by affairs, experiencing unexpected divorce and broken families. One of our patients was informed by her spouse after 33 years of marriage that he no longer wanted a conventional marriage and suddenly left the family home. Within weeks, her weight plummeted and by the second month of separation, AN had again consumed her daily life. Twenty-five years earlier, she spent 6 weeks in residential treatment for AN following the births of her two children and the departure from her professional career. Adjusting to an unforeseen marital separation at the age of 56 reactivated the former coping strategies of restricting food, obsessing about weight and shape, and neglecting healthy self-care practices.

Among the women presenting for treatment at midlife and later, we see professional women, including health-care providers, educators, technology experts, and other demanding careers. Like our younger patients, they are remarkable and resourceful, really "the best and brightest." Some, after decades of achievement and accomplish-ment, are preparing for end of career and retirement. Admitting there may be something wrong or that they may need help is like speaking a foreign language. They know how to work hard but not how to tune into their inner experiences or to depend on others. Jobs, families, and a feeling that the world depends on them all create significant obstacles to treatment of any sort. Just taking the time to attend an evaluation or engage in outpatient therapy is difficult to manage, making a higher level of care at best a remote possibility.

MEDICAL ISSUES

As with younger patients, eating disorders affect every system in the body for adult women. Electrolyte imbalances can lead to cardiac arrhythmias and arrest, while endocrine dysfunction contributes to menstrual irregularities, decreased bone mineral density, increased risk for osteopenia and osteoporosis, and a compromised immune system (Mehler and Andersen 2010; Zerbe 1999). In addition to shared risks, eating disorders also cause some unique medical issues in adult women. Depleted fat stores exacerbate the declining estrogen level, intensifying menopausal symptoms. Older patients may experience a greater or more rapid cognitive impairment secondary to dieting (Lewis and Cachelin 2001). Dieting causes muscle-wasting and reduces the metabolic rate, accelerating the natural neuromuscular decline associated with aging (Holt 2005). In adults with eating disorders, long-term medical stability and normal laboratory values can turn quickly with a rapid acceleration of medical complications and even sudden death (Herzog et al. 1997). Although often overlooked, dieting is especially risky for elderly patients (Gupta 1995; Lewis and Cachelin 2001), as the mortality risk associated with low weight is greater as people age (Miller and Wolfe 2008; Tayback et al. 1990). For older adults, a higher BMI is actually associated with greater longevity (Dolan et al. 2007).

Most of our adult patients report that no medical provider ever asked questions related to eating disorders and body image issues. We suggest that the following questions be incorporated into intake assessments and routine medical follow-up:

- Has your weight fluctuated during your adult years?
- Are you trying to "manage" your weight? If so, how?
- What did you eat yesterday?
- How much do you think or worry about weight, shape, and food? (Maine 2010)

ADULT EDs THROUGH THE LENS OF RCT

RCT provides an optimal framework for understanding and treating eating disorders in adult women, conceptualizing them as disorders of disconnection, with the therapeutic remedy being to reestablish connections with the self, the body, and other people. According to RCT, an eating disorder emerges as a means of self-protection in response to empathic failures, pain, and disappointments, intending to help them to avoid further pain, and to regain control (Tantillo et al. 2013). The eating disorder basically replaces and competes with interpersonal relationships.

While traditional theories emphasize the importance of individuation and autonomy in psychological growth, RCT stresses relationships and empathy. RCT posits that people grow through and toward relationships throughout their life span and that culture powerfully impacts relationships. Key concepts include mutuality and fluid expertise, conveying that both client and clinician bring wisdom and knowledge to treatment. In contrast to the medical model, RCT builds a mutual understanding of the eating disorder and creates new pathways toward recovery, in a "power with" the client—not a traditional "power over"—model (Maine 2009). One of the most frequent deterrents to help-seeking is the deep sense of shame women with eating disorders experience. Guided by RCT, we examine the meaning and function of the eating disorder with a nonjudgmental and empathic tone. This allows the patient to take risks to connect with another person, to move out of shame, and to reignite hope and self-compassion. Relational resilience, the capacity to move back toward reestablishing connection, refers to the ability to connect, reconnect, or resist disconnection. Movement toward empathic mutuality is at the core of relational resilience and provides the capacity to acquire new skills for recovery (Samuels and Maine 2012).

According to Tantillo (2004), women will be able to "let go of eating disorder symptoms as [they are] able to (a) identify the connections between [their] relationships with food and [their] relationships with the self and others, and (b) develop mutually empathic and empowering relationships with others inside and outside the therapy office." As they learn self-empathy, they begin to recognize the links between their eating disorder behaviors and their self-care behaviors (Trepal et al. 2012). Self-empathy allows for the possibility for more connection.

Psychiatrist Amy Banks has integrated the groundbreaking research on the brain's development and functioning into relational neuroscience. This cutting edge work demonstrates that human beings are truly hard wired for connection and that the human brain is built to operate within a network of caring human relationships. Isolation causes our brains to atrophy, so relational interventions, like RCT and RCT-informed group therapy, are essential to restoring health. Instilling the hope that all adult women with eating disorders need, she writes: "Your brain can change, and most important . . . your brain can change its patterns of relating to people. You can teach your new brain to be calmer, more accepting, more resonant, and more energetic—to bolster . . . pathways that relate to growth-fostering relationships" (Banks 2015).

RCT, GROUP THERAPY, AND ADULT EATING DISORDERS

The research assessing treatment interventions on adult eating disordered women is limited. A recent review of interventions addressing body image and disordered eating in women aged 35–55, however, found sustained improvements with multisession, therapeutically based group interventions emphasizing the context of midlife and age-related changes to self-worth, body acceptance, and self-care. The authors stressed that group cohesion is a "necessary precondition for other factors to function optimally, feel accepted and supported" (Lewis-Smith et al. 2016). Given the double stigmatization in older populations—the eating disorder itself and social attitudes that consider it a disease of youth—group therapy provides practical support and important sharing of resources (Gonidakis and Karapaylou 2014). Again, adult eating disorders are best understood and addressed through a biopsychosocial and relational framework that can be used in various modalities. Relational group therapy can be particularly useful for adult women.

Due to increased interest and requests for a dedicated group, one of the authors (KS) leads an eating disorder therapy group for women, ages ranging from 45 to 60. Collectively, they have lived hundreds of years with various aspects of their eating disorders. These women represent decades of secrecy, shame, and suffering alone. Social withdrawal and avoidance of contact with others is frequently identified as the precursor to intensified eating disorder symptoms (Samuels 2015). They come together to heal and learn in connection. Early on in the group's formation, KS introduced the concept derived from the work of Karen Laing (1998): "Isolation is the glue that holds oppression in place." With adult women, "isolation is the glue that holds an eating disorder in place." This refrain is often mentioned during the group meetings.

This midlife eating disorder therapy group has been meeting for almost 5 years, representing a range of experiences. Everyone reports that challenges with disordered eating began in their teens. Onset of one woman's eating disorder was age 12, not diagnosed or specifically treated until age 45. Another woman went for residential treatment in her 20s and considered her eating disorder in remission until her mid-50s when life events triggered relapse along with associated significant medical concerns. Another woman reports a strong genetic predisposition, as she is the third generation of women in her family to experience a clinical eating disorder. She returned to treatment as her daughters approached adolescence, determined that the cycle not continue yet another generation.

While rarely bitter or upset, each woman shared her understanding that ongoing struggles with the symptoms and consequences of the eating disorder were "unmentionable." They consider eating disorders a teenager's problem and believed that they were "beyond help." For most, their adolescent years were full of disordered eating, weight preoccupation, dangerous methods of restriction, binging and purging, excessive exercise, and related symptoms. Despite prior psychotherapeutic experiences, most commented that their eating disorder had not been addressed or had been minimized. As one woman stated "I understood my problems were anxiety and major depression, and was assured the eating disorder would resolve when my mood disorder was better managed." Another woman described her spouse's decade of sobriety and continued involvement in 12-step meetings and fellowship. She "longed for something similar" for herself. These women were eager to meet and develop a "safe environment" to share their concerns, support one another, and seek recovery. They could empathize with one another's disordered eating, changing and aging bodies, and the desire to live with more peace and improved health.

Relational-cultural group therapy focuses on teaching the importance of an interpersonal perspective by emphasizing that group members apply the skills of empathy: to listen carefully; to be curious; to resonate with others; and, especially, to identify the distorted cognitions related to the eating disorder. Group members learn to appreciate another's experiences and feelings and to receive authentic responses such as "I/we see you and know you so very differently." They are encouraged to relinquish self-loathing beliefs and receive input from other group members. It is a coordination of mental processes moving from an other-centered orientation to create a "we" rather than just a "you" or "me" perspective. "Group members learn to listen to each other and appreciate how the other individual's perceptions compare and contrast with their own: uniquely different experiences from what each individual has previously known. Beginning to glimpse the impact they have on others, new understandings unfold, old rigid beliefs begin to recede, and new emotional experiences arise" (Jordan and Dooley 2000). The healthy self-in-relation to others emerges, rather than the self-in-relation to isolation, despair, and long-held negative self-referencing beliefs.

Through shared group perceptions and understanding, idealized relational images of perfection are shattered. "Group members fully listen to each other and think about how the other individual's perceptions compare and contrast with their own, a new experience emerges . . . uniquely different from what each individual has previously known." Beginning to glimpse the impact they have on others, "Old emotional experiences become understood in context with current relationships that are uniquely individual and simultaneously relational. In doing so, we create a place that belongs to no one in particular and yet it belongs to each and all—a creative place of relationship" (Eskine 2009). RCT shifts the primary models of psychology from an emphasis on the "separate self" to an appreciation of the centrality of relationship in our lives. Shifting this paradigm from separation to connection transforms the group experience, both in the therapy room and in the broader culture and society (Jordan 2010). Empathy is understood as a cognitive-affective resonance, joining with others in a shared state of human connection. Compassion increases as the suffering of isolation declines. Mutual empathy moves us toward one another, out of isolation (Jordan and Dooley 2000). The concept of the "central relational paradox" recognizes that the yearning for and fear of connection may directly cause one to "disconnect," to employ strategies of survival—like eating disorders—as coping, as self-protection. The group dynamic allows for healing to occur when mutual empathy empowers growth-fostering relationships (Comstock et al. 2002). This particular group seeks to develop, implement, and encourage the experience of mutual empathy, both in the sessions and woven through their lives.

After years of RCT informed therapy, these women have witnessed and welcomed the relational group support through the passages of life: menopause, major illness, challenges of relationships and divorce, deaths of family members and friends, career changes, new business ventures, sending children to college, graduations, marriages, and births of grandchildren. The rates and progress in managing disordered eating symptoms vary. Overall, this group demonstrates significant remission of eating disorder symptoms and relief from medical risk factors, but the resounding centerpiece of each meeting remains to prioritize self-care, self-empathy, and mutuality in connections. This response, to no longer withdraw into preoccupation with harmful symptoms of the eating disorder, has been replaced with motivation to connect, reminders of strategies discussed in group, and self-soothing practices. The relational "we" is the chorus in these group therapy meetings: we do understand, we see and hear your struggles, we appreciate that recovery may appear different as menopause challenges the loss of status in a youth-obsessed world. Essentially, these women do not want their "sisters" to go through the healing process alone. Breaking the cycle of withdrawal is the goal.

Many times these women have dedicated themselves to the service of others. To claim their strides forward, to receive the empathy and resonance of the group members, and to share the sense that "we are no longer alone, but in this together" creates meaning and context (Seligman 2011). Next is the challenge of asking for time to discuss their personal difficulties and challenges. Adult women frequently are reluctant to ask for such time and attention. The group encourages and invites one another to reveal their recovery roadblocks, impediments to self-efficacy, as well as success. The practice of mutuality in relationship, self and other-empathy, especially pertaining to their disordered eating, becomes another layer of relational learning and growth fostering connections (Miller and Stiver 1997). Each session ends with a didactic handout. These include homework exercises (cognitive-behavioral therapy, dialectical behavioral therapy, and emotionally focused therapy-based), recommendations for recovery related to seasonal or holiday demands, recent articles related to adult women with eating disorders, and text that highlights recurring group discussion topics (Binge Eating Disorder Association n.d.; National Eating Disorders Association n.d.).

Another strategy of recovery support is challenging one another to practice exposure to feared stimuli: These women have learned to "share a meal" via phone, text, and Skype using technology to incorporate much needed encouragement amid busy and demanding lives. The concept of "text support" when faced with potential relapse triggers has become the "language of recovery." During the holiday season 1 year, each group member presented simple handcrafted gifts, fostering a sense of "connection" that could be maintained between sessions.

Jean Baker Miller describes the "five good things" of growth-fostering relationships: zest, sense of worth, clarity, productivity, and a desire for more connection (Miller 1986). The women gathered together in this relational eating disorder group describe these five and more. A recent discussion about the nuanced nature of recovery for women postmenopause brought a collective sigh of relief. Recently, when the group was asked about adding new members, the resounding response was "Yes! We suffered alone for too many years."

CASE STUDY 12.1

Ella

One group member agreed to share her story to recovery for this chapter. Growing up in a suburb of London, Ella studied dance at a conservatory from age 12 to 18. Always slim, her eating disorder went undetected during these years of endless hours in the studio. Battling low weight, depression, anxiety, and a myriad of injuries from dance studies, she never put the "face and name of anorexia" to her restrictive eating and battle with her maturing body. Prior psychotherapy addressed her mood disorder. At the age of 45, she returned to psychotherapy following the death of her father. The therapist concentrated on early trauma and the recurring patterns of depression since puberty. Steadily dropping weight again, she was confronted with "having an eating disorder" and directed to enter a 4-week residential program 5 hours from home. Her daughters were 8 and 12, and she could not fathom leaving them in the care of her husband, 20 years her senior, now retired. At the eating disorder program, she expected to be informed she did not belong there. Quite the contrary, her team was dedicated to weight and meal restoration and addressing over 30 years of body hatred and despair. Upon her return home, her therapist resumed work on grief and childhood sexual trauma. Within months, her weight plummeted again, and she could not afford to use more of the family's life savings to return to treatment. As for most, financial planning for retirement and children's college education never included money earmarked for residential eating disorder treatment.

Terrified, she changed therapists to an eating disorder specialist and joined the adult women's eating disorder group. Two years after her initial entrance into residential treatment, the depression worsened, weight dropped, and she was urged to return to a higher level of treatment. Although decades of denial had convinced her that treatment was not necessary, a group

(Continued)

meeting finally convinced her that it was. The other women expressed fear for her survival and admitted they were terrified she would not be alive by the next group's session. They encouraged and supported her during residential care, sending countless cards and messages. Upon her return from intensive treatment, she was welcomed and supported by her group, treatment team, family, and peers. Some 3 years later, she attributes the strength of these connections, working with a specialized treatment team, and acquiring relational skills as the keys to her stabilization and recovery. Coming back from treatment the second time to a strong network of women offering relational engagement contributed to Ella's health and healing. She describes the value and benefit of finding trust, safety, and "acceptance without judgement": "Knowing that as an adult, I am no longer alone and silent, with no one in my life or family who got my eating disorder: this has made a great difference, and been a relief to find understanding and acceptance from our group. There is also wisdom shared about the nature of recovery and life's challenges, such as relationships, loss, and menopause."

CASE STUDY 12.2

Diane

Diane represents an excellent example of a genetic predisposition to develop an eating disorder. Her mother and maternal grandmother both suffered from AN across their life spans. Diane's mother became medically compromised and asked a friend to raise her daughter, who was just a toddler, in another family with no history of eating disorders. Eventually adopted, Diane grew up aware that her birth mother suffered from an eating disorder and was repeatedly warned: "Don't get an eating disorder." When molested at age 10, she was too afraid of further abandonment, disappointment, and shame in her adoptive family to share this trauma. By age 12, symptoms of food restriction and binge eating emerged, accompanied by success in competitive sports. Driven to perform athletically, Diane managed to keep secret the increased disordered eating and preoccupation with weight gain as her adolescent female body developed. Simultaneously, she excelled on the soccer field.

   At university, she competed as a collegiate athlete and suffered from BN and exercise compulsion. She studied health sciences as determinedly as she pursued athletics while also being acutely aware of the health impact of anorexia and bulimia in her family of origin. Orthorexia and the Female Athlete Triad (low energy availability, amenorrhea or oligomenorrhea, and osteoporosis; Thompson and Sherman 2010) followed, with rigid eating rules, making weight for competitions, and intense training schedules. Remarkably, in her later 20s she married and managed

(Continued)

CASE STUDY 12.2 (*CONTINUED*)

to carry two healthy pregnancies to term. Postpartum brought a renewed commitment to rigorous sports involvement including training for marathon and triathlon competitions. Eventually, she qualified for the Olympic marathon trials but was unable to participate due to numerous injuries, the consequence of years of disordered eating, amenorrhea, and overtraining.

Diane had sought counseling a decade earlier but not with a specialized eating disorder team. Her older daughter, now 15, began to struggle with extreme dieting, sudden weight loss, preoccupation with restrictive eating, and body image despair. Alert to these early warning signs, Diane immediately scheduled psychological treatment for her daughter. The ensuing family counseling sessions revealed how often family meals revolved around Diane's restrictive eating, exercise training regimen, and "disappearance" after meals when she would self-induce vomiting. Diane's daughter stabilized and returned to normal eating, weight restoration, and mood management. An alarm sounded for Diane, who recalls her insight: "I can't give her what I don't have . . . and I don't want this eating disorder to pass to another generation." At age 43 she came into treatment with a renewed focus on recovery.

An initial challenge to her treatment was living the paradox: she remained a highly sought after personal fitness trainer and competitive running coach but struggled secretly with bulimia. Frequently asked for nutrition advice and the secret to her physique, she described "feeling like a fraud." Diane's spouse encouraged her to make a change. It was not until she discontinued her work as a personal fitness trainer that she fully embraced her own dedication to recovery.

Diane's journey to discontinue 30 years of bulimia, orthorexia, and exercise abuse gradually shifted in focus. Several key factors influenced her healing. She included her spouse in treatment as a key member of her treatment team. She began to study yoga, and eventually moved from a studio with mirrors and heated classes to one without mirrors. She wrote a letter to her closest friends sharing her struggles with bulimia. She told her family, immediate and extended. She started yoga teacher training but was forced to withdraw from her studies following another physical injury. Months later, healthier, with renewed focus, she resumed her studies. For the first time, instead of approaching her recovery like training for another athletic competition, Diane shifted toward a lifelong healing practice, moving away from her intense focus on fitness and training toward well-being and health.

Slowly Diane began to restore weight. She stopped competing in sports and began to practice meditation daily. She talked to her family and asked for their patience and forgiveness for years of absence. Then 1 day she discontinued purging. Three years later, Diane speaks publicly about the dangers of eating disorders. A yoga teacher, she runs her own studio, without mirrors or heaters. She volunteers in community outreach to educate about the risks and challenges of disordered eating. Although she knows her birth mother still struggles terribly with an eating disorder into her 70s, Diane is working hard to be better equipped to guide her children into adulthood.

SUMMARY AND CONCLUSIONS

Triggered by life transitions, onset or worsening symptoms, and the numerous adjustments and losses that accompany midlife and later years, more and more adult women are seeking treatment for eating disorders. Ashamed to have a condition associated with adolescent and college-aged girls, too often they are literally hopeless, doubting that they can get better or that they deserve to get better. Eating disorders interfere with the natural longing for and need for nourishment, rest, meaningful relationships, and health. When they need them most, women with eating disorders actually turn away from relationships.

As clinicians, we not only need skills to empower their healing, we also need to instill hope and a belief in the possibility of recovery. RCT provides that framework and guides our work with women at midlife and beyond. As Amy Banks and relational neuroscience have demonstrated, only when we are safely connected to others can our neural pathways operate optimally, allowing us to be calm, resilient, and productive. Change is possible, even after decades of the suffering eating disorders cause in the lives of adult women.

At midlife and later, women with eating disorders require care delivered by informed health-care providers. Medical and mental health professionals must understand the unique female bodily experiences at and beyond midlife that create risk for eating disorders. These patients deserve more specifically adult-focused treatment options than are typically available. Adult women have more barriers to treatment given the needs of their families, work, financial resources, and competing demands. Leaving these responsibilities for extended residential treatment may not be feasible. Additional challenges include insurance reimbursement, especially when the diagnosis is OSFED, BED, or a subclinical eating disorder, and access to an appropriate level and type of care. The eating disorder field is in urgent need of longitudinal research that would identify effective outreach, assessment, and treatment for adult women, especially at menopause and postmenopause. Opportunities abound both in the clinical and research domains for those interested in adult eating disorders.

Long interested in eating disorders in later life, feminist psychiatrist Kathryn Zerbe reminds us that, beyond the assessment, psychoeducation, and clinical treatment offered, the eating disorder health-care team must ask patients for the narrative details of their lives (Zerbe 2013). When we understand the role the eating disorder has played, the human cost over decades to both these clients and their loved ones, adult eating disorders will move from the shadows to the forefront of women's health care—not a moment too soon for those suffering.

APPENDIX

The following questions were developed by the authors. This type of inquiry offers a window to adult women's experience of eating disorders and how their attitudes, beliefs, behaviors, and feelings evolve over time. The questions provide opportunities for insight and for relational contact and healing.

Engaging Questions:

- What are the variables that have changed in midlife that promote increased motivation for recovery from the eating disorder?
- What has been helpful to move you over the line toward recovery?
- What occurs in your relationships that leads you to disconnect or distance yourself from the other person? What happens?
- Does the eating disorder help you to disconnect from other people? What happens?
- Does the eating disorder ever help you connect with other people? In what way? What happens? (Koehn 2010)
- What do you now know that you did not know or understand as a child or teen when the eating disorder began?
- What would you tell your child self from the vantage point of today?
- What do you feel contributed to the development of your eating disorder when you were younger? Are those things different from what kept it going into adulthood?
- What do you value most in your relationship with your partner, mother, father, sibling, best friends. . .?
- What is one thing you wish could be different in your relationship with your partner, mother, father, best friends, . . .?
- When you and your _____ experience conflict, what does that look like?
- How do you and your _____ resolve conflict?
- How does your _____ express love and caring for you?
- How do you express love and caring for your _____?
- What have you found most helpful as an adult in moving toward recovery?
- Who has been most helpful to you in recovery thus far?
- What are the challenges still to be faced in order to recover and/or to continue your recovery?

REFERENCES

Banks, A. *Four Ways to Click Rewire Your Brain for Stronger, More Rewarding Relationships.* New York, NY: Penguin Random House, 2015.

Binge Eating Disorder Association (n.d.). Available at www.bedaonline.com

Bulik, CM, and Reba-Harrelson L. A novel collaboration between *Self Magazine* and the University of North Carolina at Chapel Hill: Patterns and prevalence of disordered eating in a probability sample of American women ages 25–45. In Presentation at the International Conference on Eating Disorders. 2008, Seattle, WA.

Clarke, LH. Older women's perceptions of ideal body weights: The tensions between health and appearance motivations for weight loss. *Ageing and Society* 22, (2002): 751–773.

Comstock, DL, Duffey T, and St. George H. The relational-cultural model: A framework for group process. *Journal for Specialists in Group Work* 27, no. 3 (2002): 254–272.

Dolan, CM, Kraemer H, Browner W, Ensrud K, and Kelsey JL. Associations between body composition, anthropometry, and mortality in women aged 65 years and older. *American Journal of Public Health* 97, no. 5 (2007): 913–918.

Dunn, TM and Bratman, S. On orthorexia nervosa: A review of the literature and proposed diagnostic criteria. *Eating Behaviors* 21, (2016): 11–17.

Easton, J, Confer JC, Goetz CD, and Buss D. Reproduction expediting: Sexual motivations, fantasies, and the ticking biological clock. *Personality and Individual Differences* 49, no. 5 (2010): 516–520.

Elran-Barak, R, Fitzsimmons-Craft EE, Benyamini Y, Crow SJ, Peterson CB, Hill LL, Crosby RD, Mitchell JE, and Le Grange D. Anorexia nervosa, bulimia nervosa, and binge eating disorder in midlife and beyond. *Journal of Nervous and Mental Disease* 203, no. 8 (2015): 1–8.

Eskine, RG. Relational group psychotherapy: The healing of stress, neglect and trauma. In Keynote Address at the 4th International Integrative Psychotherapy Association Conference, April 2009, Lake Bled, Slovenia.

Forliti, A. Associated Press. Doctors treating older anorexics. *Washington Post*. 23 July 2007.

Gagne, DA, Von Holle A, Brownley KA, Runfola CD, Hofmeier S, Branch KE, and Bulik CM. Eating disorder symptoms and weight and shape concerns in a large web-based convenience sample of women ages 50 and above: Results of the Gender and Body Image (GABI) study. *International Journal of Eating Disorders* 45, no. 7 (2012): 832–844.

Gonidakis, G, and Karapaylou D. Eating disorders in late life: Implications for clinicians. Psychiatric Times. 27 November 2014. Available at http://www.psychiatrictimes.com/eating-disorders/eating-disorders-late-life-implications-clinicians/page/0/1

Gupta, MM. Concerns about aging and a drive for thinness: A factor in the biopsychosocial model of eating disorders? *International Journal of Eating Disorders* 18, no. 4 (1995): 351–357.

Herzog, W, Deter HC, Fiehn W, and Petzold E. Medical findings and predictors in long-term physical outcome in anorexia nervosa: A prospective, 12-year follow-up study. *Psychological Medicine* 27 (1997): 269–279.

Holt, M. Eating disorders in the adult population. *SCAN'S (Sports, Cardiovascular and Wellness Nutritionists) Pulse* (Winter 2005): 8–9.

Institute for Women's Policy Research. The Gender Wage Gap: 2014 Fact Sheet. 7 December 2015. Available at www.iwpr.org

Jordan, J. *Relational–Cultural Therapy*. Washington, DC: American Psychological Association, 2010.

Jordan, JV. The role of mutual empathy in relational/cultural therapy. *Journal of Clinical Psychology* 56, no. 80 (2000): 1005–1016.

Jordan, J, and Dooley C. Relational Practice in Action: A Group Manual. Project Report No. 6. Wellesley, MA: Stone Center for Developmental Services and Studies, 2000.

Koehn, CV. A relational approach to counseling women with alcohol and other drug problems. *Alcoholism Treatment Quarterly* 28, no. 1 (2010): 38–51.

Laing, K. Catalyst leadership workshop. In *Pursuit of Parity: Teachers as Liberators*. Boston, MA: World Trade Center, 1998.

Lewis, DM, and Cachelin FM. Body image, body dissatisfaction, and eating attitudes in midlife and elderly women. *Eating Disorders: Journal of Treatment and Prevention* 9, no. 1 (2001): 29–39.

Lewis-Smith, H, Diedrichs PC, Rumsey N, and Harcourt D. A systematic review of interventions on body image and disordered eating outcomes among women in midlife. *International Journal of Eating Disorders* 49, no. 4 (2016): 5–18.

Maine, M. Beyond the medical model: A feminist frame for eating disorders. In *Effective Clinical Practice in the Treatment of Eating Disorders: The Heart of the Matter*, edited by M Maine, WN Davis, and J Shure, pp. 3–17. New York, NY: Routledge, 2009.

Maine, M. The weight-bearing years: Eating disorders and body image despair in adult women. In *Treatment of Eating Disorders: Bridging the Research-Practice Gap*, edited by M Maine, B McGilley, and D Bunnell, pp. 285–300. London: Elsevier, 2010.

Maine, M, and Bunnell DW. A perfect biopsychosocial storm: Gender, culture, and eating disorders. In *Treatment of Eating Disorders: Bridging the Research—Practice Gap*, edited by M Margo, B McGilley, and D Bunnell, pp. 3–16. London: Elsevier, 2010.

Maine, M, and Kelly J. *Pursuing Perfection: Eating Disorders, Body Myths, and Women at Midlife and Beyond.* New York, NY: Routledge, 2016.

Maine, M, Samuels K, and Tantillo M. Eating disorders in adult women: Biopsychosocial, developmental, and clinical considerations. *Advances in Eating Disorders: Theory, Research and Practice* 3, no. 2 (2015): 133–143.

Mangweth-Matzek, B, Hoek HW, Rupp CI, Kemmler G, Pope HG Jr, and Kinzl J. The menopausal transition: A possible window of vulnerability for eating pathology. *International Journal of Eating Disorders* 46, no. 6 (2013): 609–616.

Mangweth-Matzek, B, Hoek HW, Rupp CI, Lackner-Seifert K, Frey N, Whitworth AB, Pope HG, and Kinzl J. Prevalence of eating disorders in middle-aged women. *International Journal of Eating Disorders* 47, no. 3 (2014): 320–324.

Mangweth-Matzek, B, Rupp CI, Hausmann A, Assmayr K, Mariacher E, Kemmler G, Whitworth AB, and Biebl W. Never too old for eating disorders or body dissatisfaction: A community study of elderly women. *International Journal of Eating Disorders* 39, no. 7 (2006): 583–586.

Margo, M, Samuels K, and Tantillo M. Eating disorders in adult women: Biopsychosocial, developmental, and clinical considerations. *Advances in Eating Disorders: Theory, Research and Practice* 3, no. 2 (2015): 133–143.

Mehler, P, and Andersen A. *Eating Disorders: A Guide to Medical Care and Complications.* Baltimore, MD: Johns Hopkins University Press, 2010.

Miller, JB. *Towards a New Psychology of Women.* Boston, MA: Beacon Hill, 1986.

Miller, JB, and Stiver IP. *The Healing Connection: How Women Form Relationships in Therapy and in Life.* Boston, MA: Beacon Press, 1997.

Miller, SL, and Wolfe RR. The danger of weight loss in the elderly. *Journal of Nutrition, Health and Aging* 12, no. 7 (2008): 487–491.

National Cancer Institute. Breast Cancer Risk in American Women. 13 September 2015. Available at www.cancer.gov/cancertopics/types/breast/risk-fact-sheet

National Eating Disorders Association (n.d.). Available at www.nationaleatingdisorders.org

Northrup, C. *Women's Bodies, Women's Wisdom: Creating Physical and Emotional Health and Healing.* New York, NY: Bantam Dell, 2006.

Overweight and Weight Loss Statistics. (n.d.). Available at http://www.worldometers.info/weight-loss/

Samuels, K. Eating Disorders in Adult Women: A Long Term Therapy Group through the Lens of Relational-Cultural Theory. May 2015. Available at http://www.edcatalogue.com/eating-disorders-in-adult-women/

Samuels, K, and Maine M. *Treating Eating Disorders at Midlife and Beyond: Help, Hope, and the Relational Cultural Theory.* Work in Progress: No. 110. Jean Baker Miller Training Institute at the Wellesley Centers for Women. 2012.

Seligman, M. *Flourish: A Visionary New Understanding of Happiness and Well-Being.* New York, NY: Free Press, 2011.

Sheehy, G. *Passages: Predictable Crises of Adult Life.* New York, NY: Ballantine Books, 2006.

Tantillo, M. The therapist's use of self-disclosure in a relational therapy approach for eating disorders. *Eating Disorders* 12, no. 1 (2004): 51–73.

Tantillo, M, Sanftner J, and Hauenstein E. Restoring connection in the face of disconnection: An integrative approach to understanding and treating anorexia nervosa. *Advances in Eating Disorders: Theory, Research and Practice* 1, no. 1 (2013): 21–38.

Tayback, M, Kumanyika S, and Chee E. Body weight as a risk factor in the elderly. *Archives of Internal Medicine* 150, no. 5 (1990): 1065–1072.

Thompson, RA, and Sherman RT. *Eating Disorders in Sport.* New York, NY: Routledge, 2010.

Trepal, H, Boie I, and Kress, V. A relational cultural approach to working with clients with eating disorders. *Journal of Counseling and Development* 90, no. 3 (2012): 346–356.

Wolf, N. *The Beauty Myth.* New York, NY: William Morrow, 1990.

Zerbe, KJ. Late life eating disorders. *Eating Disorders Review* 24, no. 6 (2013): 3–5.

Zerbe, KJ. *Women's Mental Health in Primary Care*. Philadelphia, PA: W. B. Saunders, 1999.

Zhao, Y, and Encinosa, W. An update on hospitalizations for eating disorders, 1999–2009. In *Healthcare Cost and Utilization Project (HCUP) Statistical Brief #120*. Rockville, MD: US Agency for Health Care Policy and Research, 2011.

13 Eating Disorders in Sexual and Gender Minorities

Jonna Fries, PsyD

CONTENTS

LEARNING OBJECTIVES

After reading this chapter the reader should be able do the following:

- Explain the influence of the dominant culture on the expression of eating disorders among sexual and gender minority persons
- Integrate recommendations into an eating disorder treatment plan for sexual and gender minority persons with eating disorders
- Understand the impact of multiple minority statuses on sexual and gender minority and ethnoracialized persons

INTRODUCTION

People who identify as lesbian, gay, bisexual, and/or transgender (LGBT) are under-represented in eating-disorder research. As in other areas of research, the default assumption is that participants are heterosexual and cisgender. Many studies do not require sexual orientation identification as part of demographic information collection and ascribe to binary gender categorization. Of the studies that do ask for greater detail, many do not obtain enough participants in each cell (i.e., lesbian, gay, bisexual, transgender) to make ethical generalizations to these populations. Consequently, there is a dearth of information about eating disorders in people who identify as LGBT.

What is known is that eating disorder risk factors for LGBT persons include harassment, victimization, substance use, homelessness, childhood abuse, having fewer opportunities for partnered relationships, double or multiple minority identities, sexual abuse, violence/physical assault (with transgender people experiencing the most violence), discrimination, and feelings of vulnerability (Committee on LGBT Health 2011). Lesbian women and gay men are known to experience higher rates of childhood sexual abuse and rape, well-established as significant risk factors in eating disorders (Balsam et al. 2005; Brennan et al. 2011; Moulton et al. 2015). Over 50% of transgender individuals experienced unwanted sexual touch as a minor, and over half of this group experienced having been forced to have sex (Committee on LGBT Health 2011).

Protective factors for developing eating disorders include certain strengths that may be developed in response to being a sexual or gender minority including resiliency, inner strength, overcoming adversity, self-reliance, legal and financial caution, and potentially having chosen a supportive family (Armistead Maupin, one of the first writers to address acquired immune deficiency syndrome [AIDS], is credited with coining the term "logical" family, as opposed to a biological family; Committee on LGBT Health 2011).

Disordered eating behaviors typically begin in adolescence; therefore it is helpful to understand emergent eating-disordered behaviors in the LGB population compared with the heterosexual population (there were no comparable rates found for transgender youth). As demonstrated in Table 13.1, unhealthy weight control

TABLE 13.1
Prevalence Rates of Disordered Eating Behaviors in Sexual Minority Youth

	Heterosexual Youth	Gay or Lesbian Youth	Bisexual Youth
Starved for 24 hours or more for weight loss purposes	10.3%	26.6%	25%
Took diet pills, powders, or liquids for weight loss purposes	4.8%	17%	13.8%
Vomited or took laxatives for weight loss purposes	4.5%	17.5%	15.8%
Obesity	10.6%	17.1%	13.8%
Overweight	16.1%	16.4%	19.3%

Source: Kann, L. et al., *Surveillance Summaries*, 60, 1–133, 2011.

behaviors are more prevalent in sexual minority female and male youth compared with their heterosexual peers, with one-third of sexual minority youth engaging in hazardous weight control behaviors (Hadland et al. 2014).

EATING DISORDERS AMONG GAY AND BISEXUAL MEN

Gay and bisexual men have higher rates of eating disorders than their heterosexually identified male counterparts (Feldman and Meyer 2007), particularly anorexia nervosa (AN) and bulimia nervosa (BN) (Table 13.2; Committee on LGBT Health 2011). Eating disorder prevalence rates of sexual minority men were found to be higher than heterosexual women (Diemer et al. 2015).

Pressure to Adhere to Hegemonic Masculinity and Hegemonic Gay Norms as Primary Risk Factor for Eating Disorders among Gay and Bisexual Men

Relative to heterosexual men, gay and bisexual men have been found to experience higher body dissatisfaction and more pressure to be thin; both are primary factors known to contribute to disordered eating (Brennan et al. 2011; Committee on LGBT Health 2011; Feldman and Meyer 2007). These negatively valenced body image cognitions in gay and bisexual men have been attributed to, in large part, the media's portrayal of the masculine ideal and dynamics experienced by these men, which cofunction to produce disordered eating symptoms (Committee on LGBT Health 2011; Feldman and Meyer 2007).

Hegemonic masculinity "...embodied the currently most honored way of being a man, it required all other men to position themselves in relation to it, and it ideologically legitimated the global subordination of women to men" (Connell and Messerschmidt 2005). Gay and bisexual men and other men who have sex with men (MSM) have been branded as feminine and are thus tainted by the stigma of misogyny, a type known specifically as homophobia or homonegativity. This type is defined by negative attitudes and behaviors directed toward those who either do not appear to be heterosexual or who overtly identify as non-heterosexual (Morrison 2012). In response to the implied or overt threats associated with homonegativity, gay, bisexual, and MSM often feel pressured to adhere to the hegemonic, heteronormative conceptualization of the masculine

---

TABLE 13.2

Prevalence Rates of Eating Disorders in Sexual Minority Men

	Anorexia Nervosa	Bulimia Nervosa	Binge Eating Disorder
White gay or bisexual men	1.5%	4.6%	1.5%
Black gay or bisexual men	1.6%	4.7%	4.7%
Latino gay or bisexual men	0%	9.4%	9.4%

Source: Feldman, MB, and Meyer IH, *International Journal of Eating Disorders*, 40, 218–226, 2007.

---

ideal. Many behaviors and dysfunctional thoughts may be involved in attempts to avoid the consequences of homonegativity, including others' (Halkitis 2001) and one's own internalized homonegativity. For example, it has been suggested that increased sexual risk-taking among gay men is derived from the pressure to adhere to the masculine norm (Connell and Messerschmidt 2005). As it pertains to eating disorders, the emergence of human immunodeficiency virus (HIV) and AIDS and their devastating impact on the health of sexual minority men gave further impetus to emphasize vitality by striving for the appearance of physical strength (Halkitis 2001). Further elements compelling gay and bisexual men to strive for muscularity and thinness are hegemonic gay norms that value the currency of a slim, muscular, youthful, and White body. Other factors contributing to overall stress include navigating a sense of belonging among sexual peers, frequent decisional pressure regarding sexual status disclosure in various domains and interpersonal situations, and experiencing homonegativity (Brennan et al. 2011).

Drive for Thinness and Muscularity among Gay and Bisexual Men

Similar to women's experience of the dominant culture, and their all-too-common adherence-at-all-cost response to it, in Western gay culture, there is typically pressure to be youthful, slim and/or muscular, and attractive (Williamson 1999). In a study of eating disturbance, body dissatisfaction, drive for thinness, drive for muscularity, and low self-esteem in 246 men (41% gay and 9% bisexual) who were 71% Caucasian, it was found that gay men reported significantly more body dissatisfaction and eating disorder symptoms than heterosexual men; yet heterosexual and gay men did not differ in drive for thinness, and contrary to previous research, gay and heterosexual men did not differ in self-esteem or drive for muscularity (Yean et al. 2013). Bisexual men reported less body shape distress than gay men. It was found that drive for thinness had a different impact on gay and bisexual men relative to heterosexual men in that gay and bisexual men are more likely than straight men to engage in disordered eating to achieve thinness and muscularity, even though their desire for this body type was similar. For bisexual and gay men, drive for thinness may be a driving force in determination of self-esteem, body image distress, and disordered eating (Yean et al. 2013; Brennan et al. 2011). Another study found gay and bisexual boys were more likely to attempt to align their looks to the masculine ideal than engage in drive for thinness (Committee on LGBT Health 2011).

While rates of AN and BN are overall lower for men than for women, gay males represent a large proportion of men with eating disorders. Risk factors for gay men include internalized homonegativity; negative feelings about one's sexuality leading to direct or indirect abuse and neglect of one's body; lack of support and adaptive coping skills; lack of specific gay-friendly and gay-affirming interventions; body comparisons between self and peers, endorsing the "Ganymede archetype" gay ideal of being slim, boyish, and attractive; a sense of alienation; and a desire to look healthy to avoid the appearance of having HIV which takes on different meanings for men depending on seronegative or seropositive status (Williamson 1999).

The principles of hegemonic masculinity and the dominant gay culture contribute to the development of eating disorders by way of appropriating the definition of an ideal man and promoting individual comparisons against these ideals. It follows that using healthy coping skills or rejecting these ideals as capable of defining one's worth are protective factors (Jones 2015).

INTERSECTIONALITY, BODY IMAGE ISSUES, AND EATING DISORDERS AMONG GAY AND BISEXUAL MEN

Ethnoracialization, an oppressive process which occurs when ethnic and racial stereotypes are expected based on phenotype, is particularly burdensome for gay and bisexual men (Brennan et al. 2013). Among gay and bisexual men, ethnoracialization issues include the masculine ideal typically being represented in the media as Caucasian with depictions of the masculine body hair atypical for one's phenotype, being eroticized or fetishized for one's phenotype based on stereotypes about one's race or ethnicity, beliefs about penis size or sexual prowess based on stereotypes, and Whiteness being associated with wealth and status. These aspects of ethnoracialization may lead some to engage in disordered eating such as vomiting or refraining from eating to modify one's body type (Brennan et al. 2013). Among 193 White, Black, and Latino gay and bisexual men with eating disorders, approximately one-third experienced childhood physical and sexual abuse, which creates a significant underlying vulnerability to develop an eating disorder. This childhood sexual abuse predicted both subclinical and fully diagnostic eating disorders (Committee on LGBT Health 2011). Although another study found that White gay, bisexual, and men who have sex with men were at greater risk for disordered eating symptoms than their Asian or Black peers (Brennan et al. 2011), it is important for treatment providers to assess for eating disorders regardless of ethnicity to avoid health outcome disparities in non-White groups.

EATING DISORDERS AMONG LESBIAN AND BISEXUAL WOMEN

In the 1990s, studies confirmed earlier findings that lesbian women were more likely to binge eat than diet (Heffernan 1996; Striegel-Moore et al. 1990), though one study found that lesbians followed binge eating with dieting at rates higher than a non-lesbian sample (Heffernan 1996). While BN rates among lesbian women were similar to heterosexual women, rates of binge eating were two times higher for lesbian women who were also twice as likely to meet criteria for binge eating disorder (BED; Heffernan 1996). During this time, no differences were found in the body esteem between lesbian-identified and heterosexual-identified college women (Striegel-Moore et al. 1990). It was hypothesized that "lifestyle lesbians"—those who rejected narrow interpretations of lesbian appearance—were creating a pathway for a new lesbianism to emerge, thus producing younger generations of lesbian women who were inspired to self-acceptance by feminism and the older generations of lesbian women, yet who were also embracing style and appearance in greater rates than the older generation of lesbians. This focus on appearance generated a renewed vulnerability to body image disturbance and eating disorders, further complicated by the lesbian cultural disapproval of dieting as it is reminiscent of the desire to gain men's approval. Shame, secrecy, and anger toward self often follow disapproval. Relative to heterosexual women, lesbian women scored higher on constructs of interpersonal distrust, interoceptive awareness (awareness of one's internal body sensations), and feelings of general ineffectiveness, hypothesized to be a consequence of living in a homophobic society. Therefore, it was theorized that reasons for bingeing might differ between heterosexual and lesbian women (Striegel-Moore et al. 1990).

Among lesbian women, bingeing to assuage negative affect was a likelier reason for a binge than body dissatisfaction and restraint, the most common binge reasons for heterosexual women. Stigma against lesbian women may account for this increase in binge eating motivated by negative affect. Interestingly, overweight was not as tied to lower income for lesbian women as it was for heterosexual women. However, childhood sexual abuse was found to be a significant risk factor for obesity among lesbian women (Committee on LGBT Health 2011). Weight was listed as the least important part of a partner's attractiveness, signaling that within the greater social milieu there is more pressure to conform to the heteronormative thin ideal than within lesbian relationships (Heffernan 1996).

Merely holding a critical stance against traditional female roles and rights does not necessarily protect lesbian women from negative attitudes and behaviors regarding weight and appearance (Heffernan 1996). Weight and appearance concerns among lesbian women may be exacerbated by wanting to disprove stereotypical ideas that lesbians are fat, unattractive, and not feminine, or believing that being attractive might compensate for not feeling acceptable as a lesbian. A sense of belonging within a lesbian community may be a protective factor associated with body acceptance. Involvement in lesbian/gay activities has been associated with a decrease in unhealthy weight concern, and being out has been associated with an increase in body acceptance. Differing from heterosexual women, among lesbian women who exercised, health was cited as the most influencing factor in dieting, and weight loss/weight control was the least influencing factor.

BODY IMAGE CONCERNS AMONG LESBIAN WOMEN

Studies have shown varied results evidencing that lesbian women have higher or similar levels of body satisfaction relative to heterosexual women, with no studies showing lower lesbian body satisfaction relative to heterosexual women (Huxley et al. 2011). This should not be construed as proof that sexual minority women have insignificant body image concerns. It may be mistakenly assumed that lesbian women do not care about their appearance because lesbian women are not trying to please men (Brand et al. 1992), because their partners are more accepting of the natural female form, that social support and feminist ideology protect lesbian women from body image dissatisfaction (Striegel-Moore et al. 1990), and because standards of beauty are different or less than the dominant culture (Watson et al. 2015). It appears that body image issues may gain momentum over time in sexual minority women as cultural pressures build. Lesbian and bisexual girls were found to experience less pressure than heterosexual girls to look like the dominant feminine ideal (Committee on LGBT Health 2011). Later in life, within-group butch-femme dichotomous lesbian identities were found to drive lesbian and bisexual women to use their bodies, clothes, body posture, weight, and movements to align with these image-based constructs of self-expression. These outwardly expressed identities may help lesbian women find and more easily define one another. At the same time, they constrict and put pressure on women to adhere to a specified image, especially when young or when forming their lesbian identity and its outward expression (Kelly 2007). When concerns of physical, emotional, relational, and financial safety may be jeopardized or alleviated by outward appearance, special consideration must be given in treatment. One might feel pressured to appear traditionally feminine due to fear of physical or verbal hate crimes and discrimination. Alternatively, yet motivated by this same fear, one might align with other lesbian women for group protection by visibly signifying one's lesbian identity. While it is evident that the external expression of lesbian identity has numerous social repercussions, to the heteronormative eye lesbian identity expression may obscure issues of power in intimate relationships. Because same-sex partners do not generally have the same differentiated relationship role expectations, it is unclear who is objectifying whom and for what purpose (e.g., sexually, economically, responsibilities at home, etc.; Peplau et al. 2004). Historically, it is thought that the butch-femme dichotomy involved an assumption of and role-playing a traditional male/female role. Later, lesbian feminist critiques of this adherence to hegemonic gender norms shifted the culture of gendered roles within lesbian communities to value androgyny and challenging gender norms, and more recently to prizing a full circle of acceptance of butch-femme signifiers as radical resistance to normative roles for women and signifiers of lesbian sexual desire (Huxley et al. 2011).

Lesbian women reported higher drive for muscularity than heterosexual women and lower internalization of the thin ideal, while experiencing similar levels of body image dissatisfaction and drive for thinness. Higher drive for muscularity may be due to many lesbians wanting to appear butch or less traditionally feminine as a means to externalize a renouncement of heteronormative feminine ideals and be more easily accepted within communities of lesbians. Although experiencing lower internalization of the thin ideal, lesbian women still desired to be thin; this may explain why lesbians did not differ from heterosexual women in disordered eating and eating disorder symptoms. Together, this suggests that self-objectification and disordered eating are not solely the purview of women desiring to attract men (Yean et al. 2013).

After examining how heteronormative society and the lesbian community influenced lesbians' perception of body image, a factor analysis was used to explain the findings, resulting in the overarching construct of *body silence* (Kelly 2007). Participants' BMI ranged from 19.5 to 50.4, and 14 of the 20 participants identified as White with the remainder as Hispanic American, Asian American, Black American, and Western Indian. All had been in a committed relationship at some point since identifying as lesbian. Lesbian women reported opposing views on externalizing lesbianism through appearance, with some wanting to display visible signs of lesbianism and others striving to hide it. The pressure to align with the dominant culture's image of beauty and the lesbian subculture pulling for an externalized lesbian identity promote opposing mandates, with adherence to one group's mandate provoking disdain from the other. This double bind may lead to greater distress as lesbian women continue throughout the life span to externalize a shifting expression of selfhood.

The concept of body silence provides clear and nuanced insights into the impact of oppression and homophobia, the navigation of an external expression of lesbian identity, and challenges in discussing and soliciting body-related feedback in relationships (Kelly 2007). Several components of body silence will be explained. *Lesbian invisibility* promotes body silence via the pressure lesbian women feel to choose to forgo external signs of lesbianism, leaving them invisible to a community of support. In the struggle to decide upon level of lesbian visibility, androgynous lesbians considered that other lesbian women could identify them while non-lesbians might wonder about their sexuality. Femme-identified lesbians tended to struggle with feeling accepted by other lesbians and felt stigmatized by the lesbian community for not being lesbian enough and enjoying a hegemonic identity; furthermore, they tended to have more difficulty with others not believing they were lesbian. *Fear of mistrust of intent* captures the difficulty lesbian women face when desiring to discuss body and body image. In contrast to the commonality of heterosexual women discussing bodies, lesbian women tended to be concerned that discussing bodies would lead others to assume a sexual intent, further fostering body silence. *Discomfort during intimacy* denotes body silence arising from wanting to avoid sexual intimacy due to negative perception of one's body. Although desiring positive feedback about the attractiveness of one's body, lesbian women tended to hide their bodies from their partner's view which gives rise to body silence. *Questionable feedback* captures the mistrust lesbians harbored about the authenticity of their partner's positive feedback about their bodies, typically promoting further body silence. *Body image and sexual identity* strengthens body silence by virtue of the dominant culture's belief that a woman's sexual identity is formed by men's interest or disinterest, that more effort toward a feminine appearance would cure a woman of lesbianism, and that being lesbian despite being attractive to men is a waste of mainstream beauty (Kelly 2007).

Although no significant differences were found in body dissatisfaction between lesbian and heterosexual women (Committee on LGBT Health 2011), it has been proposed that within same-sex partnered relationships, lesbian and bisexual women have a complex mix of factors positively and negatively influencing their perceptions of their bodies and their partner's bodies (Huxley et al. 2011). Seven themes were factored in a qualitative study on lesbian and bisexual women's body image within same-sex partnered relationships. The first theme, *Women's Appearance in Partner Relationships*, indicates that appearance is not as important in same-sex relationships as it is in heterosexual relationships, and that previous male partners put both subtle and overt pressure on women to manipulate their appearance. One woman expressed the belief that women's perception of men's critical gaze is far more critical than men's actual gaze and that women are more appreciative of diversity in women's body shape and size than are men. *Acceptance and Understanding* alludes to the belief that women are more understanding and accepting of the natural changes females' bodies undergo than are men. *Same-Sex Attraction* fosters trust in the notion that one's same-sex partner was attracted to them; however, this may be mediated by somewhat concealed anti-fat/thin ideal elements that were also captured within this construct, with women discussing preference for thinness as a health concern. *Comparisons between Same-Sex Partners* holds that women tend to compare their bodies with each other's body parts, leading to heightened or lowered confidence and self-consciousness. *Transference and Influence* represents the belief that lesbian couples evolve a confluent physical presentation, and that this merging of external appearance emanates from being influenced by a partner's appearance ideas and attitudes. *Stereotypical Expectations* arise from heterosexual and lesbian communities, with both making comments or asking questions in an attempt to categorize same-sex partners into gendered roles, and with women in same-sex relationships feeling both a freedom and a constraint due to lack of appearance norms. *Concern about Men's Opinions* illuminated differences among bisexual women, some of whom felt pressure to be perceived as attractive under the male gaze and some of whom experienced a resistance to this pressure, while some lesbian women expressed that within lesbian social milieus, sexual desire followed by attention to one's attractiveness is expected, thus eliciting similar "gaze" pressures felt in hetero spaces (Huxley et al. 2011).

Heterosexism and internalized heterosexism tend to negatively influence sexual minority women's perceptions of the body and eating disorder symptomatology (Watson et al. 2015). Lesbian women are immersed in both cultures and face oppression in the dominant culture, with overt stigmatizing messages flowing at a steady rate. Judgments of worth based on body size and shape, skin tone, and hair texture have been instilled in women and men regardless of sexual identity.

EATING DISORDERS AND BISEXUALITY

Bisexual women were found to indicate lower self-esteem compared with lesbian and hetero-identified women who did not differ in self-esteem levels. This may be due to self-objectification being more complex for bisexual women than for lesbian and heterosexual women (Yean et al. 2013). There are no external signifiers of bisexuality which leaves bisexual men and women with neither the pressure nor the support garnered by gay men and women who choose to align with gay and lesbian groups through coded appearance (Huxley et al. 2011). "Out" bisexual women were found to have twice the rate of eating disorders relative to lesbian and heterosexual women (Committee on LGBT Health 2011). Along with gay and lesbian youth, bisexual youth had higher rates of eating disorders, and gay and bisexual youth had higher rates of purging throughout their adolescence. If sexually active with both sexes, bisexual youth are at greatest risk for eating disorders compared with gay and lesbian youth with only same-sex partners (Committee on LGBT Health 2011). The dominant Western heteronormative culture is more forgiving of men who are explicitly and implicitly taught to attempt to attract women with power, where women typically attempt to attract men with sexuality (Williamson 1999); these biases, when internalized, become difficult to navigate for bisexual individuals who experience shifts in modes of attracting different gendered partners and may feel pressured to embody all manner of attracting romantic partners.

EATING DISORDERS AND TRANSGENDER PERSONS

Rates of eating disorders comorbid with gender dysphoria are unclear. As of 2003, only three reported cases were found of AN among adults with gender identity disorder (currently referred to as gender dysphoria) and one case in a child. Commonalities included the desire to have a feminine body, which appeared to strongly influence the desire to lose weight (Winston et al. 2004). Recently, attention has been paid to the issue of eating disorders among those with gender dysphoria and those who identify as transgender persons. Transgender people have been found to have a higher risk of eating disorders, twice as high as heterosexual women (Diemer et al. 2015).

Compared with female control participants, both male-to-female and female-to-male transgender persons endorsed higher levels of weight and shape concerns, restrained eating, body dissatisfaction, and body checking compared with male controls, with female-to-male transgender persons evidencing higher rates of drive for thinness, BN, and eating concerns (Vocks 2009). The direction of gender transition has been found to influence different manifestations of eating disorders, with male-to-female transgender persons at higher risk of cognitive and behavioral disordered eating symptoms (Vocks 2009).

Gender identity may have some fluidity in some transgender persons. When an individual shifts from identifying with male or female gender, he or she might use disordered eating to attempt to align his or her body with attributes of gender ideals, at times attempting to strive for muscularity and at other times striving for thinness given the female thin ideal. Excessive cardiovascular exercise and undereating might take precedence when attempting to align with the feminine ideal and muscle-building exercise along with increased food intake, or binge eating might take precedence when attempting to align with the masculine ideal.

Eating disorder risk factors specific to male-to-female transgender individuals may include equating femininity to being thin and wanting to undereat to suppress libido and adhere to a hyperfeminine ideal, and wanting to relate to women with amenorrhea secondary to anorexia. Adolescence is a critical phase in the development of eating disorders, and for transgender persons, the timing collides with the expression of secondary sexual characteristics (Caldarera et al. 2016). Female-to-male transgender people may undereat to reject feminization, reduce breast size (in overweight or obese persons), and suppress puberty and its role in the development of secondary sexual characteristics and menarche (Cooney et al. 2016; Hepp and Milos 2002; Murray et al. 2014); conversely, in overweight female-to-male transgender people there may be an avoidance of weight loss or desire for weight gain to reduce the ratio of breast and hip size to abdominal size or to avoid attracting sexual attention from men attracted to women (Vocks 2009). Furthermore, it is important to understand that many do not identify at the polar ends of gender identity–male or female–and that this may contribute to body image distress or dysphoria or a non-gendered identity may be a healing factor that is empowering.

Transgender clients may use *strategies of disconnection* to maintain relationships by denying important parts of self. Paradoxically, hiding the self leads to a pervasive sense of alienation from others. In attempts to align with dominant culture and avoid the pain of rejection, criticism, or worse, transgender people often internalize others' fear and hatred of difference, and strive to either repress gender identification or align one's gender expression to the dominant culture's ideals and expectations, possibly through disordered eating. The dominant culture even dictates norms in reconstructive surgery. While endorsing liposuction, rhinoplasty, and correction of birth defects, the dominant culture is confused by and judgmental about the desire to reform genitalia (Girshick and Green 2009) leaving those desiring sex reassignment surgery with another psychological hurdle to overcome.

An interesting finding was that men had twice as many somatostatin-expressing neurons in the bed nucleus of the stria terminalis as cisgender women, and male-to-female transgender persons had similar levels as cisgender women while a female-to-male transgender person had similar levels as cisgender males (Kruijver et al. 2000). The bed nucleus of the stria terminalis has been implicated in fear, stress, and anxiety (Walker et al. 2003) and in autonomic, neuroendocrine, and behavioral responses (Crestani et al. 2013), and the release of somatostatins is associated with depression (Lin and Sibille 2015). Corticotropin-releasing factor in the bed nucleus of the stria terminalis has been found to have a meaningful role in frustration and stress-induced binge eating (Micioni Di Bonaventura et al. 2014). Future research may shed light on whether this is meaningful in gender identity and rates of eating disorders in some transgender people.

RECOMMENDATIONS FOR WORKING WITH LGBT CLIENTS WITH EATING DISORDERS

There are many terms used to describe various aspects of gender and sexuality, too many to be defined here. It is important for clinicians working with sexual and gender minority youth and adults to use the appropriate language and attitudes conducive to healing. Glossaries of terminology are easily available online. Clinicians' updated vocabulary will lend credibility to expressions of empathy; conversely, using outdated terminology is likely to decrease feelings of emotional and physical safety that may be transferred onto the rest of the team and clinic. The vocabulary for sex and gender is growing rapidly and is further complicated by region, age, current events, fluidity in identity for some people, and educational and exposure levels. Key to rapport building is to use terms and labels offered by clients and not to impose labels or identities on people.

LGBT-identified youth are four times more likely to die by suicide than hetero-identified youth. If their parents are homonegative, their LGB children are 8.4 times more likely to die by suicide than LGB youth with low family rejection (American Psychiatric Association 2013; Ryan et al. 2009). Therefore, educating the family of LGBT clients should be a high priority. In eating disorder treatment, families are often incorporated in therapy, and this presents an opportunity to add LGBT psychoeducation and diversity training to families of LGBT clients. Family members can be taught empathy, compassion, and social consciousness, and can be taught to recognize, advocate against, and avoid perpetrating heterosexist, homonegative, and transphobic microaggressions (Nadal 2013).

When treating transgender clients, it is important to consider that disordered eating behaviors may be thought of as essential for survival. Due to discrimination and stigma, "passing" as cisgender may ensure physical safety, job security, and avoidance of bullying and harassment (Gordon et al. 2016). Multidisciplinary team members should share the client's preferred pronouns and preferred name. Calling a transgender client by the name on their chart rather than their preferred name may instantly damage rapport. It is important for clinicians to conceptualize gender assignment as an individual right and to conceptualize discrimination as a social and cultural problem, not a problem within the client. It is important to treat a client's gender dysphoria and support surgical transition if desired by the client; however, sex reassignment surgeries may not resolve dysphoria and suicidality may continue, abate, or worsen (American Psychiatric Association 2013). Social and internalized stigma are intra- and interpersonal problems. By addressing them as such, transgender clients will benefit from the development of coping and self-advocacy skills, rather than treatment team providers focusing on changing the desire for egosyntonic gender assignment (American Psychiatric Association 2013).

Treatment teams that challenge each other to confront bias will be more likely to identify eating disorders in sexual minority clients and provide competent and compassionate treatment. Assessments and screenings may need to be modified to include items sensitive to all gender identities, and assessors are recommended to be mindful of mistaken beliefs that sexual minority clients are not at risk of certain eating disorders (Bankoff 2014). It is recommended that psychotherapists and other treatment team providers maintain awareness of prejudice, its impact on sexual minority and ethnoracialized sexual minority clients' body image disturbance, and its expression through disordered eating behaviors. Engage clients with body image concerns in discussions pertaining to sexual power. Validate gender and sexual identities as well as cultural and gender dynamics. Address the impact of heterosexist and objectifying societies. Engage in discussions regarding the impact of body image on those whose sexual and gender identities are other than heteronormative and cis. With female clients, discuss the tension between desire to adhere to conflicting feminist and culturally imposed feminine ideals (Chmielewski and Yost 2013). Hints of advocacy such as posters and magazines in the office geared toward support and normalization of lesbian, gay, bisexual, transgender, queer, intersex, asexual (LGBTQIA) will likely contribute to recovery of eating disorders.

CONCLUSION

Hegemonic masculinity, the dominant culture's feminine and masculine ideals, homophobia and homonegativity, and transphobia collude to create a hostile environment toward those identifying as anything other than cisgendered and heterosexual. This stigma makes its way through the minds of those identifying as LGBTQIA and manifests in some functional (advocacy, community building, pride, etc.) and some dysfunctional patterns, including manifesting as body image distress and eating disorders. Empowering clients to resist objectification (Chmielewski and Yost 2013), exploring and addressing pressures exerted by culture on those with multiple stigmatized identities (Brennan et al. 2013), and advocating for the client's right to experience and express their gender and sexual identity will help assuage the pressures that lead to disordered eating.

CASE STUDY 13.1

Malaya

Malaya is an 18-year-old Filipina international student studying at a large metropolitan American university. She sought treatment at her university counseling center to address difficulty concentrating in class and when studying. She feared she might have to drop her classes which would jeopardize her ability to remain in the United States and would require informing her parents who were paying for her education. She was well aware that her cycles of bingeing, purging, and starving were somehow related to her difficulty in concentrating but did believe it was possible to change these behaviors.

(Continued)

Malaya could not remember a time when she felt comfortable in her body. She was teased for being big as a child and began bingeing, purging, and starving herself from ages 9 to 12, "I always hated my body." At intake she was bingeing 1–3 times per week, vomiting 4–6 times per day and starving most of the day 1–3 days per week with very low caloric intake. Malaya reported that she always knew she was a lesbian, she was out to her parents and friends, and was active in campus LGBTQIA event programming. Malaya stated that her coming out process was eased by her wealthy aunt's coming out as lesbian and her large family's general acceptance of her aunt's sexual identity. Her therapist referred Malaya to the Office for Students with Disabilities to obtain temporary academic accommodations for the sequelae of her eating disorder. Disability services provided her with a note taker, permission to record lectures, and extra time to complete tests. She dropped one class allowing her to ease her academic load and retain her status as an international student. She was referred to the Student Health Center for a physical and to the nutritionist in Health Education and Promotion. Malaya signed a consent to release information so her psychotherapist could communicate with each person providing services on campus. Additionally, she was referred to a free off-campus LBGT support group at a large LGBT community center. A referral to a longer term provider was made, but Malaya requested to be seen by the university counseling center due to the concern that her parents would be made aware of her seeking counseling if she used her insurance to pay for therapy. She did not yet feel comfortable disclosing help-seeking or her disordered eating to her parents.

Over the next few months, Malaya began to acknowledge to himself that he had always felt male and desired to be male. He changed his name to Nico and requested that male pronouns be used when addressing him. This was noted on his chart so that other health center treatment providers would be made aware. He rejected the label of transgender; it was experienced as a barrier to attuning to his somewhat in-flux gender identity. Nico disclosed a history of childhood sexual abuse, which led to confusion and shame as he questioned its influence on his sexual and gender identification. He was treated with eye movement desensitization and reprocessing (EMDR) over the course of 10 sessions—the counseling center's limit—and was then referred to a local therapist to continue treatment. At the time of termination, his purging had decreased by 75% and he had begun to strive for muscularity rather than thinness. His ability to concentrate in school had improved. He began to understand the impact of the stigma which had perplexed him and caused him shame since he had his family's emotional support and believed that should suffice. Although he had an advocate's understanding of the impact of hegemonic masculinity, heteronormativity, and multiple minority statuses, he was able to personalize the impact and relate it to his symptoms, demystifying his behaviors. He disclosed his body image and disordered eating in the off-campus multicultural LGBT support group, which sparked a focus for the entire group session and normalized his response to cultural pressures. Processing the trauma of childhood sexual abuse served to further improve insight into the development and maintenance of his disordered eating behaviors. His insights permitted him to disclose without shame his gender identity, eating disorder, and history of sexual abuse to his parents.

REFERENCES

American Psychiatric Association. *Diagnostic and Statistical Manual of Mental Disorders* (5th ed.). Washington, DC: Author, 2013.

Balsam, K, Rothblum E, and Beauchaine T. Victimization over the life span: A comparison of lesbian, gay, bisexual, and heterosexual siblings. *Journal of Consulting and Clinical Psychology* 73, no. 3 (2005): 477–487.

Brand, P, Rothblum E, and Solomon L. A comparison of lesbians, gay men, and heterosexuals on weight and restrained eating. *International Journal of Eating Disorders* 11, no. 3 (1992): 253–259.

Brennan, DJ, Asakura K, George C, Newman PA, Giwa S, Hart TA, Souleymanov R, and Betancourt G. "Never reflected anywhere": Body image among ethnoracialized gay and bisexual men. *Body Image* 10, no. 3 (2013): 389–398.

Brennan, DJ, Crath R, Hart TA, Gadalla T, and Gillis L. Body dissatisfaction and disordered eating among men who have sex with men in Canada. *International Journal of Men's Health* 10, no. 3 (2011): 253–268.

Caldarera, A, Brustia P, Gerino E, Dimitrios L, and Rollè L. Co-occurrence of gender dysphoria and eating disorders: A systematic review of the literature. *European Psychiatry* 33, (2016): S188–S189.

Chmielewski, JF, and Yost MR. Psychosocial influences on bisexual women's body image: Negotiating gender and sexuality. *Psychology of Women Quarterly* 37, no. 2 (2013): 224–241.

Committee on LGBT Health. Committee on Lesbian, Gay, Bisexual, and Transgender Health and Research Gaps and Opportunities, Board on the Health of Select Populations: Institute of Medicine of the National Academies. In *The Health of Lesbian, Gay, Bisexual and Transgender People: Building a Foundation for Better Understanding.* Washington, DC: National Academies Press, 2011.

Connell, RW, and Messerschmidt JW. Hegemonic masculinity: Rethinking the concept. *Gender and Society* 19, no. 6 (2005): 829–859.

Cooney, M, Kaufman M, Birken C, Dettmer E, and Toulany A. Impact of adolescent gender dysphoria on treatment uptake obesity management. *Journal of Pediatrics*, 176 (June 2016): 207–209.

Crestani, C, Alves F, Gomes F, Resstel L, Correa F, and Herman J. Mechanisms in the bed nucleus of the stria terminalis involved in control of autonomic and neuroendocrine functions: A review. *Current Neuropharmacology* 11, no. 2 (2013): 141–159.

Diemer, EW, Grant JD, Munn-Chernoff MA, Patterson DA, and Duncan AE. Gender identity, sexual orientation, and eating-related pathology in a national sample of college students. *Journal of Adolescent Health* 57 (2015): 144–149.

Feldman, MB, and Meyer IH. Eating disorders in diverse lesbian, gay, and bisexual populations. *International Journal of Eating Disorders* 40, no. 3 (2007): 218–226.

Girshick, L, and Green J. *Transgender Voices: Beyond Men and Women.* Lebanon, NH: University Press of New Hampshire, 2009.

Gordon, AR, Austin SB, Krieger N, White Hughto JM, and Reisner SL. "I have to constantly prove to myself, to people, that I fit the bill": Perspectives on weight and shape control behaviors among low-income, ethnically diverse young transgender women. *Social Science and Medicine* 165 (2016): 141–149.

Hadland, SE, Austin SB, Goodenow CS, and Calzo JP. Weight misperception and unhealthy weight control behaviors among sexual minorities in the general adolescent population. *Journal of Adolescent Health* 54 (2014): 296–303.

Halkitis, PN. An exploration of perceptions of masculinity among gay men living with HIV. *Journal of Men's Studies* 9, no. 3 (2001): 413–429.

Heffernan, K. Eating disorders and weight concern among lesbians. *International Journal of Eating Disorders* 19, no. 2 (1996): 127–138.

Hepp, U, and Milos G. Gender identity and eating disorders. *International Journal of Eating Disorders* 32, no. 4 (2002): 473–478.

Huxley, C, Clarke V, and Halliwell E. "It's a comparison thing, isn't it?" Lesbian and bisexual women's accounts of how partner relationships shape their feelings about their body and appearance. *Psychology of Women Quarterly* 35, no. 3 (2011): 415–427.

Jewell, LM, and Morrison AM. Making sense of homonegativity: Heterosexual men and women's understanding of their own prejudice and discrimination toward gay men. *Qualitative Research in Psychology* 9 (2012): 351 -370.

Jones, RG. Queering the body politic: Intersectional reflexivity in the body narratives of queer men. *Qualitative Inquiry* 21, no. 9 (2015): 766–775.

Kann, L, Emily O'Malley Olsen, Tim McManus, Steve Kinchen, David Chyen, William Harris, and Howell Wechsler. Sexual identity, sex of sexual contacts, and health-risk behaviors among students in grades 9-12—Youth risk behavior surveillance, selected sites, United States, 2001-2009. *Surveillance Summaries* 60, no. SS07 (2011): 1–133.

Kelly, L. Lesbian body image perceptions: The context of the *body silence*. *Qualitative Health Research* 17, no. 7 (2007): 873–883.

Kruijver, F, Zhou J-N, Pool C, Hoffman M, Gooren L, and Swaab D. Male-to-female transsexuals have female neuron numbers in a limbic nucleus. *Journal of Clinical Endocrinology & Metabolism* 85, no. 5 (2000): 2034–2041.

Lin, LC, and Sibille E. Somatostatin, neuronal vulnerability and behavioral emotionality. *Molecular Psychiatry* 20, no. 3 (2015): 377–387.

Micioni Di Bonaventura, MV, Ciccocioppo R, Romano A, Bossert JM, Rice KC, Ubaldi M, St Laurent, R, Gaetani S, Massi M, Shaham Y, and Cifani C. Role of bed nucleus of the stria terminalis corticotrophin-releasing factor receptors in frustration stress-induced binge-like palatable food consumption in female rats with a history of food restriction. *Journal of Neuroscience* 34, no. 334 (2014): 11316–11324.

Moulton, S, Newman E, Power K, Swanson V, and Day K. Childhood trauma and eating disorder psychopathology: A mediating role for dissociation and emotion regulation? *Child Abuse and Neglect* 39, (2015): 167–174.

Murray, SB, Boon E, and Touyz, SW. Diverging eating psychopathology in transgendered eating disordered patients: A report of two cases. In *Current Findings on Males with Eating Disorders*, edited by L Cohn and R Lemberg. New York, NY: Routledge, 2014.

Nadal, K. *That's So Gay! Microaggressions and the Lesbian, Gay, Bisexual, and Transgender Community*. Washington, DC: American Psychological Association, 2013.

Peplau, A, Fingerhut A, and Beals K. Sexuality in the relationships of lesbians and gay men. In *The Handbook of Sexuality in Close Relationships*, edited by J Harvey, A Wenzel, and S Sprecher. Mahwah, NJ: Lawrence Erlbaum Associates, 2004.

Ryan, C, Huebner D, Diaz R, and Sanchez J. Family rejection as a predictor of negative health outcomes in white and Latino lesbian, gay, and bisexual young adults. *Pediatrics* 123, no. 1 (2009): 346–352.

Striegel-Moore, R, Tucker N, and Hsu J. Body image dissatisfaction and disordered eating in lesbian college student. *International Journal of Eating Disorders* 9, no. 5 (1990): 493–500.

Vocks, S, Stahn C, Loenser K, and Legenbauer T. Eating and body image disturbances in male-to-female and female-to-male transsexuals. *Archives of Sexual Behavior* 38, no. 3 (2009): 364 -377.

Walker, DL, Toufexis DJ, and Davis M. Role of the bed nucleus of the stria terminalis versus the amygdala in fear, stress, and anxiety. *European Journal of Pharmacology* 463, no. 1–3 (2003): 199–216.

Watson, L, Grotewiel M, Farrell M, Marshik J, and Schneider M. Experiences of sexual objectification, minority stress, and disordered eating among sexual minority women. *Psychology of Women Quarterly* 39, no. 4 (2015): 458–470.

Williamson, I. Why are gay men a high risk group for eating disturbance? *European Eating Disorders Review* 7 (1999): 1–4.

Winston, A, Acharya S, Chaudhuri S, and Fellowes L. Anorexia nervosa and gender identity disorder in biologic males: A report of two cases. *International Journal of Eating Disorders* 36, no. 1 (2004): 109–113.

Yean, C, Benau E, Dakanalis A, Hormes J, Perone J, and Timko CA. The relationshp of sex and sexual orientation to self-esteem, body shape satisfaction, and eating disorder symptomalogy. *Frontiers in Psychology* 4, no. 887 (2013).

RESOURCES

Competencies for Counseling Transgender Clients. Association for Lesbian, Gay, Bisexual, and Transgender Issues in Counseling. The Center for Counseling Practice, Policy, and Research. 703-823-9800, x324. https://www.counseling.org/docs/defaultsource/competencies/algbtic_competencies.pdf?sfvrsn=8.

GLAAD Media Reference Guide—Transgender Issues. https://www.glaad.org/reference/transgender.

Guidelines for Psychological Practice With Transgender and Gender Nonconforming People. http://www.apa.org/practice/guidelines/transgender.pdf

It Gets Better Project. http://www.itgetsbetter.org/

LGBT National Hotline. http://www.glbthotline.org/

Practice Guidelines for LGB Clients. Guidelines for Psychological Practice with Lesbian, Gay, and Bisexual Clients. http://www.apa.org/pi/lgbt/resources/guidelines.aspx.

The Trevor Project. http://www.thetrevorproject.org/.

Index